Contents

The Midwife's Labour and Birth Handbook

Edited by

Vicky Chapman
RGN, RM(Dip) MA

Blackwell
Science

Editorial Offices:
Blackwell Science Ltd, 9600 Garsington Road, Oxford OX4 2DQ, UK
Tel: +44 (0) 1865 776868
Blackwell Publishing Inc., 350 Main Street, Malden, MA 02148-5020, USA
Tel: +1 781 388 8250
Blackwell Science Asia Pty, 550 Swanston Street, Carlton, Victoria 3053, Australia
Tel: +61 (0)3 8359 1011

First published 2003

5   2007

ISBN: 978-0-632-05943-0

Library of Congress Cataloging-in-Publication Data
The midwife's labour and birth handbook/edited by Vicky Chapman.
    p. cm.
    Includes bibliographical references and index.
    ISBN 0-632-05943-5 (alk. paper)
    1. Midwifery—Handbooks, manual, etc.   2. Midwives—Handbooks, manuals, etc.
    3. Childbirth—Handbooks, manual, etc.   I. Chapman, Vicky.

RG960.M54 2003
618.2—dc22

                                                                                      2003058357

A catalogue record for this title is available from the British Library

Set in 9.5/12pt Palatino
by DP Photosetting, Aylesbury, Bucks
Printed and bound in Singapore
by Markono Print Media Pte Ltd

The publisher's policy is to use permanent paper from mills that operate a sustainable forestry policy, and which has been manufactured from pulp processed using acid-free and elementary chlorine-free practices. Furthermore, the publisher ensures that the text paper and cover board used have met acceptable environmental accreditation standards.

For further information on
Blackwell Publishing, visit our website:
www.blackwellpublishing.com

Preface

As a practicing midwife I wanted to have information to hand that would help me provide care to women in a variety of intrapartum situations. I also wanted a book with a positive midwifery bias that included a variety of complex labour and birth information in one place.

To this end, *The Midwife's Labour and Birth Handbook* has been written specifically by experienced, practicing midwives and combines the latest evidence, knowledge and midwifery practice. This book is an effective reference for any midwife providing care during labour and birth, ensuring the woman remains at the centre of that care.

Section 1 of the handbook follows a consistent format with each topic's introduction being followed by factual points and applicable midwifery care. Each chapter finishes with a summary of the chapter's main points. Certain chapters cover areas of midwifery practice that are solely the midwife's domain – notably normal labour, home birth and waterbirth. In addition, midwives are increasingly the lead in preventing labour dystocia; they may be the sole carer of a woman birthing a breech baby (planned or unplanned); or they may assist a woman with the aid of a ventouse. Certain labour-based situations, such as pre-eclampsia, pre-term or stillborn babies, involve the multidisciplinary team and this book also covers those situations as a reassuring *aide memoire*. Midwives are often at the 'front line' when childbirth emergencies occur, and the text describes various options available, taking into account that the birth may not be in hospital.

Section 2 covers a wide variety of intrapartum support information and essential reference material which practitioners may use on a daily basis, including a pharmacopoeia and blood reference ranges. Some chapters use illustrations as visual prompts, for example, when interpreting cervical dilation and fetal position from vaginal examinations, diameter of the fetal skull, knot tying and the latest suturing techniques.

This book will be a valuable reference for busy practitioners. The chapters take a critical midwifery viewpoint towards 'standard' care and present alternatives where evidence or controversy exists. Midwives should find the content relevant and useful. In addition, the reference section at the end of each chapter contains useful organizations with website links and many chapters contain suggestions for further reading.

Acknowledgements

I would like to thank all those friends, family and colleagues who have supported and assisted me in the production of *The Midwife's Labour and Birth Handbook*. My biggest thanks must go to my husband and honorary midwife, Kelvin, for his huge support, patience, generous amounts of time and with his technical input with the artwork, and also to my sister, Sue Chapman, for her all-round help and support.

Thank you also to all those who proof-read work, especially Janet Gwillim and Jo

Cotton who spent many, many hours reading chapters. Both have been inspirational midwives and amazing role models. Thanks also to Cathy Charles, Kate Collett, Julie Davis, Dr Phil Barnardo, Sarah Crawshaw and all the library staff at Frimley Park Hospital. Thanks to Grace Page (my grandmother) for her interest and encouragement, and also to Pip Tanton, Anna-Marie Tuite, Angela Higgs and Jean Cooper for their interest and practical help.

Vicky Chapman

The editor, authors and publisher have taken every care to ensure the book is correct and up-to-date at the time of going to press. However, as new evidence emerges, practice guidelines may change. Hence this book is intended as a guide only and midwives are advised to confirm any uncertainties by referrng to local protocols and unit guidelines, the Midwife's Rules and Code of Practice.

Contributors

The Editor

Vicky Chapman *RGN, RM(Dip), MA*
As a midwife Vicky has worked in a variety of hospitals and in the community setting. She has an interest in normal birth, waterbirths and home births and worked in a pioneering and dynamic Midwifery Group Practice in South East Kent, JACA-NES. Vicky is presently a full-time mother, part-time bank midwife and takes an active role in local childbirth classes.

Contributors

Annette Briley *SRN, RM, MSc*
Annette is a clinical trials midwifery manager within the Maternal and Fetal Research Unit at St Thomas' Hospital, London. She was a clinical midwife for many years, working in all areas of maternity provision, including obstetric ultrasound. Annette joined the St Thomas' research team in 1997 and was involved in a major study on vitamins in pre-eclampsia. She has since worked on numerous pregnancy-related research projects. Annette has worked with Tommy's, the baby charity, and Parentalk, a charity that aims to inspire and aid parents, and has written a book with Tim Mungeam, Parentalk's CEO, about the first six weeks of parenthood.

Nick Castle *DipIMC, RCS(Ed), RGN, ENB 100, SRParamedic, MSc(Dist)*
Nick is a nurse consultant in resuscitation and emergency care in a large district general hospital and undertakes a wide range of training, research, audit and clinical duties. Nick is married with twin girls.

Cathy Charles *RGN, RM, BA(Hons), BSc(Hons)*
Cathy is a midwife and clinical audit/risk management co-ordinator for the West Wiltshire Primary Health Care Trust. Cathy has been a midwife since 1991 and a ventouse practitioner since 1998. In the area in which Cathy works, 1500 out of 5000 births take place in one of seven stand-alone midwife-led community units or at home. Having worked in low-intervention settings for the past eight years Cathy believes that women should, wherever possible, achieve the birth they want, and realises the importance of midwifery skills to help achieve this aim. Cathy is training as a supervisor of midwives and also teaches Aquanatal classes at her local leisure centre.

Julie Davis *RGN, RM*
Julie Davis qualified as a midwife in 1994. She is a mother of two children and works part time at Frimley Park Hospital in Surrey.

Janet Gwillim *RGN, RM, ADM*
Janet trained as a general nurse in 1968 and a midwife in 1969. After suspending her career to have two children, she returned to midwifery and completed the Advanced

Diploma in Midwifery and the Supervisor of Midwives course. Janet attended the first woman to have a waterbirth in East Kent, and she has been an enthusiastic teacher and resource on water and homebirths. Following the Changing Childbirth Report in 1993, Janet helped to change the way midwives work in south-east Kent by gaining funding for a pilot scheme for a midwifery group practice called JACANES, which provided choice and continuity for midwives and women. Janet retired from midwifery in February 2002.

Virginia Howes *RM, BA(Hons)*
Virginia is the mother of four children and an independent midwife who works in partnership with another independent midwife in the Kent Midwifery Practice. She also provides research-based care in East Sussex and southern Essex. Virginia is passionately committed to keep childbirth normal and to the right of women to choose the way they give birth. She recognises the benefits to women and their families of continuity of care before, during and after the birth.

Barbara Kavanagh *RGN, RM*
Barbara is married with two children. She has been an SRN since 1976, a midwife since 1978 and a community midwife since 1980. She also has an interest in bereavement issues and spent 5 years as a Cruse counsellor before deciding to take the Diploma in Bereavement Counselling. Barbara also works as a family planning nurse in a young people's clinic.

Lesley Shuttler *RN(Dip), RM, BSc(Hons)*
Lesley is married with two daughters. She is an antenatal teacher and tutor with the National Childbirth Trust and has been a midwife since 1995. Lesley strongly believes in women's innate ability to birth their babies, and the need to promote and support informed choice at all times.

List of abbreviations

AFE	Amniotic fluid embolism
AFI	Amniotic fluid index
AIDS	Acquired immunodeficiency syndrome
ALT	Alanine transaminase
APTT	Activated partial thromboplastin time
ARM	Artificial rupture of the membranes
AST	Aspartate transaminase
BBA	Born before arrival
BLS	Basic life support
BP	Blood pressure
bpm	Beats per minute
BVM	Bag-valve-mask (device)
CPD	Cephalopelvic disproportion
CRP	C-reactive protein
CTG	Cardiotocograph/cardiotocography
CVP	Central venous pressure
DIC	Disseminated intravascular coagulation
ECV	External cephalic version
EDTA	Ethylenediamine-tetra-acetic acid
EFM	Electronic fetal monitoring
ET	Endotracheal
FBC	Full blood count
FBS	Fetal blood sampling
FHR	Fetal heart rate
FSE	Fetal scalp electrode
GA	General anaesthesia
GBS	Group B Streptococcus
Hb	Haemoglobin
HBV	Hepatitis B virus
HCV	Hepatitis C virus
HELLP	Haemolysis, elevated liver enzymes, low platelets
HDN	Haemorrhagic disease of the newborn
HIV	Human immunodeficiency virus
IA	Intermittent auscultation
ICV	Internal cephalic version
IM	Intramuscular
ICU	Intensive Care Unit
INR	International normalized ratio
IUGR	Intrauterine growth restriction
IV	Intravenous

IVI	Intravenous infusion
lpm	Litres per minute
LOA	Left occipitoanterior
LOP	Left occipitoposterior
MAP	Mean arterial pressure
MCV	Mean corpuscular volume
MRI	Magnetic resonance imaging
MROP	Manual removal of the placenta
MSU	Mid-stream specimen of urine
MVP	Midwife ventouse practitioner
NICU	Neonatal intensive care unit
OA	Occipitoanterior
OP	Occipitoposterior
PCR	Polymerase chain reaction
PCV	Packed cell volume
PIH	Pregnancy-induced hypertension
POP	Persistent occipitoposterior
PPH	Postpartum haemorrhage
PPROM	Preterm prelabour rupture of the membranes
PROM	Prelabour rupture of the membranes
PT	Prothrombin time
RBC	Red blood cell
RCT	Randomized controlled trial
RDS	Respiratory distress syndrome
ROA	Right occipitoanterior
ROP	Right occipitoposterior
SCBU	Special care baby unit
SLE	Systemic lupus erythematosus
SOM	Supervisor of midwives
SROM	Spontaneous rupture of the membranes
STI	Sexually transmitted infection
TENS	Transcutaneous electrical nerve stimulation
USS	Ultrasound scan
UTI	Urinary tract infection
VBAC	Vaginal birth after caesarean
VE	Vaginal examination
VF	Ventricular fibrillation
VT	Ventricular tachycardia
WBC	White blood cells

Section 1
Midwifery care during labour and birth

1 Labour

Introduction

Evidence-based practice, midwifery skills and a woman's personal preferences should be the basis for providing good midwifery care. Many midwives practice in a political environment where they have to manage excessive workloads and balance their midwifery skills against those of medicalized protocols. Often, these areas can conflict and having the confidence to take a particular course of action (or inaction) may be fraught with difficulties. Thus, women do not necessarily receive the care that they want; rather they receive the care that midwives are encouraged to provide. Stewart (2002) advises midwives who feel restricted and unable to provide flexibility and choice to remind their managers that their professional body, The Nursing and Midwifery Council, requires that midwives provide care that is responsive to their clients' needs (NMC, 2002).

Each woman is different and each of her birthing experiences will be unique. This is why the care described in the following chapter is based on the available evidence and can be used as a *guide* for women in normal labour. As with all care, the woman's wishes are paramount and the provision of care should be interpreted with flexibility according to each situation. For women with particular problems closer monitoring may well be advisable.

Signs that precede labour

Women often describe feeling 'different', 'restless' or 'odd' prior to going into labour. Burvill (2002) suggests women experience a shift in their priorities as the birth becomes imminent, evidenced by spurts of energy and nesting activities. Physically, women may suffer an upset stomach and diarrhoea, may have a show, while others experience frequent leaks of liquor, or spontaneously rupture their membranes (see below). For days, even weeks, before labour, many women (particularly multiparous women) experience repeated contractions that eventually disappear. They may experience lower backache and deep pelvic discomfort as the baby descends in the pelvis.

Midwifery care

- Not all women seek advice at this stage. For those who do, the role of the midwife role is to give positive reassurance, to answer queries, and to advise that these signs can be normal when awaiting the onset of labour.
- Avoid using negative terms such as 'false labour' and explain that discomfort is normal and common, and usually precedes the onset of labour.

Prelabour rupture of the membranes at term

Some women experience prelabour rupture of the membranes (more commonly referred to as PROM) at term and a number of factors can be used in determining this condition (see Box 1.1).

Most women with PROM will go into labour spontaneously and have a good outcome. However, the hazards associated with ruptured membranes include underlying

Box 1.1 Diagnosing prelabour rupture of the membranes (PROM).

Woman's history
- Walsh (2000a) suggests this is usually a conclusive diagnosis in itself.
- Ascertain an accurate time and diagnosis of the amniotic fluid loss from the woman's description of events.

Visualization of liquor
- If the membranes have ruptured, the woman's sanitary pad will usually be damp or soaking with clear, occasionally, pinkish, fresh smelling fluid. (If none is visible, then ask the woman to walk around for an hour, less if she feels wet, then re-check her pad for any liquor.)
- The *pad test* can confirm the diagnosis of ruptured membranes without limiting the option of expectant management (Atalla *et al.*, 2000).

Speculum examination
- There appears to be a lack of consensus as to whether a speculum examination offers any advantage over either the woman's history or the less invasive 'pad test'. If the pad test is not conclusive, a speculum examination is not likely to clarify the situation any further and may simply undermine the woman's history (Walsh, 2000a).
- Some policies advise screening for infection (by vaginal or cervical swabs) which would need to be taken via a speculum examination.
- The examination after gently inserting the warmed, lubricated speculum, if there is no visible liquor then ask the woman to cough. Liquor may then trickle from the cervix and collect in the dip of the speculum.
- *Amni sticks* (nitrazine test) are sometimes used to try to detect liquor. However, these have high false-positive rates, testing positive to vaginal infection, urinary contamination, semen or contact with the endocervix (Atalla *et al.*, 2000).

---

infection, cord prolapse, iatrogenic, ascending infection from vaginal examinations (DoH, 2001) and the need for induction or augmentation of labour with associated interventions and morbidity (NICE, 2001a).

Incidence and facts

- 6–19% of women spontaneously rupture their membranes prior to labour (NICE, 2001).
- Onset of labour: 86% of women go into spontaneous labour within 24 hours of PROM and thereafter at a rate of approximately 5% per day (NICE, 2001).
- Hindwater or forewater leaks are indistinguishable and therefore, suggests Grant & Keirse (2000), should be treated the same.
- Ultrasound scan (USS) for oligohydramnios is a non-invasive, accurate method of diagnosing ruptured membranes (Grant & Keirse, 2000).
- As the time between rupture of the membranes and onset of labour increases, so does the risk of infection. Therefore, expectant management (Box 1.2) should not exceed 96 hours (NICE, 2001).
- For women with ruptured membranes who are not in labour, vaginal assessments should be avoided or kept to a minimum and when undertaken should be done so with appropriate aseptic precautions (DoH, 2001).

Box 1.2   Expectant management of prelabour rupture of membranes (PROM).

Await labour
   The woman can await labour onset in the comfort of her own home (away from iatrogenic infections and potential interventions).

Check temperature
   Frequency: 2 to 3 times a day. Report any rise above 37°C (NICE, 2001).

Observe the amniotic fluid
   Observe the colour and smell of the amniotic fluid (NICE, 2001a). It should be clear or cloudy, or a little pinkish, and should smell clean and fresh (Davis, 1997).

Report if unwell/flu-like symptoms
   Symptoms may include fever, flushing, shivers (NICE, 2001a) or uterine tenderness (a late and serious signs of intrauterine infection [Grant & Keirse, 2000]) and should be reported urgently.

Note baby's movements
   The woman should keep a note of her baby's movements and activity, reporting any concerns, including excessive or very infrequent movements.

General care
   • Advise the woman not to put anything into the vagina and to wipe from front to back after having her bowels opened.
   • The woman should drink plenty of fluids and foods rich in vitamin C to help promote the body's natural resistance to infections (Davis, 1997).
   • Finally, if the woman is concerned about anything she should telephone for advice.

Midwifery care

- Ascertain whether or not the membranes have ruptured (Box 1.1).
- Ensure that mother and baby are well.
- **Abdominal palpation/assessment**. By performing an abdominal palpation the midwife can ensure the presenting part is engaged and the fetal heart rate (FHR) satisfactory, as well as monitor fetal movements. A non-engaged presenting part is of concern if the membranes have ruptured, because cord compression or prolapse is a possibility. A period of monitoring the fetal heart and hospital admission should therefore be strongly recommended.
- **Visualization of liquor**. Check the woman's sanitary pad for liquor, which should be clear, cloudy or pinkish. Pink usually suggests the cervix is effacing or shortening, a positive sign (Note: it can also be pink or blood stained following a vaginal examination). Brown or green stained liquor is suggestive of the passage of meconium and is more common if the pregnancy is post-dates. This requires closer monitoring of the FHR because of its association with fetal compromise.
- **Check for signs of infection**. A woman with ruptured membranes who develops a fever and/or tachycardia should be carefully assessed by senior staff and commence appropriate antibiotics while awaiting the results of bacterial specimens (DoH, 2001). Signs of infection include:
  ○ maternal pyrexia
  ○ maternal tachycardia
  ○ fetal tachycardia

- ○ 'abnormal' urinalysis (positive to protein, blood or nitrates) is suggestive of infection, and an urgent urine specimen should be sent for testing (see also Chapter 9 on maternal infection).
- ○ *serious* signs of infection include an offensive vaginal loss and uterine tenderness or if the mother feels unwell.

The woman's choices for care

The woman should be aware of her choices and that she has a right to decline or accept care based on current evidence (NICE, 2001a). The two care options are:

(1) Induction of labour.
(2) Wait and see (known as expectant management, Box 1.2).

If the woman has not gone into labour after 4 days, induction is strongly recommended (NICE, 2001a).

First stage of labour

Taking on a woman's care and documentation

When taking on a woman's care (including taking over from a colleague) some basic information on the woman's physical and emotional well-being should be gleaned in advance and documented as necessary. Chapter 14 also covers information on record keeping.

The midwife is expected to keep contemporaneous records of the care provided during labour and birth (UKCC, 1998).

- Ensure you are familiar with the woman's birth plan and how she and her partner prefer to be addressed.
- Check the woman's ultrasound scan for placental location and to confirm the gestation.
- Ensure you have the woman's blood group and a recent haemoglobin result.
- Document any allergies the woman may have.
- Look for relevant risk factors, complications or indications of any problems.
- Be familiar with the woman's previous history, any previous pregnancies, labours and births the woman may have had.

The partogram

The partogram is a graphical representation of the physical elements in a woman's labour and includes documenting contractions, vaginal examinations, the woman's observations (temperature, pulse, blood pressure, urinalysis), any drugs administered and so on. It is usually commenced when the woman is in active labour. Observational studies (Buchmann, 2000) and a large trial in Southeast Asia, conducted by the World Health Organization (WHO, 1994) found that the partogram offered advantages in the recognition of prolonged labour and encouraged referral and appropriate action. This was found to result in a reduction in perinatal mortality, emergency caesareans and the need for augmentation (Buchmann, 2000).

For many midwives the action and alert lines of the partogram may be 'too rigid'. The focus can become medicalized and care become regimented instead of focusing on the woman's needs and wishes in labour. However, the partogram does offer an immediate impression of the overall *physical* condition of the woman. This can be beneficial in the hospital setting, where midwives may be caring for more than one woman and where staff change shifts and hand over a woman's care. Many community and independent midwives may find such a record unnecessary, particularly where the woman is personally known to them.

THE LATENT PHASE

The latent phase is the stage when the woman's body starts to go into labour. While official definitions mark the official start of labour from the active phase onwards, experience tells us that labour has already started by then. For women planning a hospital birth, probably the best place to spend the latent phase is at home and not in the hospital environment, where fear and anxieties are likely to inhibit labour and attract interventions (Walsh, 2000a). Midwives based in the community will know from experience that this phase can vary dramatically in length and, in the absence of complications, for most women home is the best place to be.

Contractions and cervical dilatation

Contractions are usually mild to moderate, increasingly uncomfortable, and some-times painful. The contractions become regular and closer as labour progresses, eventually occurring every 5 minutes or more apart and usually lasting up to 45 seconds. The cervix starts to efface and soften, moving from posterior to anterior and cervical dilatation is between 0 and 4 cm. This stage of labour is notoriously difficult to diagnose by medical criteria alone. The limitations of the medical model suggests Burvill (2002), undermines the importance of the experience of the midwife, her observation and interpretation of each woman's unique behaviour.

Women's characteristic behaviour

Women may be excited or may be anxious. They usually want confirmation of what is happening to their body as well as seeking reassurance and a rapport with their midwife. Women whose first language is not English may need extra reassurance, careful explanations and sensitivity to personal and cultural preferences. A translator that the woman is comfortable to be with should be arranged well in advance of labour. Ideally the translator should be female and not a family member, unless the woman specifically prefers otherwise.

Primigravidas in their excitement and inexperience of strong labour can sometimes overestimate their progress; they need their excitement and fears acknowledged (Simpkin & Ancheta, 2000).

Midwifery care

As a student midwife I recalled my mentor answering her telephone to women in possible labour. She would always sound enthusiastic and say 'Wow, how exciting . . . how are you feeling?' As a student midwife I learnt from her how important it is to always greet a woman positively and make her feel special.

- Assessment of a woman at home in early labour is preferable to an assessment in hospital as it reduces the time spent on the labour wards. This has been found to reduce subsequent interventions, resulting in a reduction in augmentation, reduced analgesia use (including epidurals) and reduced caesarean sections. Women have also reported an improved birth experience and an improved feeling of control (McNiven, 1998; Walsh, 2000a; Lauzon & Hodnett, 2002).
- Observe, listen, acknowledge the woman's excitement and give a realistic view of the early stage of the labour. This may be the woman's first contact with a midwife and provides a perfect opportunity to discuss her expectations, feelings and birth plan.
- Easing the discomfort. A woman in the latent phase may not advance into estab-lished labour for several days and contractions may come and go (Burvill, 2002). Gently explain to the woman that she is not in strong labour yet and, if it is night time, suggest she try a warm bath and attempt go back to sleep (or rest if she is too excited or uncomfortable to sleep). During the daytime, women should try to relax, gain comfort in warm baths or try distractions such as shopping, walking or watching a film.
- If the woman has sought direct contact, then following a normal physical check she should be left at home (or discharged home if in hospital) to establish in labour. The woman should be encouraged to eat and drink freely and to try not to focus on labour and coping techniques too early on, instead she should try to get on with everyday life (Simpkin & Ancheta, 2000).
- The physical check includes:
  - ○ blood pressure (BP), pulse, temperature and urinalysis
  - ○ abdominal palpation to ascertain presentation, position and descent, and the fetal heart listened to for several minutes. Check that the presenting part is engaged or low and finally check that the woman feels happy with her baby's movements
  - ○ a vaginal examination is not usually warranted (unless the woman specifically requests one) particularly since contractions are usually 5 minutes or more apart and typically less than 60 seconds in duration during this phase.

THE ACTIVE PHASE (ESTABLISHED LABOUR)

The active phase is usually taken from when women experience regular, progressing contractions from around 4 cm dilated until the cervix is fully dilated.

Contractions and cervical dilatation

Contractions tend to be regular, are moderate to painful, and occur usually approximately once every 2–5 minutes, and last between 45 seconds to well over 60 seconds. As labour becomes more powerful, the cervix will dilate further and contractions become stronger and increasingly painful (once every 2–3 minutes lasting 60 seconds or more).

The cervix is mid to anterior, soft, effaced (not always fully effaced in multiparous women) and 4 cm or more dilated.

Women's characteristic behaviour

In the earlier stages of labour, the woman may contiue to eat and drink (Box 1.3), or laugh and chat excitably between contractions. As the labour advances the woman is less inclined to eat or chat, and she will become quieter and behave more instinctively as the primitive parts of the brain take over (Ockenden, 2001).

Box 1.3   Eating and drinking during labour.

Fasting in labour can lead to:
- Poor progress.
- Unpleasant hunger sensations.
- A rise in urinary ketones.
- The diagnosis of dystocia and a cascade of interventions, culminating in a caesarean birth (Johnson *et al.*, 2000).

Aspiration of gastric contents/Mendelson's syndrome
- Aspiration is a problem associated with poor anaesthetic technique when administering a general anaesthetic and not with having food in the stomach.
- Aspiration of gastric contents still occurs with general anaesthetics administered to women who have fasted (Johnson *et al.*, 2000).
- Maternal deaths from gastric aspiration with general anaesthetic have decreased despite more liberal attitudes towards eating and drinking in labour.
- There were no reported direct maternal deaths from gastric aspiration at caesarean section in the report on the Confidential Enquiries into Maternal Deaths (DoH, 2001).

Women at high risk of emergency caesarean – with attendant anaesthetic risks
- Such women should be offered regular antacids/hydrogen ion inhibitors (such as ranitidine, cimetidine). These encourage rapid emptying of the stomach contents, as well as reducing the acidity of the stomach.
- Evidence supports the use of antacids/hydrogen ion inhibitors as conferring possible benefit should an emergency anaesthetic be required (Johnson *et al.*, 2000).

In stronger labour the woman is usually more focused and withdrawn from idle chatter, she is described as having 'gone into herself'. As labour becomes stronger, the woman is less mobile, holding on to something during a contraction, or standing legs astride and rocking her hips. As the woman's labour advances further, she may close her eyes and her breathing usually becomes heavier and more controlled (Burvill, 2002). She may moan or occasionally call out during the most painful contractions. Women can often be observed to curl their toes as the contraction peaks.

If the woman talks it will be brief, such as 'water' when wanting a drink or 'back' to instruct someone to rub her back. This is not the time to talk to her, or to draw her out from herself. Midwives are usually adept at reading the woman's cues, unlike those unfamiliar with women's typical behaviour in labour (such as students, the woman's partner and sometimes doctors). Others attending may need explanations and guidance so as not to disturb the woman, particularly during a contraction. When the midwife needs to check the FHR, she should first speak in a quiet voice, or simply touch the woman's arm prior to doing that task, and depending on her relationship with the woman, not always expect an answer.

Midwifery care

Between providing essential support, monitoring the FHR and completing documentation, it is hard for the midwife to find the opportunity to leave the woman's side. This intense relationship, hour upon hour, can be physically and mentally demanding. Involvement of the woman's birth partner, or a doula, can both support the midwife as well as enhance the quality of support the woman receives. Midwives who offer good-quality support will find that they personally are the best form of analgesia and their client is less likely to need pharmacological or epidural pain relief (Hodnett, 2002). Boxes 1.4 and 1.5, and Chapter 15 give more information on support in labour.

Below is an outline of the basic care for a woman in labour. Most of the information below is covered in greater depth at the end of this chapter and in the second section of this book.

The fetal heart rate

- The fetal heart rate (FHR) should be auscultated every 15 minutes for a period of 60 seconds, following a contraction.
- In the event of the woman developing any risk factors, or if any abnormal FHR is audible, including having a baseline below 110 bpm or above 160 bpm, or decelerations, NICE (2001b) advises continuous monitoring of the FHR.

Box 1.4　Advantages of continuous support (after Hodnett, 2002).

Advantages of continuous support
- Reduced need for pharmacological analgesia and fewer epidurals.
- Reduction in instrumental deliveries.
- Reduction in caesarean sections.
- More 5-minute Apgar scores greater than 7.
- Reduced perineal trauma.

Women's experiences
- Labour better than expected.
- A more positive overall experience for women.
- Women more likely to be breastfeeding at 6 weeks.
- Less depression at 6 weeks.
- Less difficulty in mothering.

Box 1.5   Support in labour.

General support in labour
- Encourage the woman's birth partner to support her. Show him/her practical ways of doing this.
- Facilitate others, preferably women, to attend in an active support role. This should be discussed during the antenatal period. Many couples are not aware that they can have additional supporters during labour.
- Encourage and reassure.
- Provide physical support such as giving drinks, rubbing the labouring woman's back, helping her move about, mopping her brow, etc.
- Ensure continuous support, someone should be there all the time, holding her hand, offering comfort.
- Communicate the woman's needs to the midwife/doctor/others.

Good midwifery support
- The continuous presence of the midwife (when wished by the mother) with maintenance of eye contact as appropriate.
- Hands on comfort – touch, massage.
- Verbal encouragement, praise, explanations of what is happening and information sharing.

Contractions/progress

For details on the various alternate methods of assessing a woman's progress please refer to 'Assessing progress in labour' on pages 22–5.

- The assessment of progress can be made by various means: abdominal palpation (Stuart, 2000), the woman's contractions and her response to them (Stuart, 2000; Burvill, 2002), the purple line (Hobbs, 1998) as well as by the traditional vaginal examination.
- The contractions should be assessed and documented regularly (half hourly to hourly) and should appear stronger and more frequent, and 'painful', as each hour passes (Sallam *et al.*, 1999).

Observations

- Assess and record a baseline set of observations.
- Temperature, pulse, BP and urinalysis are repeated as necessary according to the individual woman's circumstances (see 'Observing signs of maternal well-being' under the heading 'Maternal and fetal well-being and progress in labour' later in this chapter).

General points

- Encourage the woman to keep her bladder empty by taking regular trips to the bathroom. This can be an opportunity to discreetly ask to check the woman's sanitary pad for any vaginal loss/liquor, for any signs of meconium (the latter can be associated with fetal compromise), for excess blood loss (indicating possible

rapid cervical dilatation or a serious placental abruption) or for any obvious offensive smell (this being highly suggestive of serious infection).
- Ensure the woman eats and drinks as desired (Johnson *et al.*, 2000; Box 1.3) and provide both her and her attendants with refreshments.

Analgesia and the birth environment

- Ensure that the birth environment is as relaxed as possible with low lighting, minimal interruptions and music playing. This is particularly important in a hospital environment where general noise, including the sounds of other women giving birth, can be distressing for the woman in labour.
- Offer interventions for coping with painful contractions. Possible options include a hot water bottle for back or lower tummy ache, a warm bath/water tub, transcutaneous electrical nerve stimulation (TENS) machine, massage, and facilitating mobility and position changes with aids such as beanbags, wedges, low stools or birthing balls (Figs 1.1, 1.2).
- Facilitate informed choice about the available forms of pharmacological analgesia available should the woman request something stronger.

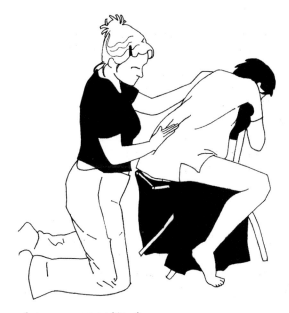

Fig. 1.1   Hands on comfort – massage and touch.

Support

- As labour advances and the contractions become increasingly painful, women usually benefit greatly from having the continuous support of their midwife (Hodnett, 2002) (see 'Support and comfort in labour', p. 29, Boxes 1.4, 1.5).

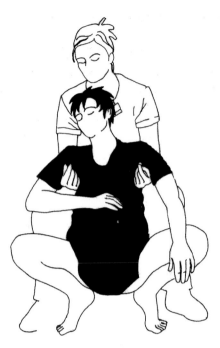

Fig. 1.2 Supported squatting position.

- As appropriate the midwife may rub the woman's back, talk the woman through each contraction if necessary, tell the woman how well she is coping and offer explanations as well as words of encouragement.
- Part of giving good support is to *listen* to the woman and respond to her verbal and non-verbal body language.
- Sensitivity is required as this can be a time of 'flashbacks' for women who have been victims of childhood sexual abuse (considered also in Chapter 16).

Documentation

- The midwife should accurately document all care in the woman's records including the FHR, the contractions and any observations taken as well as how the woman is coping.
- The partogram is usually updated half hourly, or as soon as is practical.
- Additionally any interventions, problems or referrals should also be clearly documented and signed in the woman's records (see also Chapter 14 for details on record keeping).

TRANSITION

Transition is a phase that commonly occurs at the end of the first stage of labour. While Kitzinger (1987) suggests it can last a few contractions, for some women it lasts much longer than this. This stage is thought to be the most painful and certainly the most distressing for the woman. Labour stress hormones are at their peak, which Odent (1999) suggests has a positive physiological effect on labour, and the woman experiences a surge of energy needed to push her baby out.

> 'The diagnosis of the transitional stage moves on observation to a higher level, as it is a far more women centred and subjective skill. The diagnosis of the transitional stage is essentially a midwifery observation and as such is dependent on knowing the woman, her behaviour and recognising any changes in her behaviour. Progress can thus be diagnosed without the need to resort to a vaginal examination.' (Mander, 2002)

Contractions and cervical dilatation

Contractions seem to almost merge and labour is at its most intense and painful. Many women may have a sensation to bear down during the peak of the contraction and the cervix is almost completely dilated.

Women's characteristic behaviour

The woman experiencing the 'extreme pain' of transition has a decreased ability to listen or concentrate on anything but giving birth (Leap, 2000). The woman becomes frank and honest in vocalizing her needs and dislikes, 'unfettered by politeness'. This should not be mis-interpreted as rejection or rudeness by the midwife or birth partner (Robertson, 1996).

Typical characteristic behaviour includes:

- Distressed or panicky statements:
  - 'I want to go home now'
  - 'Get me a caesarean/epidural...'
  - 'I've changed my mind'.
- Non-verbal sounds:
  - groaning or shouting out
  - involuntary pushing.
- Body language:
  - panicky, restless, toes curling
  - closed eyes due to intense concentration (Leap, 2000)
  - withdrawing from the activities and conversations of the people around her (Leap, 2000; Burvill, 2002).

Midwifery care

> 'It's a lot more work for a midwife to be interacting with somebody who's making a lot of noise and being very demanding. Then you have to be with her all of the time, you can't go out and have cups of tea or whatever...' (Leap, 2000)

This stage of labour can be the most distressing time for the woman and her partner. They need reassuring that this is normal and that it usually heralds the end of labour and the approaching birth of their baby. The birth partner and midwife may feel least adequate and helpful during transition.

The woman's partner can become stressed and want something 'done' to help his/her partner. This is a common response which is sometimes met with the woman receiving inappropriately timed analgesia (Mander, 2002) merely to make the woman's partner or the midwife feel as if they are doing 'something'. This can be a difficult situation for the midwife to judge.

Try changing the dynamics if women panic, like suggesting you go for a walk, go out to the toilet, try a position change or try focusing on her breathing (see also Chapter 15 for skills in helping women cope in labour).

Monitor the FHR, maternal observations, contractions and progress as previously described in the active phase of labour.

Second stage of labour

The second stage of labour is defined as being from the full dilation of the cervix and is complete following the birth of the baby. In the majority of cases, the actual time of onset of second stage is uncertain (Walsh, 2000b). The second stage is characterized by the urge to push, which is spontaneous and can precede full dilatation or occur during or sometime after it. All of these situations can be normal (see 'Promoting normality during the second stage of labour', p. 18).

Restricting time limits in the second stage of labour to 2 hours for primigravida and 30 minutes for multiparous women is not uncommon and is *not supported by the evidence* (Sleep *et al.*, 2000; Walsh, 2000b). Current debate suggests that arbitrary time limits on second stage should be abandoned, providing there are no fetal or maternal problems and progress is occurring (Sleep *et al.*, 2000; Walsh, 2000b). Terminating a prolonged second stage with instrumental delivery increases maternal and fetal morbidity and does not improve the outcome (Sleep *et al.*, 2000). For more information see Chapter 4, in particular the heading 'Prolonged second stage'.

Contractions

While there can be a lull in contractions sometimes lasting over half an hour, some women go straight into powerful, expulsive contractions every 2–3 minutes, lasting over 60 seconds.

Women's characteristic behaviour

Some women take the opportunity to doze as their contractions temporarily stop and this has become known as the 'rest and be thankful' stage or the latent phase of the second stage. Some women may have an increasing urge to push and may make a distinctive throaty pushing sound at the peak of a contraction, some women may verbalize that they are pushing.

Natural, spontaneous pushing

This is involuntary and characterized by:

- Short inspirations (Thompson, 1995).
- Short periods of breath-holding (never more than 6 seconds) (Sleep *et al.*, 2000).
- Followed by an expiratory grunt (Thompson, 1995).
- The woman pushes only after the contraction has built up. The earliest part of the contraction pulls the vagina taut, preventing it from being pushed down in front of the descending presenting part (Gee & Glynn, 1997).

Early physical signs around the second stage of labour

- Spontaneous rupture of the membranes.
- Rectal pressure, the sensation of needing to have the bowels opened during a contraction.
- Vomiting.
- A show or bright red vaginal loss.
- A purple line extending from the anus, to reach the nape of the buttocks (Hobbs, 1998).
- Slowing of the FHR at the peak of a contraction.

Signs of advancing second stage

- The perineum bulges, the vagina gapes and the anus flattens. Often the woman opens her bowels when pushing during the contraction.
- The presenting part is visualized and continues to advance during the contraction.

Midwifery care

Kirkham (1999) and Stapleton *et al.*, (2002) have identified that many midwives are 'policed' by colleagues into practising highly ruled behaviour. Midwives feel pressured to conform to the medical protocols and confirm full dilatation with a vaginal examination. Many midwives are known to 'fudge' the results, claiming a woman may have an anterior lip, simply to allow her more time to give birth without medical interference. Bergstrom *et al.* (1997) ask midwives to think – why does the woman's knowledge of her own body not count for anything and why does the care-givers' definition of when second stage has begun take precedent, regardless of what the woman's body is instinctively doing? Bergstrom *et al.* describe how midwives expend great energy discouraging women from pushing prior to confirmation of full dilatation, then coerce the woman into exaggerated, active pushing once full dilatation has been confirmed. They suggest that the power of authoritative knowledge is not that it is correct but that it counts.

Vaginal examination

With all the 'clues' that the woman is approaching, or is in, second stage, the midwife should ask: is a vaginal examination really indicated to confirm what may be evident? Unless there is a real concern, such as an ongoing *genuine lack of progress*, a vaginal examination is not usually indicated here.

Promoting normality during the second stage of labour

- Telling women they must not push when they cannot stop themselves at the latter end of the first stage *is unnecessary and distressing for the woman* (Sleep *et al.*, 2000).
- The midwifery myth that pushing on an undilated cervix will cause the cervix to swell is not borne out by the evidence suggests Walsh (2000b).
- **Spontaneous pushing**. Natural, spontaneous pushing is described above under 'Women's characteristic behaviour'. Active pushing is contraindicated in a 'normal' birth as it involves directed, prolonged breath-holding and prolonged bearing down (Sleep *et al.*, 2000) which can result in FHR abnormalities, lower Apgars, and increases the risk of perineal trauma, episiotomy and instrumental birth (Thompson, 1995; Sleep *et al.*, 2000).
- **Upright postures**. These reduce the length of the second stage and the severity of the pain women experience (Gupta & Nikodem, 2002). Encouraging women to remain upright during childbirth is a fundamental component of good midwifery practice. Some women initially do not want to move or may not need to. Those who do move are often surprised at how much more comfortable and effective a position change can be.
- **Monitoring the FHR**. As the baby moves downwards during the second stage, the fetal heart can be difficult to locate and the woman may find monitoring invasive and uncomfortable. Changes in the FHR often herald the onset of the second stage. Early decelerations become more common, sometimes advancing to late decelerations or even an end stage bradycardia. NICE (2001b) recommend auscultation of the FHR following a contraction for one minute repeated every 5 minutes in the second stage of labour.
- **Time limits**. Arbitrary time limits on the duration of second stage should be abandoned (Sleep *et al.*, 2000; Walsh, 2000b). There is no link between time per se and poor neonatal outcome (Sleep *et al.*, 2000; Walsh 2000b).
- **Verbal support**. As appropriate, the midwife can give lots of quietly spoken, soothing words, explanations (if needed) and praise.

As the birth approaches

- **Low lighting and privacy**. Avoid staring or focusing a light on the woman's perineum while she pushes as this puts the pressure and focus on the woman's perineum not on her; this can be embarrassing and unpleasant for any woman. It can be particularly voyeuristic and distressing for women who have been sexually abused (Kitzinger, 1992).
- **Preparation**. As the vertex is near crowning, it can be reassuring for the woman to know she is virtually there, allaying any anxieties. Explain that you will be making a little rustling noise from opening the birth pack/gloves.
- **Analgesia**. A woman who is using entonox should be able to continue to use it as it will not hinder her ability to push. However, if appropriate, avoid using entonox at the moment of birth so that the mother is aware, in control and, importantly, will be able to remember her baby's birth afterwards.

See also Box 1.6 for specific evidence-based care to preserve the perineum at birth.

Box 1.6   Specific evidence-based care to preserve the perineum at birth.

Applying a hot or cold pad
- This can be soothing if the woman wishes. The evidence suggests this is associated with lower rates of perineal trauma (Jackson, 2000).

Avoiding episiotomy
- There is evidence that this procedure is only indicated, and therefore justifiable, in cases of fetal compromise or when the perineum is unyielding and therefore responsible for a lack of progress (Sleep *et al.*, 2000).
- A truly rigid perineum is uncommon and anecdotally is associated with unusual cases where women have highly toned pelvic floors muscles, such as found in horse riders or athletes (ARM, 2000b).

Slow, gentle birth
- A birth in an atmosphere that is relaxed and unrushed is a simple practice that can reduce perineal trauma (Jackson, 2000).
- At the moment of birth, the midwife can encourage gradual delivery of the head by suggesting the woman breathes gently, pants or gives gentle, small pushes.
- The midwife usually has her 'hands on' or 'hands poised' ready to prevent rapid extension of the baby's head in order to prevent ensuing trauma (McCandlish *et al.*, 1998).

Be patient, await restitution before gently assisting the shoulders
- While a few babies are in a hurry, most will pause, await the final contraction and then restitution will take place. The midwife will see the baby's head turn to right itself with its shoulders and then the shoulders should gently emerge.
- The midwife may assist the anterior shoulder with gentle lateral traction.
- The general opinion varies as to whether to check for the cord as most women find this painful. If the cord is present the baby usually delivers easily and then it can easily be untangled following birth (ARM, 2000a).
- On the rare occasion that a baby will not deliver because the cord is literally holding it back, apply two clamps to the cord and cut between them. This can be difficult as the cord is usually very tight, and clamping and cutting the cord usually results in the baby being born with lower Apgars.

Third stage of labour

The third stage of labour follows the birth of the baby and involves the uterus contracting and reducing in size. As the placenta is non-compressible, it shears off the uterine wall and is then expelled via the vagina.

A physiological third stage

A woman experiencing a physiological third stage uses her contractions, upright postures and maternal pushing efforts to aid expulsion of her placenta. If the woman has had a positive birth followed by unhurried, quality contact with her newborn this will facilitate oxytocin release (Odent, 1999), a hormone that stimulates contraction of the uterine muscles. Breastfeeding, while not essential, if initiated will again increase natural, circulating oxytocin.

Contractions

These mild, irregular period cramps are not usually noticed by the mother until sometime after the birth. A physiological third stage can occasionally last over an hour, but is usually shorter in multiparous women and averages 20 minutes (Begley, 1990).

Women's characteristic behaviour

By this stage, most should be enjoying skin-to-skin contact with their newborn and most are oblivious to their placenta *in situ*. For further information on the benefits of skin-to-skin contact see Box 8.1.

Some women do groan or go suddenly quiet if they are having strong uterine cramps, usually preceding the passing of the placenta, a clot or blood loss. This sensation may be accompanied by a mild urge to push, to expel the placenta.

Active management of the third stage of labour

Any woman who is at significant risk of a postpartum haemorrhage should be advised to choose *active management* of the third stage of labour. This involves the administration of an oxytocic injection following birth. Delivery of the placenta is performed by the midwife who guards the uterus with one hand and applies controlled traction to the cord with the other, typically several minutes after the administration of the oxytocic agent. A list of oxytocic agents is given later in Table 23.5.

Midwifery care

Benefits of a physiological third stage

The woman should have had a physiologically 'normal' labour and birth. Box 1.7 shows the indications and possible benefits of a physiological third stage.

Box 1.7 Indications and possible benefits for a physiological third stage.

Informed choice
- Women may request a physiological third stage, particularly if they have laboured and birthed without any drugs or analgesia.

Benefits of physiological third stage
- Leaving the cord unclamped and attached is thought to offer important clinical benefits, including transfusing significant blood volume to the baby, in the order of 20–50% (Prendiville & Elbourne, 2000), which increases the baby's haemoglobin and haematocrits without any significant increase in symptomatic polycythaemia or postpartum jaundice (Mercer, 2001).
- Delaying cord clamping is proven as beneficial for women who are Rhesus negative, in terms of reducing feto-maternal transfusion (Prendiville & Elbourne, 2000).

Avoid the potential side effects of active management
- Women may wish to avoid the side effects of oxytocics (nausea, vomiting, severe after-birth pains, headaches) (Begley, 1990). See also Table 23.5 for a more extensive list of oxytocic side effects.
- There is no clear data to rule out the possibility that administering a routine oxytocic for the third stage can increase the risk of retained placenta (Prendiville & Elbourne, 2000).

Conduct of a physiological third stage

The midwife should be skilled in 'doing nothing' and competent in facilitating a physiological third stage.

- **'Watchful waiting'. Do nothing!**
  - do not administer oxytocic agent (as used in active management)
  - do not palpate the uterus
  - do not apply cord traction
  - do not cut the cord.
- **Monitor blood loss and observe for signs of separation by:**
  - cord lengthening
  - possible trickle of blood/ passage of small clots
  - the woman may have an urge to push or 'achy' tummy pain
  - the placenta may be visible at the vagina.
- **Following separation (or after 20–30 minutes) assist the mother to birth her placenta:**
  - assist the woman into an upright position, such as kneeling. Alternatively, try sitting on the toilet, or a bedpan which may be more comfortable than squatting
  - the woman may find any expulsive/pushing efforts are usually more effective if timed with a contraction (this is usually felt as a period type-ache/pain)
  - if the placenta does not emerge after several attempts relax and wait a while before trying again.
- **When the placenta emerges – have a bowl ready to catch it**. The cord can now be clamped and cut. The woman or her birthing partner may wish to do this.

Possible problems and subsequent care

- **If the baby requires intensive resuscitation**. Clamp and cut the cord but leave the maternal end unclamped and free to bleed. This is recommended by Levy (1990) so that the uterus can contract and the placenta compress, with excess blood escaping via the maternal end of the cord.
- **If the placenta does not emerge**. If the woman has tried pushing, utilizing gravity, position changes, breastfeeding and has passed urine, the midwife may wish to check that the placenta has actually separated. Using a clean glove, the midwife inserts two fingers gently into the vagina, where a partially or totally separated placenta can be felt in the os or vagina. If the placenta has separated but not delivered then, although controversial, many midwives use gentle cord traction in conjunction with maternal bearing down efforts (Begley, 1990). If pulling the cord or maternal pushing results in fresh bleeding then stop, the placenta is still partially adhered. If there is no active bleeding, then encourage the baby to nuzzle and feed at the breast. Encourage the woman to relax and try to do the same!
- **If the placenta is delivered, but the membranes remain stuck**. Avoid pulling on the cord. Suggest the mother gives a few hearty coughs, this usually releases the membranes and they slide out. It also possible to gently twist the placenta round and around, up down and coax them out (Davis, 1997).
- **If vaginal bleeding appears heavy, gushing or continuous**. Proceed to active management (see also Chapter 11). Syntocinon® is preferable to Syntometrine® as

the later causes the cervical os to close, which could complicate the situation if the bleeding continues and the placenta remains undelivered (Crafter, 2002).

Maternal and fetal well-being and progress in labour

Monitoring the fetal heart rate

For the majority of women in normal labour, intermittent auscultation (IA) is the recommended choice for monitoring the FHR in labour (NICE, 2001b) (see also Chapter 17).

The NICE (2001b) guidelines for 'low-risk' women are:

- The admission trace should be abandoned.
- Low risk women should be offered intermittent auscultation.

In the event of the woman developing any 'risk factors', see also Appendix E, or if an abnormal FHR is detected, NICE 2001b advise recommending to the woman the continuous monitoring of her baby's heart rate.

The NICE (2001b) guideline for women deemed 'high-risk' is:

- Electronic fetal monitoring (EFM) should be offered to 'high-risk' cases.

Recommendations for intermittent auscultation (NICE, 2001b) are:

- The FHR should be auscultated after a contraction for one minute:
  - every 15 minutes in the first stage of labour
  - every 5 minutes in the second stage of labour.

NICE (2001b) FHR guidelines for *intermittent auscultation* are based on 'medical expert committee reports/opinion', and are neither evidence based (as there were no randomized controlled trials [RCTs] for NICE to base their recommendations on) nor do they come from a strong midwifery perspective. This means they have a medical bias which can be restrictive and inflexible in practice (Beech Lawrence, 2001), particularly during the early stages of labour.

Assessing progress in labour

It is important for midwives to gain confidence in their midwifery skills of observation and minimal intervention in order to assess maternal well-being and progress. Midwives are accountable and responsible for their own actions and, as such, they should not be pressured to adhere to protocols with a medical bias and an obstetric lead, particularly in low-risk births where they remain the lead professional.

Kirkham (1999) and Stapleton *et al.* (2002) have identified that midwives practising in the hospital environment are policed and pressured by colleagues into highly ruled, conforming behaviour. Midwives may find conflict between providing choice for women, their own opinions and conforming to the medical model of care. For a midwife to state she is happy with a woman's progress, because the woman's contractions are more frequent and painful than a couple of hours ago, may or may not be met with understanding! In contrast, repeated vaginal examinations in labour have become the corner stone of assessing progress under the medical model of childbirth.

Yet vaginal examinations are not always reliable, they are an invasive, subjective intervention and remain of unproven benefit (Crowther *et al.*, 2000).

Stuart (2000) suggests that it is through the acquisition of practical knowledge that midwives can use midwifery skills to ascertain progress and make clinical decisions without needing to resort to interventions such as routine vaginal examinations. She recalls that during her training in the 1970s labour progress was assessed by contractions and abdominal palpation.

Methods of assessing progress in labour include:

- Vaginal examination.
- Contractions/woman's behaviour.
- Abdominal palpation.
- Purple line.

Vaginal examination

Timing of vaginal examinations should be relevant to each individual woman in order to permit adequate assessment of her progress and should not be performed too frequently or for the sake of 'routine' (Crowther, 2000b). These assessments and definitions of progress vary greatly between units and in the literature (Crowther, 2000b).

A cervical dilatation rate of 0.5 cm per hour may be more appropriate as a lower limit for defining progress within the context of maternal well-being (Crowther, 2000b). This may lead to fewer unnecessary interventions than the more commonly used assessment of progress by 1 cm per hour.

Contractions/woman's behaviour

Burvill (2002) describes how midwives can assess a woman's progress by her verbal and non-verbal response to the various stages of labour. The woman's behavioural response to contractions varies according to their strength, and thus severity, and this can be used as an indicator of progress.

Sallam *et al.* (1999) identify, in one study, what most midwives know through personal observation, there is a direct correlation between frequency and strength of contractions, and cervical dilatation and progress in labour (Table 1.1).

It can be useful to ask 'Do the woman's contractions seem as frequent as an hour ago? Do they appear more painful than an hour ago?'.

Abdominal palpation

Stuart (2000) describes how performing abdominal palpation every 2–3 hours can monitor descent, and thus determine if the head is engaged or deeply engaged (Fig. 1.3). Landmarks used to assess descent and flexion are the pelvic brim, the sinciput and the occiput of the fetal head. Stuart described developing a 'feel' for these landmarks, which feel different abdominally. However, some women may find this examination too painful, particularly in advanced labour.

Table 1.1   Assessing contractions.

Criteria	Cervical dilatation (cm)				
	0–3	3–4	4–7	7–9	9–10
Contractions increasing in length, frequency and strength/pain (Stuart, 2000)	Tight uterus, with painless, contractions Sometimes irregular and may stop	2 in 10 minutes Increasingly regular, lasting 20–40 seconds	3 in 10 minutes Regular, usually with bearable pain, lasting around 60 seconds or more	3 or 4 in 10 minutes Regular with increasing pain	4 or 5 in 10 minutes Regular and at their most painful. May experience an increasing urge to push
Breathing and conversation (Burvill, 2002)	May have exaggerated panic-like breathing Chatty, speaks quite excitedly		Deeper breathing like a sigh, controlled pronounced start of voice breathing	Focused The woman becomes quiet and conversation stops Focused on breathing, which slows down with a contraction Makes grunting throat sounds, cries out with expiration	
Movement and posture (Burvill, 2002)	Moves during contractions		Grasps abdomen and bends forward	Less mobile overall and stops during a contraction eventually staying still even between contractions Holds on to something during a contraction	

Purple line

Hobbs (1998) has described the visualization of the 'purple line' from the woman's anal margin, which gradually extends to the nape of the buttocks relative to the dilatation of the cervix. Just below the sacrococcygeal joint, where the coccyx starts to curve inwards, the nape of the buttocks can be found. She describes the start of the purple line just above the anal margin at between 0 and 2 cm cervical dilatation. Hobbs explains that the line does not seem to rise in strict proportion: there is a longer gap between 4 and 7 cm dilatation than there is both before and after. She suggests that when it reaches the nape of the buttocks the woman is full dilated, allegedly.

For some women, such as those who are overweight, or still in early labour, checking the purple line can be quite invasive and this form of assessment may not be appropriate for everyone.

Observing signs of maternal well-being

In normal labour, different midwives will have different frequencies of monitoring maternal progress and well-being. The usefulness of such routine observations in normal labour has been questioned and it is surprising to know that such observations

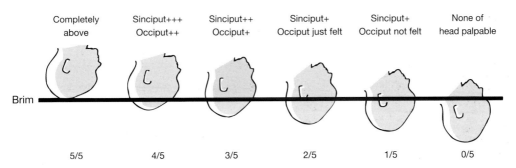

Completely above	Sinciput+++ Occiput++	Sinciput++ Occiput+	Sinciput+ Occiput just felt	Sinciput+ Occiput not felt	None of head palpable
5/5	4/5	3/5	2/5	1/5	0/5

Fig. 1.3 Abdominal palpation (Stuart, 2000).

are thought likely to serve no useful purpose (Crowther *et al.*, 2000). However, in the absence of evidence to support or disprove the benefits, some regular monitoring of maternal observations is usually undertaken (Table 1.2).

- A baseline set of observations is undertaken, against which any future observations can be compared and significant changes noted.
- Subsequent observations during labour remain at the judgement and account-ability of the individual midwife. Midwives should exercise clinical judgement and be guided by the woman's condition and circumstances. For example, if the woman is labouring in water, it is advisable to check her temperature more frequently, hourly is recommended (D. Garland, personal communication, 2002).
- Following the birth, prior to transfer to a postnatal area, or if at home prior to the midwife leaving, a further set of observations should be taken.

These are *guidelines* only. There is little evidence on which to base the frequency of such observations.

Promoting normality – the basics of midwifery care

Eating and drinking during labour

Encouraging women to fast in normal labour is not evidence based and is not recommended (Box 1.3). Studies show that women often want to eat in early labour and find enforced hunger a very unpleasant experience (Johnson *et al.*, 2000). During the more active phase of labour most women, however, do not wish to eat.

Midwives should offer women whatever they fancy to eat. This is usually possible at home or in most birthing centres but, surprisingly, large hospitals usually have a reduced selection of food to offer. Some suggested foods for labour are low-residue or high-calorie snacks and drinks such as fruit juice, tea, toast and butter, biscuits, eggs and so on (Johnson *et al.*, 2000)

Mobility and positions for labour and giving birth

Actively promoting and encouraging women to mobilize during childbirth is a fundamental component of good midwifery practice and is a safe, effective way of

Table 1.2   Maternal observations in labour.

Observations and normal range	Frequency	Interpretation of results
Blood pressure Normal range varies between women Systolic = 100–140 mmHg Diastolic = 60-90 mmHg (Baston, 2001a)	Tested at the onset of labour Subsequently tested as required for conditions such as pre-eclampsia, an epidural, haemorrhage, post delivery	Hypertension can occur in pre-eclampsia or maternal hypertension during general anaesthetia, pain, stress and anxiety *Hypertension*, with a diastolic of > 90 mmHg on two or more consecutive occasions, is usually of concern *Severe hypertension* is defined as a systolic > 160 mmHg or a diastolic $\geq$ 110 mmHg or a mean atertial pressure (MAP) > 125 mmHg (DoH, 2001) For more detail on accurate blood pressure recording, ranges and arterial MAP range see Chapter 7, Box 7.1 *Hypotension* can occur following: • An epidural/epidural top-up • Aortocaval occlusion caused by poor maternal position such as lying flat • Reduced blood volume through haemorrhage • Shock
Temperature Normal body temperature = 36–37°C (97–98.4°F)	Tested at the onset of labour Subsquently tested as required for conditions such as suspected infection, prolonged labour, waterbirth, epidural, post delivery, etc.	A *pyrexia* (temperature above 37°C) is associated with: • Infection (Baston, 2001c). • Epidurals. These can cause a low-grade pyrexia in labour, >37.2°C. This gradually increases the longer the epidural is *in situ*. • Dehydration (Baston, 2001c)
Pulse rate 55–90 regular beats per minute	Tested at the onset of labour Subsequently checked between 1 and 4 hourly during labour	Is the pulse weak, thready, bounding, tachycardic or steady? A *tachycardia*, pulse > 100 bpm, can be caused by: • Stress, pain and anxiety, hyperventilation • Pyrexia, dehydration • Obstructed labour • Exercise or exertion • Haemorrhage, anaemia and shock (Baston, 2001b) A *bradycardia*, pulse < 55 bpm, can be caused by rest, relaxation, shock, injury, and myocardial infarction (Baston, 2001b)

Cont.

Table 1.2 Continued.

Observations and normal range	Frequency	Interpretation of results
Urine Urine should be 'clear' with a pH of between 4.6 and 8.0 (Baston, 2002)	Tested at the onset of labour Subsequently tested as required for conditions such as pregnancy-induced hypertension, diabetes, prolonged labour or suspected infection	It is common to find blood and protein in the urine sample of a woman during the course of labour. This is usually by contamination of the urine sample from vaginal secretions, liquor and blood Mild *ketoacidosis* is a normal occurrence in labour (Grant, 1990) and, by encouraging women to eat and drink freely in labour, prevention of severe ketosis is possible. Strongly positive ketones may be a result of vomiting throughout labour, dehydration or prolonged labour (Baston, 2002) *Proteinurea* may suggest contamination, infection or pre-eclampsia *Blood* in the urine is usually from contamination but it may also be caused by an asymptomatic urinary tract infection *Glucose urea* can be found in diabetics. It is not uncommon to occasionally detect it during pregnancy (due to a lowered renal threshold) or following eating something high in sugar (Baston, 2002) *Specific gravity* between 1.002 and 1.030. The higher the value the more concentrated the urine (Baston, 2002) *Nitrates* may indicate infection (Baston, 2002). *Bilirubin* may indicate hepatic disease, if raised *Urobilinigen* is normally present in small amounts (Baston, 2002)

providing optimum care to healthy women (Box 1.8). It is also a simple, cost-effective way of reducing complications caused by restricted mobility and semi-recumbent postures, as well as enriching the woman's personal birth experience.

Women's experiences (MIDIRS, 1999)

In the UK today around three quarters of women spend their labours lying on their backs propped up by pillows or wedges. Most women surveyed specified that they would like to be upright for any subsequent labour and birth. For those women who were upright the first time, they specified that they would like to do the same again. The evidence suggests that they are probably better off that way.

Women's expectations of how to behave in labour, combined with unfamiliar sur-roundings, the 'bed' in the labour room, a lack of privacy and the medical model of care, all serve to restrict or inhibit their mobility in labour.

Box 1.8   The evidence for mobilization and upright postures for labour and birth.

Upright postures
- Improved frequency, strength and length of contractions.
- A reduction in the use of oxytocin to augment labour with, on average, shorter labours.
- Reduced discomfort and pain experienced in upright postures with a reduced need for epidurals and narcotic analgesia.
- Reduction in episiotomies and a small reduction in assisted deliveries.
- Improved oxygen supply to the baby/fewer abnormal heart rate patterns.
- Adversely, estimated blood loss of > 500 ml is more common in women using a birthing chair or stool which Gupta & Nikodem (2002) suggest is possibly due to the ease of catching and measuring blood loss in upright positions.

Evidence from Cochrane Review of 18 randomized controlled trials (Gupta & Nikodem, 2002).

Other evidence
- Radiological evidence illustrates that the pelvis moves and widens during birth and that the outlet diameters can increase by nearly a third in the squatting/kneeling positions (Borrell & Fenstrom, 1957; Russell, 1982).
- Upright postures have been found to improve the alignment of pelvic bones and the shape and capacity of the pelvis, optimizing the chances of a 'good fit' between baby and pelvis (Simpkin & Ancheta, 2000).
- Sutton & Scott (1994) suggest that lying down adds the weight of the uterus on the spine which reduces the angle of the uterus with the spine, resulting in poor alignment of the baby within the pelvis.
- Women express a preference to labour and birth in upright positions; this decision is not affected by the positions they have adopted in a previous labour (MIDIRS, 1999).

The supine position
The randomized controlled trials (Gupta & Nikodem, 2002) also found that there was no evidence to support the most frequently encouraged and adopted position in labour – the supine position. This position:
- Adversely affects contractions and the progress of labour.
- Is associated with an increase in abnormalities of the fetal heart rate (due to aortocaval compression) and can cause maternal postural hypotension.
- Is not what women choose.

Midwifery issues to consider

- If you are unfamiliar with assisting the mother to labour and birth in alternative positions (Figs 1.4, 1.5, 1.6) it can be useful to ask yourself 'Why?' Try to witness other midwives during deliveries or ask a colleague for support when the mother is giving birth in a non-supine position.
- Have you discussed with the woman in labour why it is important to mobilize in labour? By pointing out that labour is more likely to be shorter and less painful, you will give her 'permission' to move around freely and to do what she feels is best for her.
- Women often get 'stuck' on the bed following an examination or during continuous monitoring. It can be useful if you suggest the woman stretch her legs, get comfortable, even mobilize out to the toilet.
- Mind your back! Any birth on a bed does involve twisting which is not the opti-

mum position for your back. Any position where you face directly to the woman is better. You may need to kneel down, or temporarily squat (Fig. 1.4), as the baby is born depending on your own preference and on the mother's position.

- In hospital births, it is sensible to always leave the bed uncluttered and accessible, should you need it suddenly. If you and the woman decide to use a mattress on the floor, if possible avoid using the one from the bed.
- Should you find yourselves in a bathroom or elsewhere giving birth, think what you may need within easy reach (delivery pack, gloves, call bell), etc., particularly with multiparous women!

Support and comfort in labour

'The aims of the service should be for every woman to have a midwife with her throughout her labour, if she wishes. If possible, the same midwife should remain with the woman throughout.' (DoH, 1993)

There is clear, remarkably consistent evidence that women receiving continuous support in labour (such as from a female relative, doula, or birth attendant) benefit from a reduction in maternal and fetal morbidity (Hodnett, 2002) (Box 1.4). Historically, female support for labouring women has been established practice in most of the traditional non-western world, presumably because it is so successful.

Kind words, the constant presence of the midwife and appropriate touch are proven powerful analgesia (Hodnett, 2002). The midwifery qualities of giving support remain invisible and fellow midwives, managers and medical staff alike fail to appreciate the value of such care (Stapleton *et al.*, 2002). While midwives aim to play the support role in labour, increasing administration, medicalization, staffing levels and shift changes all contribute to the erosion of the midwife as an effective birth supporter. In several studies, midwives were observed to spend less than 10% of their time giving support and actually being with the woman in labour (Hodnett, 2002).

Summary

Latent phase

- In the absence of complications this time should ideally be spent at home.

Prelabour rupture of the membranes (PROM)

- Screen/check for infection:
  - if infection advise intravenous (IV) antibiotics and induction of labour
  - if all appears well, expectant management or induction remains the woman's choices.

Care in labour

First stage of labour

- Take a baseline set of observations including urinalysis. Repeat observations according to individual circumstances.

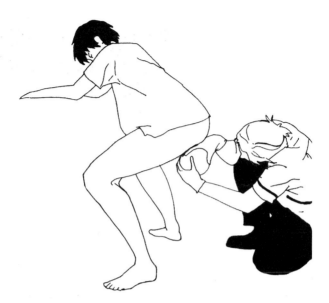

Fig. 1.4   Standing/hanging from a bed.

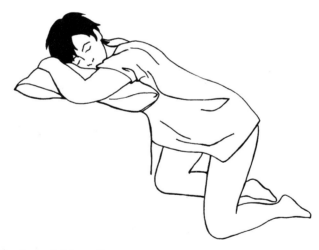

Fig. 1.5   Kneeling forwards into a pillow.

Use the equipment in the room. For example, a raised bed will enable the woman to remain upright and 'hang' from it during a contraction, a stool will enable her to sit astride and rest forward onto a bed. Utilize aids such as a beanbag (a scrunched up duvet if at home) either on the bed or off. Both can be great for supported side lying or kneeling, while a birthing ball is good for resting sitting upright, for backache or rotating the hips

Think!

'Where would you stand/kneel/squat to receive the baby?' In all fours, kneeling and standing postures, consider where the anterior and posterior shoulders lie so you are prepared should they require assistance at delivery

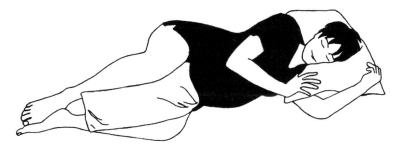

Fig. 1.6 Side lying.

- Monitor the fetal heart rate (FHR) intermittently
- Encourage mobilization and facilitate position changes.
- Eat and drink freely.
- Continuous supportive presence of the midwife is proven effective analgesia.
- Avoid arbitrary time limits in labour.
- Contractions and the woman's response: are they as strong, frequent and as long as an hour ago?
- Progress and descent felt abdominally.
- Monitoring the purple line.
- Cervix/dilatation and descent.

Second stage of labour

- Avoid arbitrary time limits if all is well.
- Assessment of maternal/fetal well-being and progress.
- Non-directed pushing.
- Encourage upright postures.
- Applying a hot or cold pad to the perineum, if the woman wishes.
- Avoiding episiotomy.
- Slow, gentle birth.

Third stage of labour

- The woman should have had a physiologically 'normal' labour and birth.
- A physiological third stage involves: 'watchful waiting' and doing nothing!
- Monitor blood loss and observe for signs of separation.
- Following separation assist the mother to birth her placenta.
- Collect the placenta in a bowl then the cord can be clamped and cut.

Useful contacts

Association for Improvements in the Maternity Services (AIMS)   AIMS Helpline: 0870 765 1433. Website: www.aims.org.uk

Doula UK   PO Box 26678, London N14 4WB. Website: www.doula.org.uk
Trained birth supporters for women.

Language Line   11–12 Northdown Street, London N1 9BN. Telephone: 0800 169 2879. www.languageline.co.uk
Interpreters and translation services for the public sector in the UK.
National Childbirth Trust (NCT)   Alexandra House, Oldham Terrace, Acton, London W3 6NH. Enquiry line: 0870 444 8707. Website: www.nct-online.org
Nursing and Midwifery Council (NMC)   23 Portland Place, London W1B 1PZ. Telephone: 020 7637 7181. Website: www.nmc-uk.org
Professional information, including *The Code of Professional Conduct*.

Recommended reading

Bergstrom, L., Seedily, J., Schulman-Hull, L. *et al.* (1997) 'I gotta push. Please let me push!' Social interactions during the change from first stage to second stage of labour. *Birth* **24** (3), 173–80.
Simpkin, P. & Ancheta, R. (2000) *The Labor Progress Handbook*. Blackwell Science, Oxford.

References

ARM (2000a) Association of Radical Midwives Nettalk: Checking for cord. *Midwifery Matters* Issue 87, 28–30.
ARM (2000b) Association of Radical Midwives Nettalk: Tight pelvic floor muscles and horse riders. *Midwifery Matters* Issue 87, 28–30.
Atalla, R., Kean, L. & McParland, P. (2000) Preterm labor and prelabor rupture of the membranes. In *Best Practice in Labor Ward Management* (Kean, L.H., Baker, P.N. & Edelstone, D.I., eds), pp. 111–39. WB Saunders, Edinburgh.
Baston, H. (2001a) Blood pressure measurement: midwifery basics. *The Practising Midwife* **4** (9), 10–14.
Baston, H. (2001c) Temperature measurement: midwifery basics. *The Practising Midwife* **4** (10), 19–22.
Baston, H. (2001b) Pulse and respiration measurement: midwifery basics. *The Practising Midwife* **4** (11), 18–21.
Baston, H. (2002) Urinalysis: midwifery basics. *The Practising Midwife* **5** (1), 32–5.
Beech Lawrence, B. (2001) Electronic fetal monitoring: Do NICE's new guidelines owe too much to the medical model of childbirth? *The Practising Midwife* **4** (7), 31–3.
Begley, C. (1990) A comparison of 'active' and 'physiological' management of the third stage of labour. *Midwifery* **63**, 3–17.
Bergstrom, L., Seedily, J., Schulman-Hull, L. *et al.* (1997) 'I gotta push. Please let me push!' Social interactions during the change from first stage to second stage of labour. *Birth* **24** (3), 173–80.
Borrell, U. & Fenstrom, I. (1957) The movements of the sacroiliac joints and their importance to changes in the pelvic dimensions during parturition. *Acta Obstetrica et Gynaecologica, Scandinavica* **36**, 42–57.
Buchmann, E.J. (2000) Monitoring progress in labor. In *A Guide to Effective Care in Pregnancy and Childbirth*, 3rd edn (Enkin, M., Keirse, M.J.N.C., Neilson, J. *et al.*, eds), pp. 281–8. Oxford University Press, Oxford.
Burvill, S. (2002) Midwifery diagnosis of labour onset. *British Journal of Midwifery* **10** (10), 600–605.

Crafter, H. (2002) Intrapartum and primary postpartum haemorrhage. In *Emergencies Around Childbirth – A Handbook for Midwives* (Boyle, M., ed.), p. 113–26. Radcliffe Medical Press, Oxford.

Crowther, C., Enkin, M., Keirse, M.J.N.C. & Brown, I. (2000) Monitoring progress in labor. In *A Guide to Effective Care in Pregnancy and Childbirth*, 3rd edn (Enkin, M., Keirse, M.J.N., Neilson, J. *et al.*, eds), pp. 218–8. Oxford University Press, Oxford.

Davis, E. (1997) *Hearts and Hands: A Midwife's Guide to Pregnancy and Birth*, 3rd edn. Celestial Arts, Berkeley, California.

DoH (1993) *Changing Childbirth. Report of the Expert Maternity Group*. Department of Health, HMSO, London.

DoH (2001) *Why Mothers Die, 1997–1999. The fifth report of the Condifential Enquiries into Maternal Deaths in the United Kingdom*. Department of Health, RCOG Press, London.

Gee, H. & Glynn, M. (1997) The physiology and clinical management of labour. In *Essential Midwifery* (Henderson, C. & Jones, K., eds), pp. 171–202. Mosby, London.

Grant, J. (1990) Nutrition and hydration in labour. In *Intrapartum Care – A Research Based Approach* (Alexander, J., Levy, V. & Roch, S., eds), pp. 58–69. Macmillan, Basingstoke.

Grant, J. & Keirse, M.J.N.C. (2000) Prelabor rupture of the membranes. In *A Guide to Effective Care in Pregnancy and Childbirth* (Enkin, M., Keirse, M.J.N.C., Neilson, J. *et al.*, eds), pp. 196–209. Oxford University Press, Oxford.

Gupta, J.K. & Nikodem, V.C. (2002) Woman's position during the second stage of labour (Cochrane Review). *The Cochrane Library* Issue 4. Update Software, Oxford.

Hobbs, L. (1998) Assessing cervical dilatation without VE's. *The Practising Midwife* **1** (11), 34–5.

Hodnett, E.D. (2002) Caregiver support for women during childbirth (Cochrane Review). *COCHRANE. The Pregnancy and Childbirth Database*. The Cochrane Collaboration. CD ROM: Issue 1. Oxford.

Jackson, K. (2000) The bottom line: care of the perineum must be improved. *British Journal of Midwifery* **8** (10), 609–14.

Johnson, C., Keirse, M.J.N.C., Enkin, M. & Chalmers, I. (2000) Hospital practices – nutrition and hydration in labor. In *A guide to Effective Care in Pregnancy and Childbirth*, 3rd edn (Enkin, M., Keirse, M.J.N., Neilson, J. *et al.*, eds), pp. 255–66. Oxford University Press, Oxford.

Kitzinger, J.V. (1992) Counteracting, not re-enacting, the violation of women's bodies: the challenge for perinatal caregivers. *Birth* **19** (4), 219–22.

Kitzinger, S. (1987) *Giving birth: How it really feels*. Gollancz, London.

Kirkham, M. (1999) The culture of midwifery in the National Health Service in England. *Journal of Advanced Nursing* **30** (3), 732–9.

Lauzon, L. & Hodnett, E. (2002) Labour assessment programs to delay admission to labour wards (Cochrane Review). *The Cochrane Library* Issue 4. Update Software, Oxford.

Leap, N. (2000) Pain in labour. *MIDIRS Midwifery Digest* **10** (1), 49–53.

Levy, V. (1990) The midwife's management of the third stage of labour. In *Intrapartum Care 1-1 A Research Based Approach* (Alexander, J., Levy, V. & Roch, S., eds), pp. 139–143. Macmillan, Basingstoke.

McCandlish, R., Bower, U., van Asten, H. *et al.* (1998) A randomised controlled trial of care of the perineum during the second stage of normal labour (HOOP trial). *British Journal of Obstetrics and Gynaecology* **105**, 1262–72.

McNiven, P., Williams, J., Hodnett, E., Kaufman, H.M. (1998) An early labour assessment program: a randomised controlled trial. *Birth* **25** (1), 5–10.

Mander, R. (2002) The transitional stage – pain and control. *The Practising Midwife* **5** (1), 10–12.

Mercer, J.C. (2001) Current best evidence: a review of the literature on umbilical cord clamping. *Journal of Midwifery and Women's Health* **46** (6), 402–14.

MIDIRS (1999) Positions in Labour and Delivery. Informed Choice Leaflet: Midwives Information and Resource Service, Bristol.

NICE (2001a) *Clinical Guideline D – Induction of Labour*. National Institute for Clinical Excellence, London.

NICE (2001b) *Clinical Guideline C – The Use of Electronic Fetal Monitoring*. National Institute for Clinical Excellence, London.

NMC (2002) *Code of Professional Conduct*. Nursing and Midwifery Council, London.

Ockenden, J. (2001) The hormonal dance of labour. *The Practising Midwife* **4** (6), 16–17.

Odent, M. (1999) *The Scientification of Love*. Free Association Books, London.

Prendiville, W. & Elbourne, D. (2000) The third stage of labor. In *A Guide to Effective Care in Pregnancy and Childbirth*, 3rd edn (Enkin, M., Keirse, M.J.N.C., Neilson, J. *et al.*, eds), Oxford University Press, Oxford.

Robertson, A. (1996) *Empowering Women: Teaching Active Birth in the 90's*. ACE Graphics, Camperdown, NSW, Australia.

Russell, J.G.B. (1982) The rationale of primitive delivery positions. *British Journal of Obstetrics and Gynaecology* **89**, 712–15.

Sallam, H.N., Abdel-Dayem, A., Sakr, R.A. *et al.* (1999) Mathematical relationships between uterine contractions, cervical dilatation, descent and rotation in spontaneous vertex deliveries. *International Journal of Gynaecology and Obstetrics* **64**, 135–9.

Simpkin, P. & Ancheta, R. (2000) *The Labor Progress Handbook*. Blackwell Science, Oxford.

Sleep, J., Roberts, J. & Chalmers, I. (2000) The second stage of labor. In *A Guide to Effective Care in Pregnancy and Childbirth*, 3rd edn (Enkin, M., Keirse, M.J.N.C., Neilson, J. *et al.*, eds), pp. 289–99. Oxford University Press, Oxford.

Stapleton, H., Kirkham, M., Thomas, G. & Curtis, P. (2002) Midwives in the middle: balance and vulnerability. *British Journal of Midwifery* **10** (10), 607–11.

Stewart, M. (2002) Respecting the individual – implications of the Code of Professional Conduct. *The Practising Midwife* **5** (10), 32–33.

Stuart, C. (2000) Invasive actions in labour. Where have all the 'old tricks' gone? *The Practising Midwife* **3** (8), 30–33.

Sutton, J. & Scott, P. (1994) Optimal fetal positioning: a midwifery approach to increasing the number of normal births. *MIDIRS Midwifery Digest* **4** (3), 283–6.

Thompson, A. (1995) Maternal behaviour during spontaneous and directed pushing in the second stage of labour. *Journal of Advanced Nursing* **22** (6), 1027–34.

UKCC (1998) *Guidelines for Records and Record Keeping*. United Kingdom Central Council for Nursing, Midwifery and Health Visiting, London.

Walsh, D. (2000a) Evidence-based care. Part 3: Assessing women's progress in labour. *British Journal of Midwifery* **8** (7), 449–57.

Walsh, D. (2000b) Evidence-based care. Part 6: Limits on pushing and time in the second stage. *British Journal of Midwifery* **8** (10), 604–608.

WHO (1994) World Health Organization partogram in the management of labour. *The Lancet* **343**, 1399–404.

2 Home birth

Janet Gwillim

Introduction

At booking all women should be given full information on the options for place of birth, including at home (DoH, 1993). It is the midwife's duty of care to provide support and care for the woman who chooses a home birth, even if the woman's pregnancy is considered not within normal parameters (UKCC, 1996).

Incidence

Home birth rates vary widely throughout the country. Around 1.8% of women delivered their babies at home during the last decade, with around 2.6% of women opting for a home birth in 2001 (NCT, 2001). It is anticipated that this will rise to around 7% by 2005 (Chamberlain *et al.*, 1994).

Attending home births

Midwives should feel confident when attending home births. Inexperienced midwives may require support from more experienced colleagues. To help gain confidence midwives should aim to attend regular home birth workshops. Home birth study days are usually inspiring as well as offering the opportunity for knowledge sharing and experience.

All midwives, especially those who practice in the community, need to keep their skills and emergency drills up to date as well as ensuring they have practised the manoeuvres for breech birth and shoulder dystocia. Midwives must be able to cannulate, resuscitate adults and the newborn, and should know how to proceed if a postpartum haemorrhage occurs.

Personal safety checklist

- Know your destination/location and how to access the woman's house/flat.
- If you are attending another midwife's client, and particularly if the woman's home is difficult to find, ensure your colleagues have given you a map, with adequate landmarks or directions.
- Carry both an Ordnance Survey and on A–Z map of your area.
- Have a system in place for informing your colleagues as to your whereabouts both day and night.
- Inform any other relevant people, such as the labour suite co-ordinator, the supervisor of midwives (SOM), the general practitioner, should they need or wish to be involved.
- If you feel threatened going somewhere take a second midwife with you.
- Mobile telephone battery charged, torch charged, car fuelled.

Supervision issues

The purpose of supervision is to protect the public by actively promoting a safe standard of midwifery practice. Supervision should be supportive and proactive.

The supervisor of midwives (SOM) meets with midwives for an annual review and also ensures that the midwife carries out safe practice. The SOM also identifies personal and professional development needs and encourages evidence-based practice (ENB, 1997).

A SOM is not normally the midwife's manager but part of the SOM support can be attending a home birth with the midwife. As a practitioner you may need your supervisor's support so build up a good rapport with them. Keep the SOM informed of impending confinements in the area, share and discuss cases.

Midwives working outside of the NHS also need supervision and support. These midwives may be working in independent practice, as a midwife teacher or employed by general practitioners as a midwife.

Essential equipment

Essential equipment for the midwife

Always keep equipment stocked, in working order, and make sure drugs and intravenous (IV) fluids are in date. For a list of equipment see Boxes 2.1 and 2.2. The list appears endless but if the equipment is always separated into the appropriate bags and boxes then colleagues become familiar with them and in an emergency it is much easier to locate the appropriate piece of equipment.

'Equipment' and preparation for the woman

In addition to a midwife's equipment, the woman intending to have a home birth should also make some preparations beforehand.

- **Protective pack**. The woman may want to make a pack to protect her birthing space consisting of a 1 metre $\times$ $1\frac{1}{2}$ metre sheet of thick polythene, then thick layers of newspapers glued or sticky taped to the polythene, and a top layer of old clean sheeting, glued, sticky taped or sewn. This can then be laid on the floor, bed, settee or wherever the woman wishes to give birth, and can then be burnt in the garden or taken to the hospital incinerator afterwards.
- **Refreshments and home comforts**. Plenty of drinks and snacks for all present at the birth. Pillows, duvet, flannels, bowls, towels for hot and cold compresses. Transcutaneous electrical nerve stimulation (TENS) machine, music, massage oils, beanbag, birth ball and candles. Birthing pool if wanting water for labour and birth.
- **Warm birthing environment**. Room thermometer and some means of heating may be necessary in the winter, to boost the room temperature. Clothes and nappies for the baby. Hot water bottle to warm whatever the woman has chosen to wrap her baby in at birth. Baby clothes, nappies and towel. Hand basin available, towels and liquid soap for the midwife.
- **Pain reflief**. Pethidine is rarely used at a homebirth because of its poor pain-relieving qualities and unwanted side effects. If the woman wishes to have pethidine 100 mg, she should get it prescribed by her general practitioner and have this dispensed ready for her use. It is the woman's property and the midwife cannot remove it from the house/flat afterwards but it is advisable to suggest that it is destroyed prior to the midwife's departure.

Box 2.1   Midwifery equipment.

Labour and birth bag	Antenatal/postnatal bag	Emergency bag
Delivery pack (small community pack) – some units combine delivery/suture packs	Thermometer	Intravenous (IV) giving set × 2 (clear fluids and blood)
Suture pack (small suture pack) and suture material	Sphygmomanometer	Grey/large bore cannula × 3
	Pinards	
	Doppler	Three-way tap
Tampon	Urine testing strips	Plaster and IV sterile fixing dressing
Urethral catheter	Tape measure	
Amnihook	Baby scales	Sterile gloves
Sterile gloves	Cord clamp remover	Unsterile gloves
Unsterile gloves	Stitch cutters	Label for drug additives
Inco pads/sanitary towels	Scissors	Razor
Water-based vaginal lubricating jelly	Plastic apron	
	Sterile gloves	Pinards
	Unsterile gloves	Plastic apron
	Glycerine suppositories	Inco pads/sanitary towels
Baby labels (some parents wish to have these)	Speculum	
	Water-based vaginal lubricating jelly	Blood bottles for cross-matching and forms
Syringes and needles	Swabs for culture including Chlamydia swabs	
Blood bottles and equipment for Rhesus negative women	Torch	Drugs/IV fluids
		Syntocinon® 40 units
		Normal saline
Drugs/IV fluids	Neonatal screening test kits	Hartmann's solution
Local anaesthetic	Paperwork for pathology laboratory and notes	Intravenous fluids
Syntometrine®	Blood bottles	
Ergometrine	Sharps container	Essential resuscitation equipment – see Box 21.2 on page 284
Vitamin K		
Plastic aprons		
Rubbish bags		

Box 2.2   Drugs and gases carried by the midwife.

Drugs carried by the midwife
  Syntometrine®
  Syntocinon® 40 units
  Ergometrine
  Oxytocics (can be kept for about 1 year in high temperatures. Advisable to discard every 6
    months [Chua *et al.*, 1993]
  Lignocaine 1% 20 ml
  Neonatal intramuscular (IM) vitamin K (1 mg in 0.5 ml) or neonatal oral equivalent preparation
  Naloxone hydrochloride for the baby if using pethidine

Gases
  Entonox
  Oxygen

Care in labour

The woman and her family are the centre of the care. This care needs to be given *sensitively*. Not all women want to give birth at home and the midwife should support her in her decision and should continue to support her if she changes her mind or the need arises to be admitted to hospital. Home birth is a very fulfilling experience for not only the woman and her partner but also for the midwife, and it is an honour to be asked to attend.

Early labour

- **First call**. When the woman contacts the midwife on call to say she thinks she may be in labour, go to her. For independent midwives distance may play its part in the decision about when to attend a woman in labour, as she may not live close, and it may be more appropriate to stay once the decision is made to visit. Perform a full antenatal check including maternal temperature and pulse. Watch for a while to see how the contractions are progressing before performing a vaginal examination. Think to yourself, is a vaginal examination necessary? Discuss the woman's plans with her again now she has started labouring.
- **Advice**. Make sure the woman and her partner know to call again if she has a spontaneous rupture of membranes or, if her membranes are already ruptured and the colour changes, has some heavy bleeding, the contractions become stronger or they are worried. Remember to document everything you have performed and your findings. Arrange a time to go back and review the situation unless she calls you back in the meantime.
- **Return at the time you arranged**. If you are going to be late make sure you tele-phone the woman to let her know. You may need to go back two or three times before she needs you to stay. Staying when you are not required does not help a labouring woman and her family.

Labour

- **Staying**. When the time comes for the midwife to stay, make sure you do not dominate the situation. It is the woman's day and *she* is going to birth *her* baby, not the midwife!
- **Equipment**. Try not to have all the equipment in the birthing space but have it handy outside the room ready if you need it. It may be threatening to the woman to see all the 'emergency' equipment at the ready as if problems are expected. If there is evidence of fetal compromise some midwives do make a discreet, newborn-resuscitation area in the corner of the room. The mother may then be asked to move towards such an area so that the baby can remain attached to its umbilical cord even if it requires resuscitation.
- **Monitoring the well-being of the woman and baby**. Observations should be performed as indicated and documented in the notes. Any deviation from the normal should be discussed at the time with the woman and her partner, and recorded in the notes. Maternal blood pressure (BP), pulse, temperature, urine output and fluid intake should be observed as well as frequent auscultation of the

baby's heart beat. The regularity, strength and length of the contractions and the dilatation of the cervix should be noted. Artificial rupture of the membranes (ARM) should be avoided at home due to the potential complications that are associated with this intervention (see also Chapter 16).

- **Blend into the background**. Most women will labour well when they have not had to move elsewhere and they remain in their own environment, in a position they wish to be in with their family and friends. Make sure you blend in with the background and enable the woman to labour, this is also recommended by the *National Birthday Trust Report* (Chamberlain *et al.*, 1994).

The birth

- **Second midwife**. Remember to call the back-up midwife before she is needed urgently. Independent midwives have challenged the routine of a having a second midwife at all home births and only call for back-up if they have a specific concern. Some independent midwives suggest that a second midwife can affect the dynamics of the relationship with the woman. If a second midwife attends, leaving the door on the latch is sensible so that the woman is not disturbed. The second midwife does not have to be present in the room, only somewhere else in the house so as not to intrude.
- **The birth**. Providing the woman feels in control and well supported, a home birth can be a deeply personal and fulfilling experience for both the woman and her partner. Do not forget hands off, enabling the woman to birth her own baby, to make as much noise as she wishes and to lift up her baby to her breast and to discover the sex. Give her time to do this, do not overcrowd her but just quietly observe until she is ready to speak.
- **The third stage**. Most babies will naturally search at the breast which encourages the natural release of oxytocin. Allow the woman to expel her placenta when she wishes. If the woman chooses to have a managed third stage of labour then an oxytocic drug should be given intramuscularly and the placenta and membranes delivered by controlled cord traction within a few minutes. The placenta is the woman's property and she may want to keep it. If the placenta is to be disposed of by the midwife a placentabin will be required for transporting it to the hospital incinerator.
- **After the third stage**. The woman may want to celebrate in a variety of ways, she may want to remain very quiet and together with her partner or she may want to enjoy champagne with her family and friends or share the moment with her other children. She may also be very hungry and want lots of fresh toast and tea. Whatever she chooses, respect her wishes.
- **Prior to leaving the house**. Midwives normally remain in the house after the third stage until the woman and the midwife feel happy that the time has come for the midwife to leave. During this time weighing, measuring and examining the baby can be performed, offering the vitamin K, completing the notes and having a cup of tea.
- **On leaving**. Make sure that the woman's uterus is well contracted, her lochia is not excessive and that she has passed urine. The woman and her family need to be given the contact numbers to call a midwife should any problems occur and a time

given for the return visit by the midwife. NHS midwives will need to complete hospital paperwork/computer details and all midwives should replenish their equipment. Any collegues who were informed of the home birth should be informed that the woman and her baby are safely delivered.

Possible transfer to hospital

When things do not go according to plan during labour or after the birth, transfer may be indicated, see Box 2.3 for a list of possible problems.

Box 2.3   Possible problems requiring transfer to hospital.

Prelabour rupture of the membranes – with no labour
  Up to a maximum 96 hours (NICE, 2001).

Liquor
  • Offensive smell.
  • Old meconium with other associated problems.
  • Obvious fresh meconium.
  • Heavily bloodstained.

Bleeding
  Bleeding causing concern.

Fetal heart rate
  • Persistent decelerations with contractions.
  • Decelerations following contractions.
  • Persistent bradycardia/persistent tachycardia.

Position of baby
  • Posterior position with no progress.
  • Breech position.
  • Complicated presentation.

Maternal observations
  • Pyrexia.
  • Raised blood pressure.

Pain
  • Woman waiting further pain control.
  • Unusual pain in labour.

Choice
  Woman changed her mind.

Dilatation
  • No progress for a length of time.
  • Swollen anterior lip of cervix for a long time.

Postpartum
  • Retained placenta.
  • Postpartum haemorrhage.
  • Third-degree tear.

Baby
  Any condition causing concern.

The midwife needs to use her judgement. If the woman is very near the onset of the second stage or is in the second stage of labour, especially if she is not a primigravida, it may not be possible or safe, to move to hospital before the birth of the baby. Think, is an emergency ambulance on the way? Has the hospital delivery suite co-ordinator been informed?

Emergency transfer to hospital

- **Dial 999**. In an emergency ask the partner to telephone 999 for the emergency services and to ask for a paramedic ambulance. Although the ambulance is alerted immediately and is on its way, the control operator will ask other questions.
- **Directions**. Directions given to the emergency person as to where and how to get to a house/flat can take a long time to explain, especially when it is dark and in rural areas as landmarks do not always show up. The partner can save the midwife valuable time in making this call so that the midwife is able to be with the woman.
- **Second midwife**. If a second midwife has not already been requested to attend, use a mobile telephone so that the woman is not left unattended. It may not be possible to do this yourself if you are busy siting cannulas, taking blood, controlling bleeding or resuscitating the baby. Make this the partner's next telephone call.
- **Inform co-ordinator**. The hospital delivery suite need to be informed so make sure the co-ordinator knows. The co-ordinator is in overall charge of the delivery suite and will assess the situation, get a room prepared and inform the relevant people, for example consultant obstetrician, registrar, paediatrician, pathology laboratory, theatre, special care baby unit (SCBU), and the supervisor of midwives (SOM) if necessary to give you support. Working as a team inside and outside the hospital counts. Remember to keep collegues informed, keep communicating.
- **Record keeping**. Write times down and remember to take the woman's notes to hospital. Take emergency bag, the personal bag and collect together other equipment.
- **Go in the ambulance with the woman**. Escort the woman in the ambulance, leave the car and get a lift or taxi back to the car later. The hospital will pay for the fare.

Non-emergency transfer to hospital

In a non-emergency situation transfer to hospital may be necessary. This may be due to a number of reasons. The usual reasons in a non-emergency are that the woman has changed her mind or that she wishes to have a form of pain control that is unavailable to her at home.

Other reasons for transfer are that the woman may have prelabour rupture of the membranes (PROM) and no labour or slow progress in labour (Davies *et al.*, 1996). Think, is the women able to travel by car or should she travel by ambulance? In a non-emergency situation the midwife may be able to travel by car and follow the ambulance to the hospital.

The woman and her partner may be extremely upset with the decision to transfer to hospital, even when the decision has been made entirely by themselves. Explain that neither of them have failed, the language used in midwifery about 'failure to progress', 'maternal distress' and the like do not help parents come to term with their decisions.

They will need to be debriefed very carefully afterwards, with the midwife who cared for them together with the notes.

Remember the woman and her partner do not have to transfer to hospital. If you have a good relationship with them and they know you would not be suggesting the transfer to them unless you were worried, they are unlikely to refuse. Remember to document everything.

- **Born before arrival (BBA)** in a term pregnancy, in a well woman with no complications of pregnancy, normally occurs because she has a precipitate labour and birth. This can be a shock to the woman and her partner. Thankfully this normally appears to happen at home with the condition of both the woman and the baby satisfactory. The midwife will need to use her judgement to decide whether the woman and her baby need to be admitted to hospital for observation. History of fresh meconium-stained liquor might indicate the need to be admitted. For a preterm birth before 35 weeks, the mother and baby will most likely need to be admitted to hospital. Often these babies are well at birth but need some extra care when they are a few hours old. Skin-to-skin contact is recommended to keep the baby warm and secure. This is preferable to an incubator should a transfer be indicated (Christensson *et al.*, 1998).
- **Unplanned home birth**. Unplanned home births also occur because either there is no time to transfer prior to birth or the mother has changed her mind in labour. These births are, generally, without their problems but all the relevant people need to be informed.
- **Unplanned breech**. Unplanned, undiagnosed breech birth at home can be a shock if the midwife arrives to find the breech presenting and descending (see also 'Labour and birth' in Chapter 5 and techniques for an assisted breech birth in Table 5.2). Again all the relevant people need to be informed and requested, the midwife must just get on and deliver the breech. Breech babies are more likely to be temporarily 'shocked' at birth and may need some basic resuscitation.
- Remember the same applies to all home births whether planned or unplanned, for NHS midwives – informing the hospital, and your colleagues.

Summary

- Know your destination and keep colleagues informed of your whereabouts.
- Always keep equipment stocked, in working order, and drugs and IV fluids in date.
- Care as per 'normal' labour.
- Avoid interventions with potential complications, such as ARM.
- Stand back, do not dominate the couple's space. Let the woman labour.
- Discuss and document any need to transfer to hospital fully with the parents.
- Have a second midwife present for the birth.
- In the event of an emergency call a paramedic ambulance. They can provide prompt, skilled hands for resuscitation and cannulation and can always leave if they are not required. Inform the labour ward co-ordinator if the woman is being taken into hospital.

Useful contacts

Association for Improvements in the Maternity Services (AIMS)   AIMS Helpline: 0870 765 1433. AIMS Homebirth Support Co-ordinator: 0870 765 1447. Website: www.aims.org.uk

Home birth reference websites   www.homebirth.org.uk and www.birthchoiceuk.com

Independent Midwives Association (IMA)   1 The Great Quarry, Guildford, Surrey GU1 3XN. Telephone: 01483 821104. Website: www.independentmidwives.org.uk

National Childbirth Trust (NCT)   Alexandra House, Oldham Terrace, Acton, London W3 6NH. Enquiry line: 0870 444 8707. Website: www.nct-online.org

References

Chamberlain, G., Wraight, A. & Crowley, P. (1994) *National Birthday Trust Report – Report of the Confidential Enquiry into Home Births*. Parthenon Publishing Group, London.

Christensson, K., Bhat, G.J., Amadi, B.C. *et al.* (1998) A randomised study of skin-to-skin versus incubator care for rewarming low risk hypothermic neonates. *The Lancet* **352**, 1115.

Chua, S., Arulkumaran, S., Adaikan G. *et al.* (1993) The effect of oxytocics stored at high temperatures on postpartum uterine activity. *British Journal of Obstetrics and Gynaecology* **100**, 874–5.

Davies, J., Hey, E., Reid, W. & Young, G. (1996) Prospective regional study of planned home births. *British Medical Journal* **313**, 1302–06.

DoH (1993) *Changing Childbirth. Report of the Expert Maternity Group*. Department of Health, HMSO, London.

ENB (1997) *Preparation of Supervisors of Midwives. Module 1.* English National Board for Nursing, Midwifery and Health Visiting, London.

NCT (2001) NCT Press Release – 19 June. National Childbirth Trust, London.

NICE (2001) *Clinical Guideline C – The Use of Electronic Fetal Monitoring*. National Institute for Clinical Excellence, London.

UKCC (1996) *Guidelines for Professional Practice*. United Kingdom Central Council for Nursing, Midwifery and Health Visiting, London.

3 Waterbirth

Introduction

'... the reason for the birthing pool is not to have the baby born in water but to facilitate the birth process and to reduce the need for drugs and other intervention.' (Odent, 2000)

Most maternity units have guidelines devised for the safe conduct of waterbirths both at home and in the hospital setting. These guidelines should be *flexible*, so that midwives can provide individualized care based on the evidence available in conjunction with the woman's birth wishes.

Facts

- Labouring in warm water increases the release of the woman's natural endorphins and oxytocin levels, catecholamine secretion is reduced (Odent, 1983; Ockenden, 2001a) and pain perception may be lowered (Ockenden, 2001b).
- A significant finding in many large studies found that women using a pool needed less additional analgesia compared to dry land births, suggesting that water is a safe, cost-effective analgesic (Brown, 1998; Garland & Jones, 2000; Otigbah *et al.*, 2000; Burns, 2001).
- Water offers a peaceful, secure environment, which helps the woman to relax. The woman's buoyancy in the water encourages her to find comfortable positions enabling and supporting her to move freely (Ockenden, 2001b).
- Women with backache and back problems appear to benefit greatly (Nightingale, 1996).
- Overall, women birthing in water were more likely to experience intact perineums or tears of a lesser severity (2nd and 3rd degree tears as opposed to 3rd or 4th degree) compared to similar births on dry land (Gordon, 1996; Brown, 1998; Garland & Jones, 2000; Burns, 2001).
- No difference in length of labour, Apgar score, or blood loss and no increased risk of infection found in mothers and babies who used a waterbirth tub (Gordon, 1996; Brown, 1998; Garland & Jones, 2000; Burns, 2001).
- Babies (unless severely hypoxic) do not gasp or inhale water when born into the tub which must be kept at body temperature for birth (Johnson, 1996).
- Water embolisms are hypothetical and none have been noted in any of the literature (Odent cited by Gordon, 1996).
- It has been found that women who spent over 2 hours in the tub, or who got in too early (usually before 5 cm cervix dilation), were more likely to find their labour progress adversely affected and their contractions weaked (Eriksson *et al.*, 1997). This should not preclude those individuals from getting in early if they really want to, or staying in more than 2 hours, but the midwife and the woman should be aware of the possibility of contractions decreasing.

Criteria for labouring in water

Each unit will have its own criteria for labouring in water but care should be individualized to meet women's requests. Ultimately, the woman makes the decision when she has been presented with all the information.

Criteria for the use of water include (RCM, 2000):

- Women's informed choice.
- Normal, term pregnancy from 37 weeks.
- Singleton, cephalic presentation.
- No systemic sedation.
- Spontaneous rupture of the membranes of less than 24 hours.

Preparation

Water temperature

The tub should be filled to an adequate depth to enable the woman's uterus to be amply covered. The temperature of the water should be between 35 and 37°C for the first stage and 37°C for the second stage and the birth. The surface temperature is often cooler than the deeper water so put the water thermometer deepish, or stir the water well to mix it. Hot water may need to be added every 30 minutes in order to regulate and maintain the temperature.

Cleansing

Local infection control policies should cover waterbirths (RCM, 2000). Following use, the tub should be rinsed of debris and cleaned with a chlorine-releasing agent which is effective against HIV, hepatitis B and hepatitis C (Burns & Kitzinger, 2001).

Equipment

- Thermometer, to check water temperature.
- Waterproof sonicaid for monitoring the fetal heart.
- Lift or aid to get the woman out of the tub in an emergency (hospital only).
- Gauntlet gloves for the midwife to wear.
- A small, portable mirror for visualization of progress during the second stage of labour.
- Low stool or step to help the woman in and out easily.
- Plenty of towels.
- Pure essential oils (aromatherapy) can be administered under the supervision of an aromatherepist. Burns *et al.* (1999) suggest using a teaspoon of full-fat milk as a dispersal agent, then adding to the bath to aid relaxation.
- Portable entonox or extended entonox tubing should allow the woman to use it freely in the tub.
- 'Cleaning' equipment.
- Sieve and bowl, to collect any matter such as bits of mucous, 'show' or faeces.

At home (in addition to the above)

- Pool liner.
- A bowl and pump if this is being used to empty the tub, labelled 'dirty'.
- Plastic sheeting (available from DIY shops) for the base of the pool.

Waterbirth at home

If a home waterbirth is planned, it is advisable for the mother to experiment and have a practice run of filling the tub. This ensures the woman knows there will be enough hot water and is able to estimate the filling time which can take in excess of an hour at home. The tub is emptied using a pump conforming to BS standards. The water can be emptied down the sink, as this goes directly into the foul drain (C. Charles, personal communication, 2002).

Home waterbirths may require additional items such as a disposable inner liner, a main liner, a pump and tubing to empty the pool, plastic matting to protect the floor and so on. A structural survey of the floor is rarely indicated but may be advisable, depending where the tub is to be placed. A full pool can weigh up to 850 kg so may be best placed on the ground floor. If unsure, the woman should seek advice from the organization from which she is hiring her birthing pool. Such organizations are usually very helpful and have a wealth of experience and literature about home waterbirths.

Most common reasons to leave the pool

In a large study by Burns (2001), 47% of primigravida left the pool at some point in labour, for a variety of reasons while 53% remained for the birth. Water was consistently rated positively irrespective of whether the woman stayed in the pool for birth or not.

- **Slow progress in the first stage**. Immersion in water at body temperature appears to facilitate the birth process for a limited length of time, usually not greater than 2–3 hours (Odent 2000 citing Eriksson *et al.*, 1997). If the woman has entered the pool too early, usually before 5 cm dilated, then contractions can slow down. If this happens the woman needs to leave the water, to mobilize, void her bladder, take some refreshments and allow her contractions to build up again (see also Box 4.1 in Chapter 4 which describes interventions to increase uterine contractibility).
- **Slow progress during the second stage of labour**. This may often be rectified by pushing while standing up in the tub, for a trial period, or by getting out and adopting a position most effective for that individual woman. If contractions are poor, time will be needed for the second stage.
- **Personal choice**. A small minority of women do not enjoy being in the water so do not stay. Others decide to get out just prior to giving birth.
- **Additional analgesia**. While women using the pool are less likely to need additional analgesia, (Brown, 1998; Garland & Jones, 2000; Burns, 2001) some women do request additional pain relief such as pethidine or an epidural and so need to leave the pool.
- **Change in the baby's condition**. Evidence of fetal compromise, such as the fresh passage of meconium or abnormal fetal heart changes.
- **Change in the mother's condition**. Any concern about maternal well-being, such as bleeding, pyrexia, hypertension.

Labour care

See also Chapter 1 for more information about care in labour.

First stage of labour

- Check the woman's temperature in the water hourly (D. Garland, personal communication, 2002).
- Allow the woman to drink freely, to avoid dehydration as diuresis increases as a result of being in water (Ockenden, 2001b).
- The water temperature should be measured and recorded on both the partogram and the woman's notes, half hourly, and should be between 35 and 37°C.
- Vaginal examinations are usually performed with relative ease in the tub.

Second stage of labour

- Monitor maternal and fetal well-being as per normal labour.
- Adjust water temperature to 37°C.
- You can submerge a small, portable mirror to visualize progress during the second stage of labour.
- Have a 'hands off' approach to delivery, it is thought that touching the fetal head underwater may stimulate the baby to try to breathe.
- Let the head deliver. The woman will usually tell you, she may instinctively put her hands down to touch. You may be able to see the dark head underwater, if you are really unsure a brief touch will confirm.
- Do not check for the cord.
- Await the next contraction. Then the woman will usually deliver the baby herself. If this does not seem to be happening, try releasing a shoulder, as you would on 'dry land'. If appropriate encourage the woman to bring her baby to the surface herself.
- If the woman is on all fours the second midwife may help pass the baby through (not around) the woman's legs, underwater, and bring it gently up to the surface in front of the woman, to avoid the cord becoming caught up (Fig. 3.1).
- Water babies do not always cry and do not always appear to breathe instantly. Check the baby's colour, be calm and if unsure check the heart rate by placing your fingers on its chest. If you are concerned, rub the baby with a towel, or lift the baby briefly into the cool air and this will usually stimulate them to cry.
- Ensure the cord is left attached and pulsating. This can continue for some time. Although not standard practice, it is advisable to routinely subtly inspect the cord at birth, to ensure it is intact, as a snapped cord could become a life-threatening emergency for the baby if unnoticed (Cro & Preston, 2002). See also 'Cord problems' below under the heading 'Emergencies'.

Third stage of labour

It is not usually necessary to ask the woman to get out of the tub for delivery of the placenta unless she so wishes or active management of the third stage is initiated.

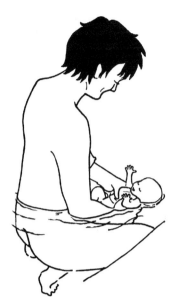

Fig. 3.1   For women who give birth in the all-fours position, the baby should be passed through the woman's legs so that the woman can receive her baby without the cord becoming caught up or restricted.

Many women find after the initial 5 minutes or so of getting to know their baby, they are ready to climb out of the water, which can be, by this point, a little murky and uninviting!

Women who chose to stay in the pool

If the woman chooses to remain in the water, keep the water warm and the baby warm by submerging the baby's body in the water and draping a towel over the woman's shoulders. Water embolisms are hypothetical and none have ever been noted in any of the literature (Odent cited by Gordon, 1996).

Odent (1998) cites one isolated case where a baby born in water received a large placental transfusion and developed polycythaemia (Austin *et al.*, 1997). Odent suggests that the cold air would stop the umbilical cord pulsating sooner on dry land (vasoconstriction being caused by exposure to the cold air) but that warm water may delay this from happening. This is a sensible point but since the problem appears to have been an isolated case midwives should be guided by the woman's preferences at the time.

It is not always easy to observe blood loss in the water; there is usually a moderate visible bleeding as the placenta separates, which tends to sink to the bottom of the tub around where the woman is sitting. If, however, the bleeding appears excessive, spreading quickly through the water, it *may* be a postpartum haemorrhage. If in doubt it is advisable to ask the woman to get out of the tub so you can better observe any blood loss.

Emergencies

- Most midwives devising guidelines for the safe conduct of waterbirths recommend that a second midwife is present for the birth.
- Midwives are likely to feel more confident if they have practised delivering babies in hypothetical emergency situations.
- In any emergency, home or hospital, call for assistance immediately.

Cord problems

Cord entanglement

The midwife does not know if the cord is holding the baby back until the baby fails to deliver, then the midwife needs to check to confirm the presence of a cord. Most babies with cord entanglement will easily deliver with the cord around the neck or body without the need for any intervention (ARM, 2000). In the rare eventuality that the cord will not give and allow the baby to deliver, do not clamp and cut it underwater but proceed as follows:

- Get the woman out the tub quickly.
- Apply two clamps to the cord and cut between them; this can be very awkward as the cord is usually very tight.
- Deliver the baby.
- Never submerge a baby if it is born out of the water.

Snapped cord

This rare event is not an emergency if it is recognized quickly. However, it is sometimes difficult to visualize a snapped cord due to murky water or the position of the mother and baby. There are several documented cases where this problem has gone unnoticed at waterbirths with serious consequences for the babies involved (Cro & Preston, 2002).

- Always lift the baby carefully into the mother's arms, being aware not to pull on a short cord (Garland, 2002).
- If the cord snaps, grasp the baby's end of the cord quickly to prevent blood leakage.
- Apply a clamp securely.
- Assess the baby and, if required, inform the paediatrician. Post-birth haemoglobin may be advised.

Shoulder dystocia

In cases of shoulder dystocia the woman should be asked to stand up to deliver. If this does not help then the woman must get out of the tub immediately. This in itself often rotates the baby in the pelvis and spontaneous delivery then occurs. Further details of dealing with shoulder dystocia are covered in Chapter 12.

Postpartum haemorrhage

It is difficult to assess blood loss in the tub. A postpartum haemorrhage is usually visible as a bright, fresh red loss spreading quickly through the water. The woman may go very quiet or complain of stomach cramps and look pale. Some loss occurs naturally as the placenta separates. If you are concerned, ask the woman to get out the tub, clamp and cut the cord promptly and pass the baby to her partner to enable this to happen more easily. The midwife should manage the third stage actively if the woman is haemorrhaging. Further details of dealing with postpartum haemorrhage are covered in Chapter 11.

The unresponsive baby

The procedure to follow for an unresponsive baby is to:

- Clamp and cut the cord.
- Transfer the baby in a warm towel to the resuscitaire, or prepared resuscitation area if at a home birth.
- Dry the baby vigorously.
- Follow the care for neonatal resuscitation given in Chapter 21 together with Fig. 21.1.

Fainting

A woman may feel faint, or actually faint. It is surprisingly easy to hold a woman who has fainted in the tub, as the water supports her weight and you can hold her head and shoulders comfortably above water. Women who faint at birth are unusual and they tend to recover without any untoward effects. However, you will require many hands to lift her out. Use the appropriate lifting aid or hoist, providing you have time. At a home birth, enlist the birth partner to help in lifting the woman out of the tub.

Midwifery issues

> 'The assistance of women to labour and deliver in water should be considered a core midwifery competence. Continuing professional development in this area should be seen as a service requirement.' (RCM, 2000)

There are various consumer reports that some managers and midwives can be obstructive towards women's requests for waterbirths, inventing excuses to deny women their wishes (Robinson, 2001). Only midwives who are supportive of waterbirth should be involved in caring for such women because they are less likely to be obstructive and are more able to meet the woman's requirements for providing care in labour. All midwives should read, observe and keep up to date on waterbirths (RCM, 2000). Otherwise, they put themselves in a dangerous professional position, should they be called upon to assist at a pool birth in the community, birthing centre or hospital. This is especially true if called upon in an emergency to help (Chapman, 1994).

Issues to consider include:

- Keep lights as low as appropriate and voices quiet.
- Mind your back. Bend from the hips if you are leaning into the tub to deliver the baby or perform a vaginal examination.
- Write your notes in black, waterproof ink.
- Do not stand constantly and peer in at the woman in the tub. Sit away from the tub, so as not to overcrowd the woman.
- Beware of the danger of water and electricity, especially at home. Trailing leads and lamps are dangerous; always have a charged torch to hand.
- Practise delivering in hypothetical emergency situations with colleagues. Do you know how to use the hoist? How would you deliver a woman who is standing up in the tub to give birth?

Summary

- Treat as normal labour.
- Allow the woman to drink freely.
- Monitor the mother's temperature hourly.
- Check and record water temperature half hourly.
  - ○ maintain it between 35 and 37°C for the first stage
  - ○ maintain it at 37°C for the second stage.
- Have a hands off birth! Only assist if necessary.
- Maintain a quiet, relaxed atmosphere.

Useful contacts

Active Birth Centre 25 Bickerton Road, London N19 5JT. Telephone: 020 7281 6760. Website: www.activebirthcentre.com

Association for Improvements in the Maternity Services (AIMS) AIMS Helpline: 0870 765 1433. Website: www.aims.org.uk

Splashdown Water Birth Services Ltd 17 Wellington Terrace, Harrow on the Hill, Middlesex, HA1 3EP. Telephone: 0870 444 4403. Website: www.splashdown.org.uk

Recommended reading

Garland, D. (2002) *Waterbirth: An Attitude to Care*, 2nd edn. Books for Midwives Press, Cheshire.

References

ARM (2000) Association of Radical Midwives Netalk: Checking for cord. *Midwifery Matters* Issue 87, 28–30.

Austin, T., Bridges, N., Markiewicz, M., *et al.* (1997) Severe polycythaemia after third stage of labour underwater. *The Lancet* **350**, 1445–7.

Brown, L. (1998) The tide has turned: audit of waterbirth. *British Journal of Midwifery* **6** (4), 236–43.

Burns, E. (2001) Waterbirth. *MIDIRS Midwifery Digest* **11** (3, Suppl. 2), 10–13.

Burns, E., Blamey, C., Ersser, S.J. *et al.* (1999) *The Use of Aromatherapy in Intrapartum Midwifery Practice. An Evaluative Study.* Oxford Centre for Healthcare Research and Development, Report No.7. Oxford Brookes University, Oxford.

Burns, E. & Kitzinger, S. (2001) *Midwifery Guidelines for Use of Water in Labour.* Oxford Centre for Health Care Research and Development, Oxford Brookes University, Oxford.

Chapman, V. (1994) Waterbirths: breakthrough or burden? *British Journal of Midwifery* **2** (1), 17–19.

Cro, S. & Preston, J. (2002) Cord snapping at a waterbirth delivery. *British Journal of Midwifery* **10** (8), 494–7.

Eriksson, M., Mattsson, L.A. & Ladfors, L. (1997) Early or late bath during the first stage of labour: a randomized study of 200 women. *Midwifery* **13**, 146–8.

Garland, D. (2002) *Waterbirth: An Attitude to Care*, 2nd edn. Books for Midwives Press, Cheshire.

Garland, D. & Jones, K. (2000) Waterbirth supporting practice through clinical audit. *MIDIRS Midwifery Digest* **10** (3), 333–6.

Gordon, Y. (1996) Waterbirth the safety issues. In *Waterbirth Unplugged. Proceedings of the First International Water Birth Conference*, (Lawrence Beech, B., ed.), pp. 135–42. Books for Midwives Press, London.

Johnson, P. (1996) Birth under water – to breathe or not to breathe. In *Waterbirth Unplugged. Proceedings of the First International Water Brith Conference* (Lawrence Beech, B., ed.), pp. 31–33. Books for Midwives Press, London.

Nightingale, C. (1996) Water and pain relief – observations of over 570 waterbirths at Hillingdon. In *Waterbirth Unplugged. Proceedings of the First International Water Birth Conference* (Lawrence Beech, B., ed.), pp. 63–9. Books for Midwives Press, London.

Ockenden, J. (2001a) The hormonal dance of labour. *The Practising Midwife* **4** (6), 16–17.

Ockenden, J. (2001b) Waterbirth. *The Practising Midwife* **4** (9), 30–32.

Odent, M. (1983) Birth under water. *The Lancet* **2**, 1476–7.

Odent, M. (1998) Use of water during labour – updated recommendations. *MIDIRS Midwifery Digest* **8** (1), 68–9.

Odent, M. (2000) Abstract, comments and updated recommendations. *MIDIRS Midwifery Digest* **10** (1), 63–4.

Otigbach, C.M., Dhanjal, M.K., Harmsworth, G. *et al.* (2000) A retrospective comparison of waterbirths and conventional vaginal deliveries. *European Journal of Obstetrics and Gynaecology and Reproductive Biology* **91**, 15–20.

RCM (2000) The use of water in labour and birth. *RCM Midwives Journal* **3** (12), 374–5.

Robinson, J. (2001) Demand and supply in maternity care. *British Journal of Midwifery* **9** (8), 510.

4 Slow progress in labour and malpresentations/malpositions in labour

Introduction

> 'The monitoring of progress in labour is still driven by a preoccupation with time
> and definitions that pathologise labour if it deviates from strict time parameters.
> This may have a place where obstetric services are vast distances from primary care
> settings and where women's health is severely compromised prior to labour.
> However, for the vast majority of women in the UK, time limits on the first stage of
> labour reflect practitioners' predisposition to distrust normal labour physiology.'
> (Walsh, 2000a)

Labour is a complex, multifaceted process where psychological and physiological
events are intertwined and inseparable. Women who are categorized as having a slow
labour should not necessarily require medical intervention. All of these factors for each
individual woman, together with her wishes, should be taken into account.

In the quest for preventing long labours, some of the direct effects of the medical
model of care – restricted mobility, enforced fasting, lack of continuity of carer or
support in labour – have surprisingly been overlooked as direct causes of labour
dystocia. While ignoring simple, preventative measures, many clinicians have adopted routine vaginal examinations, artificial rupture of the membranes (ARM) and
oxytocics to 'monitor' and 'manage' this fairly common problem. Midwives should
dedicate time and effort to the *prevention* of labour dystocia. Such care should aim to
prevent dystocia by offering continuous, caring support of the woman in labour,
encouraging women to mobilize freely and to eat and drink as desired (Keirse *et al.*,
2000).

Incidence

- The diagnosis of dystocia is open to interpretation and statistics vary between
  practitioners and units, depending upon the parameters that are used for the
  assessment of labour progress (Crowther *et al.*, 2000).
- Approximately half of women judged to have a 'slow' labour, or poor progress in
  cervical dilatation will progress equally well whether or not oxytocic drugs are
  used (Keirse *et al.*, 2000).
- Keirse *et al.* (2000) suggest that most slow labours tend to conclude favourably with
  the simple interventions of kind words, good support and encouragement to
  mobilize.

Facts

- Assessment by community midwives of women in early labour has been found to
  reduce the time spent on the labour ward. This reduces subsequent interventions,
  including reduced augmentation, analgesia and epidurals, and women are more
  likely to report an improved birth experience (Walsh, 2000a; Lauzon, 2002).
- Psychological stresses have a very physical effect on labour (see 'Stress response'
  under 'Causes of a prolonged labour' below).
- Support in labour acts as a buffer to stress in labour. This labour intervention
  consistently elicits beneficial outcomes for mother and baby (Hodnett, 2002).

- Actively promoting and encouraging women to mobilize during childbirth is a fundamental component of good midwifery practice and is a safe, effective way of providing optimum care to healthy women. It is a simple, cost-effective way of reducing labour dystocia as well as enriching the woman's personal birth experience.
- Keirse *et al.* (2000) suggest that the evidence of the effect of oxytocin stimulation on the length of labour is not clear. Even more surprisingly, trials assessing the effect of ARM on the length of labour have never been studied with women experiencing slow progress, only with women having a normally progressing labour.
- Midwives should avoid terms using negative terminology as this affects the woman's perception of herself. The language of labour dystocia is paternalistic and victim blaming (Walsh, 2000a). Avoid terms such as 'failure to progress'.

Prolonged labour

How slow is too slow?

Much has been written, predominantly by obstetricians, based on identifying the onset of labour and how to measure its progress (Walsh, 2000a). Traditionally, it was thought that a prolonged labour increased fetal morbidity. However, this view has been challenged in 'normal' labour and is not borne out by recent evidence (Walsh, 2000a). Interventions to hasten labour all carry risks and increased morbidity for mother and baby alike. However, this should not preclude midwives from being vigilant in identifying the minority of women who are not progressing and who do need help (Cluett, 2000).

Women are individuals and what is slow for one woman may be acceptable for another. The assessments and definitions of progress, and when to intervene, vary greatly (Crowther *et al.*, 2000). Crowther *et al.* (2000) suggest that a cervical dilatation rate of 0.5 cm per hour may be more appropriate (than the commonly used 1 cm per hour) as a lower limit for determining progress. Crowther *et al.* (2000) also suggest that, used within the context of maternal well-being, assessing cervical dilatation at the more moderate 0.5 cm per hour may lead to fewer unnecessary labour interventions.

It should be standard practice to share the decision-making process with the woman in labour. While some women may feel exhausted and demoralized, and will welcome assistance, others will feel they are coping well and do not want any interventions at the present time.

The evidence on assessing progress in labour

In the 1950s, an obstetrician called Friedman categorized the phases of labour as latent and active, and plotted the rate of cervical dilatation against a mean time limit (Walsh, 2000a). The use of the partogram (with alert and action lines) for assessing progress has evolved from Friedman's work. However, the decision to commence a partogram is somewhat subjective and once commenced it has the potential for routine intervention for any woman crossing the action line. Midwives should be aware that the latent and active phases of labour are artificial constructs defined purely for clinical management purposes (Cluett, 2000). Assessing the onset of labour and defining a woman's progress in labour remain inexact and vary between individual practioners, birthing units, local policies, hospitals, regions and countries.

Most of the methods used for assessing labour progress are to some degree invasive for the woman. All the methods remain unevaluated and of unproven benefit, including the almost universal practice of repeated vaginal examinations (Crowther *et al.*, 2000).

Various methods for assessing labour progress include:

- Abdominal palpation every 2–3 hours to assess descent of the presenting part and thus monitor progress (Stuart, 2000).
- The woman's response to the contractions correlated to cervical dilatation (Stuart, 2000).
- Sallam *et al.* (1999) described the direct link between the frequency and strength of contractions and cervical dilatation in labour.
- Hobbs (1998) has described the visualization of the 'purple line' from the woman's anal margin, which gradually extends to the nape of the buttocks relative to the dilatation of the cervix.
- Vaginal examinations monitor the cervical dilatation and are the most common method for assessing labour progress. See also Chapter 16 for more on vaginal examinations.
- The various methods of assessing if labour is progressing are described in more detail under 'Assessing progress in labour' in Chapter 1 on pages 22–5.

Causes of a prolonged labour

Within the context of maternal and fetal well-being, slow progress can occur for a variety of reasons and may well be 'normal' for that individual. Many preventable causes, including psychological stresses and physical problems, can result in non-progressing, inadequate contractions. Some causes are:

- Stress response.
- Fetal presentation/position.
- Cephalopelvic disproportion (CPD).
- Restricted mobility and the semi-recumbent posture.
- Enforced fasting.
- Analgesia.
- Less common physical causes.

Stress response

Psychological stresses have a very physical effect on labour. Stress hormones, such as adrenaline, interact with the beta-receptors in the uterine muscles and inhibit contractions, slowing labour down (Cluett, 2000). This is an involuntary response when a woman feels threatened or insecure, her labour 'pauses' in order for her to reach a place of perceived 'safety'.

A stress response can be triggered by external factors such as negative environmental stimuli (entering the labour ward, bright lights, unfamiliar noises, lack of privacy) or a lack of support from caregivers (midwife busy with other clients, shift changes, exposure to unfamiliar or unpleasant people). Additionally, and sometimes harder to remedy during labour, are internal factors such as deep-rooted anxieties (fear of pain, childbirth, interventions), a history of a previous traumatic delivery or previous childhood sexual abuse (see also pages 233–5).

Fetal presentation/position

Malpresentation can occur when the baby presents as breech, brow, face, or transverse lie. A *malposition* is usually associated with the baby in an awkward vertex position (deflexed or tilted head). Both can be associated with longer labours, irregular contractions and often back pain, with the presenting part usually high at the onset of labour. Malpresentations and malpositions are rarely preventable and are associated with increased interventions and maternal and neonatal morbidity (Coates, 2002) (for more information see 'Malpresentations and malpositions in labour' later in this chapter).

Cephalopelvic disproportion

Cephalopelvic disproportion (CPD) can be difficult to diagnose; pelvimetry is not a reliable indicator of pelvic adequacy (Hofmeyr, 2000). Previous uncomplicated delivery of a baby of similar or greater weight is the most reliable predictor of pelvic adequacy, and labour is the best test of pelvic adequacy in cephalic presentations (Hofmeyr, 2000). Diagnosis can sometimes only be made with the passing of time and an obvious lack of descent of the presenting part (Crowther *et al.*, 2000). Upright positions, while important for any labour, are essential for women with slow progress or borderline CPD. Some predisposing risk factors include a small woman with a suspected large baby, maternal diabetes, or a macrosomic baby. Physical manifestations are similar to those described under 'Malpresentations and malpositions in labour' on page 68 and may include irregular contractions, slow progress, back pain and again a high presenting part.

Restricted mobility and the semi-recumbent posture

In the UK, three quarters of women spend their labours lying on their backs propped up by pillows or wedges (MIDIRS, 1999). A Cochrane Review (Gupta & Nikoden, 2002) of approved trials found that immobility/the supine position has a variety of side effects including:

- Reduced natural circulating oxytocin levels.
- Adversely affecting contractions and, therefore, labour progress resulting in, on average, longer labours.
- An increased use of oxytocics for augmentation.
- Supine positions can result in a longer second stage of labour.
- Women found contractions more painful in the second stage if they were in a supine position.

Enforced fasting

Some clinicians recommend fasting in labour because of their concern over the dangers of gastric aspiration. Gastric aspiration is a problem associated with *poor anaesthetic technique* when administering a general anaesthetic and not with having food in the stomach (Johnson *et al.*, 2000). In the Confidential Enquiries into Maternal Deaths (DoH, 2001) there were no deaths attributable to gastric aspiration during caesarean section.

Enforced fasting in labour can lead to poor progress, the diagnosis of dystocia and a cascade of interventions culminating in a caesarean birth (Johnson *et al.*, 2000).

Chapter 1 also covers the question of fasting in labour under the heading 'Promoting normality – the basics of midwifery care' and in Box 1.3.

Analgesia

Epidural analgesia decreases natural oxytocin levels and relaxes the normally firm, pelvic-floor muscles. This form of pain relief is associated with a reduction in contractions and an increase in the use of intravenous (IV) oxytocin (Dickersin, 2000). Epidural increases the incidence of malrotation, delay in labour and related interventions (Dickersin, 2000). This is more marked in women who have an epidural *early* in labour.

Immersion in water in a waterbirth tub or deep bath, at body temperature, appears to facilitate the birth process for a limited length of time (Odent, 1998). If the woman has entered the pool too early, usually before 5 cm dilated, contractions can decrease. Women spending long periods in the tub, usually exceeding 2–3 hours, are more likely to find that their labour progress is adversely affected and contractions may weaken (Eriksson *et al.*, 1997).

Less common physical causes

Less common physical causes of prolonged labour include anomalies of the pelvis and cervical problems.

Anomalies of the pelvis occur in women who have suffered a fractured pelvis or have significant weight-bearing problems, such as from lower limb amputation, spina bifida, spinal injury, etc. Usually the woman would have a history taken antenatally where any of the conditions or associated problems would have been identified and discussed prior to labour.

Cervical problems may arise following cervical surgery, including a previous cone biopsy. The internal os can feel 'rough' to the touch and the cervix can feel tight and unyielding for a prolonged period (commonly during the latent phase). Simpkin & Ancheta (2000) suggest that contractions of great intensity may be required to overcome the initial resistance, following which dilatation usually occurs.

Prolonged latent phase

'Some women, having no idea what to expect from early labour, 'over-react', that is they are preoccupied with every contraction and they may rush to use learned coping techniques that are more appropriate for active labour. They often expect to be 5 or 6 cm dilated when they are first checked and are crushed when they are examined and found to be only 1 to 2 cm ... The caregiver must help to acknowledge the woman's disappointment, giving her some suggestions to reduce the intensity of the contractions and proceed to calm and relax her. She will need help to get her head back to where her cervix is.' (Simpkin & Ancheta, 2000: 33).

The latent phase of labour varies enormously from woman to woman and sometimes last for several days (Burvill, 2002). The latent phase does not respond well to medical interventions such as ARM or oxytocics (Simpkin & Ancheta, 2000). In the absence of problems, this stage requires no medical intervention other than effective explanations, reassurance and support. Good support from the midwife and a 'wait and see' course of action will do much to help a woman through a long latent phase.

Midwifery care

A prolonged latent phase can leave the woman feeling exhausted and demoralized as well as doubting her body's ability to continue to labour without problems. Offer explanations and genuine reassurance that a prolonged latent stage is not uncommon and does not mean there will be problems with her labour as it establishes (Simpkin & Ancheta, 2000).

Women may well benefit from their midwife sitting with them through several contractions, chatting, offering acknowledgement of the woman's pain, giving reassurances and suggestions for coping with contractions. Discuss practical ideas for coping with contractions such as a bath, use of transcutaneous electrical nerve stimulation (TENS), massage, or distractions such as going for a walk, cooking, watching TV and so on.

Before leaving the woman to labour, or discharging her home if in hospital, ensure she knows how to get in contact with you if she needs to. If it is night time, or the woman feels exhausted, she should aim to rest and relax for periods, even if she cannot sleep. Side lying, supported by cushions or a duvet, is preferable to lying flat on her back.

For some women prolonged, persistent pain is hard to bear and a minority request some form of pharmological analgesia or epidural. Although this has the potential to open the floodgates to medical intervention, it may be the appropriate choice for that woman in her situation. Pethidine may cause contractions to slow down, offering some respite as well as the potential for the woman to doze and relax.

For more information on the latent phase of labour, see Chapter 1 under the heading 'First stage of labour'.

Prolonged active phase

The active phase should see contractions increasing in frequency, strength and pain. For more information on the active phase of labour see Chapter 1, under the heading 'First stage of labour'. It can be useful to ask 'do the woman's contractions seem the same or more frequent, and more painful, than an hour ago?'.

Midwifery care

For women who are not progressing, refer to the checklist below. It may also be appropriate to try the interventions given in Box 4.1 to increase uterine contractibility. If there is no identifiable or physical cause for slow progress, directly ask the woman if anything is worrying her. Sharing information, explanations and offering possible solutions for specific anxieties will help. Avoid offering 'empty' reassurances ('don't worry about that, you'll be fine'), as this will do little to address her anxieties and even unintentionally suggest that the matter has been discussed and is somehow resolved!

Checklist for slow progress

- Is the woman in established labour (cervix >3–4 cm dilated) – very basic but very important!
- Address physical causes
  - bladder empty
  - hunger or thirst
  - mobilizing/upright postures.
- See also Box 4.1.
- Consider psychological needs
  - listen to the woman; ask her about her worries and fears
  - explanations, reassurances and information sharing.
- Reduce environmental stressors
  - use dim lights, music
  - maintain privacy
  - keep interruptions/shift changes to a minimum.
- Offer support by ensuring the continuous presence of the midwife (when wished by the mother) and, as appropriate:
  - verbal encouragement, praise, maintenance of eye contact
  - hands on comfort – touch, massage
  - partner support facilitated/encouraged.

Prolonged second stage

Time limits placed on the duration of the second stage vary. They are usually dictated to by the local labour ward protocols rather than the available evidence or the woman's choice. Women rarely chose an instrumental delivery.

It would appear that maternal position, non-active pushing, and avoiding arbitrary time limits in the second stage, are beneficial to improving the spontaneous vaginal birth rate, without causing harm to mother or baby. Terminating a straightforward but slow second stage with an instrumental delivery increases maternal trauma, can cause fetal trauma and has no benefit on infant outcomes (Sleep *et al.*, 2000).

Box 4.1 Interventions to increase uterine contractibility.

Support
The continuous presence and verbal support from the midwife is an invisible buffer to stress. It can help the woman to cope with labour and has been found to reduce the length of labour (Hodnett, 2002).

See also 'Support and comfort in labour' under the heading 'Promoting normality – the basics of midwifery care' in Chapter 1, Boxes 1.4 and 1.8, and Chapter 15.

Mobilization and position changes
- Mobilization increases uterine contractibility, as well as shortening the length of labour.
- Upright postures may lead to an improvement in the alignment of pelvic bones, thereby optimizing the chances of a 'good fit' between baby and pelvis (Sutton, 2000; Gupta & Nikodem, 2002).

See also Chapter 1, 'Mobility and positions for labour and giving birth' under the heading 'Promoting normality – the basics of midwifery care'.

Comforting touch
- Simpkin & Ancheta (2000) suggest that massage, stroking, handholding, etc., all increase endogenous oxytocin production, thereby stimulating uterine contractions.
- The midwife can explain the importance of physical support for the woman with her birth partner by offering practical suggestions such as massaging the woman's neck and shoulders, feet or back, or suggesting that the couple get in close together and hold each other if appropriate.
- Touch is very personal and some women do not like to be touched. This simple intervention should be used with care as it is not appropriate for everyone.

Acupressure
This is described in detail by Simpkin & Ancheta (2000).

Nipple stimulation
- The woman or her partner can lightly stroke one or both nipples, which increases uterine contractions by stimulating natural oxytocin (Simpkin & Ancheta, 2000). Most women would naturally require privacy for trying this.
- Some women may not wish to try this intervention which may be embarrassing or, after some time, uncomfortable or irritating.

Hydrotherapy/warm bath/water tub
- Water can have a dramatic effect on labour, sometimes enhancing contractions (usually in the active phase) and sometimes causing contractions to subside (occasionally if used during the latent phase) (Odent, 1998).
- Water is easy to stop using if it appears ineffectual.
- A woman who appears tense or anxious may benefit from retreating to the privacy of a warm, relaxing bath. Women who may feel self-conscious may wish to keep a T-shirt on in the water tub.

Heat applied to the fundus
Simpkin & Ancheta (2000) report that one study found that locally applied heat in the form of a hot water bottle applied to the fundus was found to increase uterine activity. A warm compress or microwave heat pack could also be used.

Contd.

Box 4.1 Contd.

Artificial rupture of membranes (ARM)

The data on the use of ARM relates solely to women in spontaneous labour (as opposed to women experiencing a slow labour). Fraser *et al.* (2002) suggest that given the evidence from these trials it is highly likely that amniotomy would also enhance progress in a prolonged labour.

- ARM results in a shorter labour, particularly in nulliparous women, by a dramatic 60–120 minutes (Rosser & Anderson, 1998).
- The available data suggests that ARM appears to forestall the need for oxytocic infusion in some women (Fraser *et al.*, 2002).
- ARM is not without contraindications, complications and acute risks, for more information see Chapter 16.

Oxytocin

Despite being widely used for slow labour, the evidence of the effect of oxytocin stimulation on the length of labour is not clear (Keirse *et al.*, 2000). Some trials suggest it has little effect on the labour length compared to the controls. In one trial, in which the controls were encouraged to get up and to move around, stand or sit as they wished, the mean duration of labour was slightly shorter in the control group than in the augmented group (Keirse *et al.*, 2000).

Comments on the use of intravenous oxytocics use include:

- In one study women described the experience as 'unpleasant' and specified that they would prefer to try without the drug when next giving birth (Keirse *et al.*, 2000).
- Over 80% of the women felt that the drug had increased the amount of pain they felt, whereas only 20% of women in the ambulant group felt that ambulation had increased their pain (Keirse *et al.*, 2000).
- Oxytocics may achieve cervical dilatation without improving the outcome (Gee, 2000).
- Where there is genuine dystocia, oxytocin will not help. However, Crowther *et al.* (2000) suggest using oxytocics may help avoid a false diagnosis of cephalopelvic disproportion (CPD).

Midwifery care

Checklist for slow progress

- Is the woman's bladder full?
- Is she experiencing the latent phase of the second stage of labour?
- Does she have a genuine urge to push? If not, pause and await events.
- Are contractions adequate? Contractions with a long gap between them will mean the woman's second stage will be longer and this must be taken into account if augmentation is not being used. Encourage the woman to adopt upright postures to enhance contractions.

Emotional dystocia

The imminent arrival of the baby may trigger many anxieties in the woman ranging from worries about the baby, to a fear of pain and tearing. Emotional 'dystocia', suggest Simpkin & Ancheta (2000), may manifest itself as the woman losing control, shouting, being aggressive or controlling caregiver's actions.

Strategies the midwife may adopt to help the situation include:

- **Survivors of childhood sexual abuse**. It may help to focus the women in the present, offering gentle reassurance that what they can feel is their baby soon to be born. Chapter 16 provides information on counteracting the re-enactment of childhood sexual abuse.

- **Acknowledging fears**. The midwife may not be able to alleviate the woman's fears, but she should aim to acknowledge them.
- **Support and control**. The midwife should offer plenty of praise and reassurance, particularly when the woman is pushing. If it helps the woman to feel more in control, the midwife could suggest that the woman hold or squeeze her hand.
- **Holding back**. A woman who is tense and holding back, possibly frightened or inhibited, needs privacy and a relaxed focus away from her perineum and towards her well-being. Keep the atmosphere calm, mellow and relaxed. Avoid stimulating the autonomic nervous system with unnecessary noise, lights, distractions, 'white coats' and interruptions. Refrain from shining a spot light on, or staring at, the woman's perineum with every contraction. If appropriate suggest the woman goes and sits privately on the toilet to push for a while, give her the call bell and be ready close by.

Physical causes of dystocia

For inadequate or incoordinate contractions:

- Try some of the measures described in Box 4.1 'Interventions to increase uterine contractibility'.
- **General mobilization** or upright and frequent position changes should help poor contractions. Moving around every 20 minutes or so is a simple intervention and yet can be the solution.
- **Maternal exhaustion**. A tired, demoralized woman may benefit from refreshments, cool drinks, a fresh flannel, cool facial spray, some music, a breeze via an open window and for sleepy, tired supporters to rally round, brighten up, wake up and give support!

For borderline CPD: (see also 'Causes of a prolonged labour' above and 'Malpresentations/malpositions in labour' below).

- In general, avoid semi-recumbent or lying back positions. A supported squat or asymmetrical postures can prove beneficial (see Figs 4.1, 4.2, 4.3).
- The old midwifery trick of encouraging the woman to walk up and down a flight of stairs or climbing on, over and off the bed a couple of times may cause a stuck baby to move its position and free the lumbar spine.
- Radiological evidence illustrates that the pelvis moves and widens during birth and that the outlet diameters can increase by nearly a third in the squatting or kneeling positions (Borrell & Fenstrom, 1957; Russell, 1982).
- It is not uncommon for women prepared for an instrumental delivery to spontaneously deliver when their legs are placed in the lithotomy position as per fig 4.4. However, this position has potential risks to the mother (including risk of DVT and perineal trauma) and it can be dangerous for the midwives back, if they support the woman's legs on their hips.
- Malpresentations are covered in more detail under the heading 'Malpresentations and malpositions in labour' on page 68.

Figs 4.1–4.4 show beneficial positions for the second stage of labour.

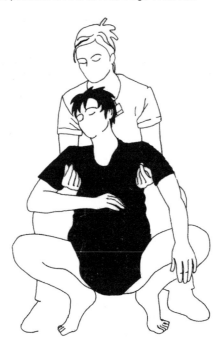

Fig. 4.1 Supported squat. Upright and frequent position changes can open up the pelvis to its maximum. Assist the woman in a supported squat or to try standing up to push.

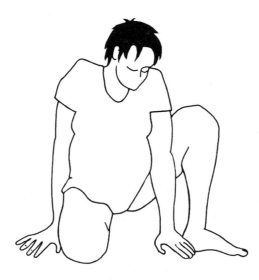

Fig. 4.2 Asymmetrical posture. Asymmetrical postures can be useful for poorly positioned babies such as in the occipitoposterior orientation or asynclitism. Give the woman plenty of reassurance and privacy, and encourage her to try different positions to see which is more effective for her.

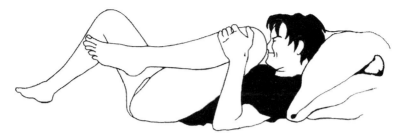

Fig. 4.3 On back with one leg raised. Also an asymmetrical posture (see Fig. 4.2).

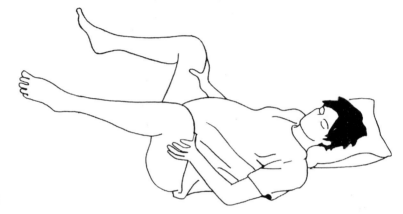

Fig. 4.4

Lithotomy style, or lying back with feet pushing against lithotomy poles should only be used as a last resort and for a short time period to see if the baby advances. This position should not be routine during the second stage and can be uncomfortable and disempowering for women if not used sensitively and appropriately.

Epidural anaesthesia

Epidurals can prolong labour and increase the need for oxytocin, particularly during the second stage of labour (Zhang *et al.*, 1999). Epidurals cause the pelvic floor muscles to relax which impedes flexion and rotation of the fetal head, often leading to delay and malrotation in the second stage of labour (Dickersin, 2000).

It is up to the midwife to be pro-active in reducing the risk of instrumental delivery. It is also important to give the woman every chance of a spontaneous vaginal delivery and again to avoid arbitrary time limits on second stage (Walsh, 2000b). With most modern epidural anaesthesia, women can still move around in labour. Some women are truly mobile and can even stand up to push. However, most will be restricted to giving birth on the bed. Encourage frequent, upright position changes, within the limitations of the woman's mobility, as this may be the key to assisting in optimal fetal positioning, rotation and descent, particularly during the second stage.

Spontaneous vaginal births with epidurals have been attributed to:

- Allowing the epidural to wear off prior to pushing (Sleep *et al.*, 2000).
- Delayed pushing, i.e. pushing only when the vertex is visible (Buxton, 1988).

- Syntocinon infusion, particularly for primigravidas, during the second stage (Heywood & Ho, 1990).
- Avoiding arbitrary time limits on the second stage (Walsh, 2000b).

Positions to try include:

- Kneeling/leaning over the back of the bed.
- In a dense epidural, side-lying positions can be comfortable and maintainable.
- Languishing in an ineffective position for too long should be discouraged. Position changes may be the key to an unassisted birth.

Malpresentations and malpositions in labour

Malpresentations are classed as any presentation of the baby other than vertex, such as breech (see Chapter 5), face or brow presentation, transverse lie or shoulder presentation. A *malposition* is a term used to describe a presentation whereby the vertex is in an abnormal position. The diameter of the skull (see Fig. 4.5) in relation to the pelvic opening is greater than normal (Chadwick, 2002), for example the occipito-posterior (OP) position, or an asynclitism, where the fetal head is tilted laterally so that the parietal bone presents first (see also Fig. 4.6).

A woman whose baby is presenting in a malposition is more likely to experience a longer labour and increased maternal and neonatal morbidity (Chadwick, 2002; Coates, 2002). Women with a malpresentation, or a malposition, need a great deal of encouragement and support to help them through a potentially prolonged and difficult labour. Midwives caring for women at home, or in a birthing centre, should be aware that when the occiput is not the denominator, labour can be slower and the birth have a variety of outcomes, any of which may necessitate transfer to a consultant unit.

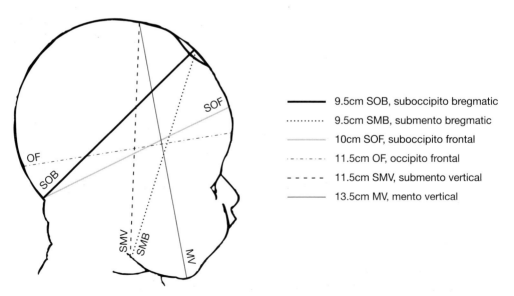

9.5cm SOB, suboccipito bregmatic
9.5cm SMB, submento bregmatic
10cm SOF, suboccipito frontal
11.5cm OF, occipito frontal
11.5cm SMV, submento vertical
13.5cm MV, mento vertical

Fig. 4.5   Diameters of the fetal skull.

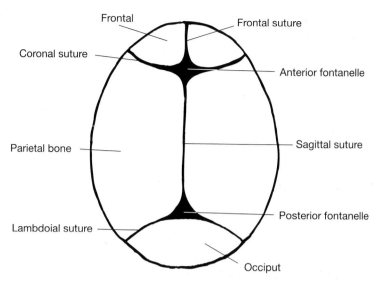

Fig. 4.6 The vault of the fetal skull.

Home birth/birthing centre

Some malpresentations, such as a brow presentation, occur or are diagnosed usually during the second stage, and are associated with a high caesarean rate. Depending on the baby's presentation or position, transfer to a consultant unit may be advisable.

Midwives need to be vigilant for presentations or complications which may necessitate transfer. If the birth is at home, or in a birthing centre, prepare the birthing area for neonatal resuscitation or postpartum haemorrhage as a precaution. Problems include failure to progress, deep transverse arrest, operative delivery and the possibility of the baby requiring resuscitation (Chadwick, 2002). There is the potential for the woman to be exhausted and the uterus less able to contract efficiently following birth, increasing the potential for postpartum haemorrhage.

Occipitoposterior position

The most common malposition is the occipitoposterior (OP) position, commonly referred to as the OP position. The fetus lies with its back against the mother's, the occiput in the posterior part of the pelvis and the head is deflexed (Coates, 1999). Gardberg & Tuppurainen (1994b) found that the OP position was linked to an increase in maternal morbidity and a higher prevalence of abnormal heart rate patterns in labour, but with no difference in Apgar scores or birth asphyxia.

Incidence

- 15% during labour.
- 5% persistent OP at birth (Gardberg & Tupparainen, 1994b).
- A study by Gardberg *et al.* (1998) suggests that two-thirds of persistent OP

positions develop through malrotation from occiptoanterior (OA) to occiptopos-terior (OP) during labour. Coates (2002) suggests that current thinking does not reflect this fact, as many midwives believe OP positions establish during pregnancy.

- More common in primigravida.

Signs and symptoms

- Spontaneous rupture of the membranes is common before the onset of labour due to the ill-fitting presenting part (Gardberg & Tupparainen, 1994b; Sutton, 2000).
- Deep back discomfort during labour with intense back pain during contractions (Sutton, 2000; Coates, 2002).
- Contractions can be irregular, often coupling with a lengthy gap before the next (Simpkin & Ancheta, 2000; Sutton, 2000).
- Long, protracted labours (Sutton, 2000; Coates, 2002).
- On abdominal palpation, the fetal back is against the maternal spine. There is usually a dip around the area of the woman's umbilicus marking the space between the baby's arms and legs. The fetal heart rate (FHR) is usually clearest well over to the side of the woman's uterus (Sutton, 2000). The woman may find abdominal palpation deeply uncomfortable as she has to lie back and such a posture usually causes intense back pain/discomfort.
- An ultrasound scan can diagnose OP positioning and may also confirm an anterior placenta which is more common with this position (Gardberg & Tupparainen, 1994a).
- Involuntary pushing is more common before the cervix is fully dilated (Walmsley, 2000) and can be very distressing for a woman, particularly if her carers are dis-couraging her from bearing down (Bergstrom *et al.*, 1997). Walmsley (2000) suggests that a premature urge to push, common in posterior position babies may be physiologically desirable because it forces the presenting part to flex, then rotate, optimizing its position, prior to full dilatation.
- During second stage labour progress can be slow due to the wide diameter of the presenting part, which also causes gaping of the vagina, before the vertex is visible.
- Vaginal examination may confirm the anterior fontanelle in the anterior of the vagina. Caput and moulding may also be present and make the diagnosis of landmarks on the fetal skull difficult (Chadwick, 2002).
- A 'shrinking' cervix, or an oedematous cervix, can be associated with the de-flexed head of the OP position baby (ARM, 2000a).

Midwifery care

Despite anecdotal practice recommendations to improve or correct fetal misalignment by rotating the fetal head to OA (Sutton, 2000), some authors stress that there is not always a 'quick fix' solution for the baby presenting in the OP position (Walmsley, 2000; Coates, 2002). Walmsley (2000) recommends that preparing the woman for a labour of indeterminate length, combined with providing good midwifery support, may be the most effective midwifery intervention.

Keeping things normal and preventing unnecessary interventions

- While labour may be longer, and progress is likely to be slow, this should not necessarily mean that medical augmentation is indicated. The woman's general condition, her ability to cope and her wishes are all-important factors here.
- Huge support, praise and words of encouragement are necessary to help the woman cope and keep a positive frame of mind.
- The woman should eat and drink as desired to avoid dehydration, ketoacidosis and subsequent slow progress (Johnson *et al.*, 2000).
- Mobilization and upright postures should be used to encourage contractions (Gupta & Nikodem, 2002).
- Ensure regular trips to the toilet to keep the bladder empty.
- Many authors argue that ARM can be detrimental as this intervention encourages descent, precludes the baby from rotating into a more favourable position and predisposes the baby to a deep transverse arrest (Chadwick, 2002 citing El Hata, 1996).

Back pain/painful contractions

- Heat can be applied locally to the woman's lower back by the use of a hot water bottle or a microwavable heat pack (Simpkin & Ancheta, 2000).
- Firm, lower-back massage or direct pressure centrally over the sacrum as directed by the woman can help ease discomfort.
- Simpkin & Archeta (2000) describe the pelvic press, suggesting it can bring relief as it alters the shape of the pelvis subsequently aiding the baby to shift its head and descend (see Fig. 4.7).
- Simpkin & Ancheta (2000) also describe abdominal lifting to improve fetal alignment and to relieve backache. The woman places her hands under her abdomen and lifts it up during a contraction while keeping her knees slightly bent and her pelvis tilted forward.
- In some cases, an epidural may bring welcome relief. While epidurals can prolong labour, particularly during the second stage (Zhang *et al.*, 1999), an epidural may be the one thing the woman needs in order to continue with a difficult labour.
- It is up to the midwife to be pro-active in reducing the risk of instrumental delivery. See 'Prolonged second stage' above for more information on delay and epidural use.

Optimizing fetal position

Women should draw benefits from adopting frequent and upright positions of comfort, preferably following their own instincts, inclinations and personal comfort. Sutton (2000), says 'as a rule of thumb; when a woman's knees are lower than her hips she is allowed ample room in her pelvis for the baby to enter'. The all-fours position is usually found to bring the greatest relief from back pain. However, this position can be difficult to maintain over long periods. The list below suggests a variety of maternal postures which anecdotal evidence suggest may aid fetal rotation and descent thus optimizing the fetal position (see also Figs 4.7–4.11). External version/internal rotation

Figs 4.7–4.11 show maternal postures which anecdotal evidence suggests may aid fetal rotation and descent.

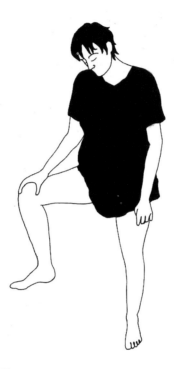

Fig. 4.7   Asymmetrical posture.

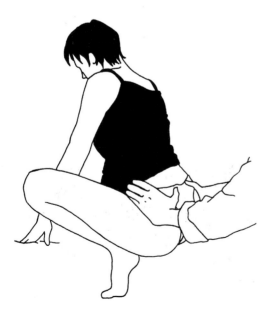

Fig. 4.8 Pelvic press. Simkin and Archeta (2000) describe this in the following way: the woman squats with her birth partner kneeling behind her. The partner places the flats of their hands over the woman's iliac crests and presses them very firmly towards each other during a contraction. Within three to four contractions there should be some evidence of rotation or decent. Do not try this if the woman has an epidural or if this causes any joint pain. Many women with backache find the pelvic press eases their back pain.

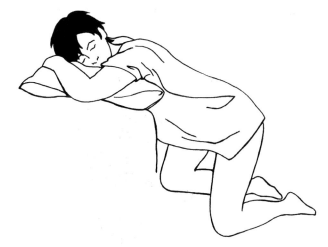

Fig. 4.9   Kneeling position.

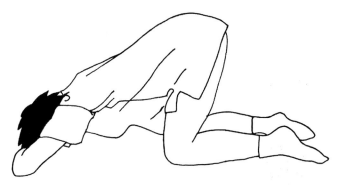

Fig. 4.10   Knee-chest position.

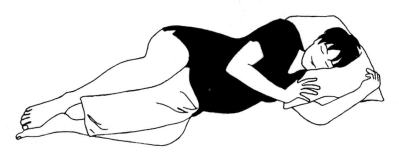

Fig. 4.11   Side lying.

to OA is described by many authors (Davis, 1997; Coates, 2002). Coates (2002) suggests that due to the lack of studies to evaluate this practice, there could be a risk in undertaking such an intervention.

- All-fours position or a kneeling/leaning forwards posture.
- Leaning forward, either sitting or standing.
- Supported positions such as an asymmetrical squat or lean.
- Lying on alternate sides. In a dense epidural, or if the woman is too tired to mobilize, side-lying positions can be comfortable and maintainable. Sutton (2000) recommends that if the baby is left occipitoposterior (LOP), the woman lies on her left side and if the baby is right occipitoposterior (ROP) she lies on her right side. This, she suggests, facilitates the chances of the fetal trunk and occiput with the aid of gravity, to pull into the correct position (see also Fig. 4.11).
- Avoid semi-recumbent or sitting back postures. Some women will adopt a 'flat on the back' legs abducted position. Providing the fetal heart is satisfactory, and this is what the woman wants to do, then this may well be the ideal position for the woman.

Face presentation

When the face is the presentation the head is hyperflexed so the occiput is in contact with the fetal back and the mentum is the denominator. In the past, causative factors included cranial vault abnormalities such as anencephaly (Bhal *et al.*, 1998). A face presentation can develop from an OP position during the second stage of labour (Chadwick, 2002). The majority of face presentations are in the mentoanterior and are usually unproblematic. Mentoposterior is uncommon and is usually undeliverable vaginally (Gaskin, 1990; AAFP, 2000/2001) because the fetal neck is shorter than the maternal sacrum and therefore cannot stretch to the hollow of the sacrum (Chadwick, 2002).

Incidence

- 0.1–0.2% of vaginal births (AAFP, 2000/2001).
- >50% are diagnosed during the second stage of labour (Bhal *et al.*, 1998).
- Two-thirds are in multiparous women (Bhal *et al.*, 1998).

Signs and symptoms

- The presenting part is usually high (Gaskin, 1990).
- Facial features can be felt. The mouth and two molar prominences can be felt as a triangle (Chadwick, 2002).
- Care must be taken not to damage the baby's eyes on vaginal examination (Chadwick, 2002).
- Dilatation of the cervix over the labour may be slower in a face presentation but second stage progress is usually good suggests Gaskin (1990).

Midwifery care

Spontaneous vaginal delivery usually occurs with relative ease (AAFP, 2000/2001). At the birth of a baby presenting as a face presentation be prepared for the possibility that there may be an underlying cause. This could include a tight, entangled or short umbilical cord and, although rare, a baby born with anencephaly is a possibility.

While such births are uncommon and may attract an audience, it is the midwife's duty of care to protect the woman's privacy and to stop uninvited people from coming into the room. The parents should be prepared and reassured that their baby will have a bruised and swollen face at birth and that this will improve significantly in the hours following birth.

Manipulation to convert the presentation to OA, or the use of a fetal scalp electrode (FSE) or vacuum (ventouse) extraction are contraindicated in face presentation (AAFP, 2000/2001). Intravenous oxytocin is usually avoided (AAFP, 2000/2001).

Brow presentation

The baby presenting by the brow has its head partially extended, with the widest diameter presenting in the mentovertical as illustrated in Fig. 4.5. A brow presentation is an unstable presentation and will usually convert to a face or vertex presentation prior to birth (AAFP, 2000/2001). Gaskin (1990) suggests this position can be associated with the cord wrapped around the baby's neck several times and this is confirmed by other authors including Bhal *et al.* (1998), who also noted higher incidence of fetal heart rate (FHR) abnormalities, meconium-stained liquor and lower Apgar scores in brow and face presentations.

Incidence

- 0.2% of vaginal births (AAFP, 2000/2001).
- >50% are diagnosed or occur during the second stage (Bhal *et al.*, 1998).
- More common in primigravida.

Signs and symptoms

- Labour may be slower, more difficult and felt by the woman as a 'back pain' labour (Gaskin, 1990).
- The vaginal examination can be difficult to interpret due to oedema and the unfamiliarity of the presenting features (AAFP, 2000/2001).
- Anterior fontanelle and frontal sutures can be felt on one side of the pelvis, orbital ridges on another; the eyes and root of the nose may also be felt (Chadwick, 2002).
- The presenting part is usually very high and the presenting diameter feels unusually large. (Gaskin, 1990).

Midwifery care

The wide diameter of a persistent brow can prove very difficult to birth but vaginal delivery is possible suggests Gaskin (1990). Gaskin (1990) suggests that the pelvic press during the second stage of labour, as well as adopting an upright or squatting posture, will improve the chances of a spontaneous birth (see Fig. 4.7).

In contradiction to Gaskin's experience, AAFP (2000/2001) suggests that a brow is undeliverable under 'normal conditions' and requires a small baby or a roomy pelvis. In the absence of conversion to a vertex presentation, or an obstructed second stage, a caesarean section would be required (AAFP, 2000/2001).

Transverse lie (shoulder presentation)

Shoulder presentation is undeliverable and occurs when the baby lies transverse and the denominator is often the shoulder (acromion process or dorsum). Causes include multiple pregnancy, polyhydramnios, placenta praevia, macerated fetus, weak abdominal muscles, uterine abnormality (Coates, 1999). External cephalic version (ECV) may be successful. Some doctors then attempt a controlled ARM. However, this is in itself is risky, particularly in early labour, as no amount of 'care' can prevent a cord prolapse if the woman is lying flat with a presenting part that is far from engaged.

Incidence

- 0.3% deliveries (AAFP, 2000/2001).
- Of those babies presenting as transverse near term only 17% will remain in a transverse lie at the onset of labour (Gimovsky & Hennigan, 1995).
- The majority of shoulder presentations occur in multiparous women (Gimovsky & Hennigan, 1995).

Signs and symptoms

- The woman's uterine shape appears wide as opposed to round and, on palpation, the fundal height is lower than would be expected for dates.
- The diagnosis of transverse lie is usually made easily by abdominal palpation, where the head is palpable on one side, the buttocks on the other and usually nothing in the pelvis (AAFP, 2000/2001). The lie is occasionally oblique but it usually becomes transverse during labour (Coates, 1999).
- Vaginal examination will firstly detect a high presenting part, sometimes the distinctive pattern of the ribs may be felt or the shoulder or even a hand and an arm.

Midwifery care

The midwife who detects a shoulder presentation during labour should summon help. If at home, or in the birthing centre, immediate transfer to hospital is indicated. If the woman is in labour it may be necessary for the midwife to attempt external and, if necessary, internal cephalic version (described below). A vaginal examination *should only be performed* if placenta praevia has been excluded (Coates, 1999).

- **External cephalic version (ECV).** Care should involve attempts to turn the baby externally by ECV, even if labour has started this can often be successful. AAFP (2000/2001) note that a second twin who presents as transverse at full dilatation can turn easily by external version, as the uterus is initially relaxed and accommodating following delivery of the first twin.

- **Internal cephalic version** is often considered hazardous for the baby and a caesarean section is often the preferred option. However, in an emergency (such as a second twin presenting transverse and the cervix fully dilated) internal version may be undertaken (AAFP, 2000/2001). This would require the clinician to grab the baby's feet (via the cervix) and pull the baby into a breech position.
- **An immediate caesarean section** is indicated if there is a:
  - cord prolapse
  - ECV is unsuccessful
  - labour has been ongoing for sometime and/or the membranes rupture (Coates, 1999) as uterine rupture is a serious complication.

Summary

Slow progress in labour

- Preoccupation with strict time definitions in labour are not evidence based.
- Prevention of dystocia is better than cure.
- Support has a positive psychological effect on the progress of labour.
- Upright positions and mobilizing have a positive physical effect on labour progress.

Interventions to increase uterine contractibility

- Continuous presence and verbal support from the midwife.
- Mobilization/position changes.
- Comforting touch.
- Acupressure.
- Nipple stimulation.
- Warm compress or hot water bottle applied to the fundus.
- Hydrotherapy/warm bath/water tub.
- ARM (not useful in OP or malpresentations).
- Oxytocin.

Recommended reading

Simpkin, P. & Ancheta, R. (2000) *The Labor Progress Handbook*. Blackwell Science, Oxford.
Walsh, D. (2000) Evidence-based care. Part 3: Assessing women's progress in labour. *British Journal of Midwifery* **8** (7), 449–57.

References

AAFP (2000/2001) *Advanced Life Support in Obstetrics*. Course Syllabus Manual, 4th edn. American Academy of Family Physicians, Leawood, Kansas.
ARM (2000b) Association of Radical Midwives Nettalk: Tight pelvic floor muscles and horse riders. *Midwifery Matters* Issue 87, 28–30.

ARM (2000a) Association of Radical Midwives Nettalk: Incredible shrinking cervices. *Midwifery Matters* Issue 87, 28–30.

Bergstrom, L., Seedily, J., Schulman-Hull, L. *et al.* (1997) 'I gotta push. Please let me push!' Social interactions during the change from first stage to second stage of labour. *Birth* **24** (3), 173–80.

Borrell, U. & Fenstrom, I. (1957) The movements of the sacroiliac joints and their importance to changes in the pelvic dimensions during parturition. *Acta Obstetrica et Gynaecologica, Scandinavica* **36**, 42–57.

Burvill, S. (2002) Midwifery diagnosis of labour onset. *British Journal of Midwifery* **10** (10), 600–605.

Buxton, E.J., Redman, C.W.E. & Obhrai, M. (1988) Delayed pushing with lumbar epidural in labour – does it increase the incidence of spontaneous delivery? *Journal of Obstetrics and Gynaecology* **8**, 258–61.

Chadwick, J. (2002) Malpositions and presentations. In *Emergencies Around Childbirth* (Boyle, M., ed.), pp. 76–9. Radcliffe Medical Press, Abingdon.

Cluett, E. (2000) The onset of labour. 2: Implications for practice. *The Practising Midwife* **3** (7), 16–19.

Coates, T. (1999) Malpositions of the occiput and malpresentations. In *Myles Textbook for Midwives*, 13th edn (Bennett, R. & Brown, L.K., eds), pp. 507–37. Churchill Livingstone, Edinburgh.

Coates, T. (2002) Malpositions and malpresentations of the occiput: current research and practice tips. *MIDIRS Midwifery Digest* **12** (2), 152–4.

Crowther, C., Enkin, M., Keirse, M.J.N.C. & Brown, I. (2000) Monitoring progress in labor. In *A Guide to Effective Care in Pregnancy and Childbirth*, 3rd edn (Enkin, M., Keirse, M.J.N.C., Neilson, J. *et al.*, eds), pp. 281–8. Oxford University Press, Oxford.

Davis, E. (1997) *Hearts and Hands: A Midwife's Guide to Pregnancy and Birth*, 3rd edn. Celestial Arts, Berkeley, California.

Dickersin, K. (2000) Control of pain in labor. In *A Guide to Effective Care in Pregnancy and Childbirth*, 3rd edn (Enkin, M., Keirse, M.J.N.C., Neilson, J. *et al.*, eds), pp. 313–31. Oxford University Press, Oxford.

DoH (2001) *Why Mothers Die, 1997–1999. The fifth report of the Confidential Enquiries into Maternal Deaths in the United Kingdom.* Department of Health, RCOG Press, London.

Eriksson, M., Mattsson, L.A. & Ladfors, L. (1997) Early or late bath during the first stage of labour: a randomized study of 200 women. *Midwifery* **13**, 146–8.

Fraser, W.D., Krauss, I., Brisson-Carrol, G. *et al.* (2002) Amniotomy for shortening spontaneous labour (Cochrane Review). *The Cochrane Library* Issue 4. Update software, Oxford.

Gardberg, M. & Tuppurainen, M. (1994a) Anterior placental location predisposes for occiput posterior presentation near term. *Acta Obstetrica et Gynaecologica, Scandinavica* **73**, 151–2.

Gardberg, M. & Tuppurainen, M. (1994b) Persistent occiput posterior presentation – a clinical problem. *Acta Obstetrica et Gynaecologica, Scandinavica* **73**, 45–7.

Gardberg, M., Laakkonen, E. & Salevaara, M. (1998) Intrapartum sonography and persistent occiput posterior presentation: a study of 408 deliveries. *Obstetrics and Gynecology* **91**, 746–9.

Gaskin, I.M. (1990) *Spiritual Midwifery*. The Book Publishing Co., Summertown, Tennessee.

Gee, H. (2000) Abnormal patterns of labour and prolonged labour. In *Best Practice in Labor Ward Management* (Kean, L.H., Baker, P.H. & Edelstone, D.I., eds), pp. 65–79. WB Saunders, Edinburgh.

Gimovsky, M. & Hennigan, C. (1995) Abnormal fetal presentations. *Current Thinking in Obstetrics and Gynaecology* **7** (6), 482–5.

Gupta, J.K. & Nikodem, V.C. (2002) Woman's position during the second stage of labour (Cochrane Review). *The Cochrane Library*. Issue 4. Update software, Oxford.

Heywood, M.A. & Ho, E. (1990) Pain relief in midwifery. In *Intrapartum Care – A Research Based Approach* (Alexander, J., Levy, V. & Roch, S., eds), pp. 70–121. Macmillan, Basingstoke.

Hobbs, L. (1998) Assessing cervical dilatation without VEs. *The Practising Midwife* **1** (11), 34–5.

Hodnett, E.D. (2002) Caregiver support for women during childbirth (Cochrane Review). *COCHRANE. The Pregnancy and Childbirth Database*. The Cochrane Collaboration. CD ROM: Issue 4. Oxford.

Lauzon, L. & Hodnett, E. (2002) Labour assessment programs to delay admission to labour wards (Cochrane Review). *The Cochrane Library* Issue 4. Update software, Oxford.

Johnson, C., Keirse, M.J.N.C., Enkin, M. & Chalmers, I. (2000) Hospital practices – nutrition and hydration in labor. In *A Guide to Effective Care in Pregnancy and Childbirth*, 3rd edn (Enkin, M., Keirse, M.J.N.C., Neilson, J. *et al*., eds), pp. 255–66. Oxford University Press, Oxford.

Keirse, M.J.N.C., Enkin, M.W., & Lumley, J. (2000) Social and professional support in childbirth. In *A Guide to Effective Care in Pregnancy and Childbirth*, 3rd edn (Enkin, M., Keirse, M.J.N.C., Neilson, J. *et al*., eds) pp. 247–54. Oxford University Press, Oxford.

MIDIRS (1999) *Positions in Labour and Delivery*. Informed Choice Leaflet. Midwives Information and Resource Service, Bristol.

Odent, M. (1998) Use of water during labour – updated recommendations. *MIDIRS Midwifery Digest* **8** (1), 68–9.

Rosser, J. & Anderson, T. (1998) Amniotomy to shorten spontaneous labour: a presentation of the main points from the Cochrane Database review on routine ARM. *MIDIRS Midwifery Digest* **8** (2), 201–202.

Russell, J.G.B. (1982) The rationale of primitive delivery positions. *British Journal of Obstetrics and Gynaecology* **89**, 712–15.

Sallam, H.N., Abdel-Dayem, A., Sakr, R.A. *et al*. (1999) Mathematical relationships between uterine contractions, cervical dilatation, descent and rotation in spontaneous vertex deliveries. *International Journal of Gynaecology and Obstetrics* **64**, 135–9.

Simpkin, P. & Ancheta, R. (2000) *The Labor Progress Handbook*. Blackwell Science, Oxford.

Sleep, J., Roberts, J. & Chalmers, I. (2000) The second stage of labor. In *A Guide to Effective Care in Pregnancy and Childbirth* (Enkin, M., Keirse, M.J.N.C., Neilson, J. *et al*., eds), pp. 289–99. Oxford University Press, Oxford.

Stuart, C. (2000) Invasive actions in labour. Where have all the 'old tricks' gone? *The Practising Midwife* **3** (8), 30–33.

Sutton, J. (2000) Occipito posterior positioning and some ideas about how to change it. *The Practising Midwife* **3** (6), 20–22.

Walmsley, K. (2000) Managing the OP labour. *MIDIRS Midwifery Digest* **10** (1), 61–2.

Walsh, D. (2000a) Evidence-based care. Part 3: Assessing women's progress in labour. *British Journal of Midwifery* **8** (7), 449–57.

Walsh, D. (2000b) Evidence-based care. Part 6: Limits on pushing and time in the second stage. *British Journal of Midwifery* **8** (10), 604–608.

Zhang, J., Klebanoff, M.A. & DerSimonian, R. (1999) Epidural analgesia in association with the duration of labour and mode of delivery: a quantitative review. *American Journal of Obstetrics and Gynecology* **180** (4), 970–77.

5 Breech birth

Lesley Shutter

Introduction

Breech presentation is where the lie of the baby is longitudinal and the baby's buttocks are in the lower segment of the mother's uterus.

Incidence and facts

- While 25% of babies adopt a breech position at some time in pregnancy, only 3–4% remain breech at term (Sweet & Tiran, 1997; Frye, 1998; Hofmeyr, 2000).
- Many babies appear to adopt a breech position for no particular reason! However, a minority will adopt a breech position because of 'problems' such as short or entangled cord, prematurity, placenta praevia or fetal abnormalities.
- Evidence suggests that external cephalic version (ECV) should be offered to all women with an uncomplicated breech baby at term (37–42 weeks) (RCOG, 1997).
- Women should be facilitated to make an informed choice about their birth options and should not be coerced into one particular mode of delivery. These discussions should include the possible differences between a 'managed' vaginal breech birth and one 'facilitated' by a skilled practitioner.
- For a woman with predisposing factors, such as diabetes, fetopelvic disproportion, a previous macrosomic baby, or a suspected large baby and poor labour progress, a caesarean section is usually advisable (Hofmeyr, 2000).
- Midwives working an all environments are likely to be the only professional around when faced with an unexpected or undiagnosed breech baby. It is, therefore, important that they are prepared to deal with this eventuality and that they have the training, knowledge and skills to assist the woman and her baby at this time (CESDI, 2000; Robinson, 2000).
- Whilst having a good heart rate, breech babies may be slower to breathe spontaneously than cephalic babies, and may require bag-and-mask resuscitation to establish breathing.

Types of breech presentation

The baby in a breech presentation will adopt a variety of positions, similar to a cephalic baby, with the sacrum being the denominator. Table 5.1, provides descriptions of different breech presentations.

Women's options and the provision of care

The midwife needs to explore her own feelings and prejudice, and ensure that she remains unbiased, non-judgemental and acts in a manner that will facilitate both informed choice and decision making as well as enabling the woman to access appropriate care.

- Explore the options – ECV, vaginal breech birth, and caesarean section; home or hospital.
- Women can choose who assists at the birth – her midwife, an independent midwife or an obstetrician.

- Discuss the possible difference between a vaginal breech birth that is 'managed' and one that is 'facilitated' by a skilled practitioner/midwife. Managed/medicalized breech birth tends to include a package of epidural anaesthesia, routine episiotomy and lithotomy position for the delivery. A facilitated birth encourages the breech baby to deliver through supporting the woman in upright postures and only intervening should a direct indication arise.
- Choice may be restricted due to 'local policy' or a lack of suitably skilled practitioners.

Self-help measures

While there is little research on self-help measures, many women may wish to try something during the antenatal period. These include postural management involving the knee–chest position and pelvic rocking. Other interventions include visualization, swimming, massage, talking to her baby as well as complementary therapies including hypnosis, homeopathy, acupuncture, acupressure, moxibustion, chiropractic or osteopathic intervention.

External cephalic version

All women should be offered information about the safety and benefits of external cephalic version (ECV) at term. While ECV statistics vary, an estimated seven out of ten babies remain cephalic presentation following the procedure (MIDIRS, 1997). Hofmeyr (2000) suggests that when a breech presentation is encountered in labour, and the membranes remain intact, the limited data available would indicate that ECV performed with tocolysis has a reasonable success rate.

Caesarean section

The use of caesarean section for breech babies, in the belief that it is safer, may become a self-fulfilling prophecy, as attendants become less skilled in vaginal breech birth. The Royal College of Obstetricians and Gynaecologists (RCOG, 1999) admit that with the increasing number of caesarean sections, there are too few doctors with vaginal breech experience. The most recent research evidence on breech babies concludes that, 'planned caesarean section is better than planned vaginal birth for the term fetus in the breech presentation' (Hannah *et al.*, 2000). It is possible that the findings and recommendations from this study will be applied to maternity care in some areas. This will further reduce the choices available to women and the opportunity for practitioners to develop skill and confidence in supporting women in vaginal breech birth. Some authors are challenging these recommendations (Robinson 2000/2001; Banks, 2001; Gyte, 2001; Lancet correspondence, 2001) and midwives are strongly advised to read and critically evaluate the study for themselves.

Table 5.1   Types of breech presentation. (Written information reproduced from Stables, 1999 with kind permission of Elsevier Science.)

Type	Description
Complete Also known as flexed or full breech 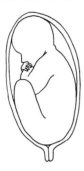	• The baby's legs are bent at the hips and knees; feet are positioned close to the baby's bottom in a cross-legged position • This position is commonest in multigravidae
Incomplete Also known as extended or frank breech 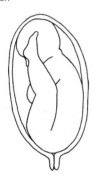	• The baby's legs are bent at the hip and lie alongside the trunk; feet are positioned near the baby's head in a jack-knifed position • This position is commonest in primigravidae, near to term, due to firm uterine and abdominal muscles restricting movement of the baby
Footling This is a rare presentation, more common in premature labour 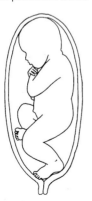	One or both knees and hips are extended with the baby's feet or foot below its buttocks

Contd.

Table 5.1 Continued.

Type	Description
Knee/Kneeling This is a rare presentation and is the least common of all	One, or both, of the baby's hips are extended and the knees are flexed; the knee(s) present below/in front of the baby's buttocks
Others	Some babies may have a combination of the incomplete presentations, e.g. one leg flexed, the other extended

Concerns and possible complications with a breech birth

Hypoxia

Hypoxia has been identified as the commonest cause of death in breech babies. CESDI (2000) suggest that the lack of recognition and prompt action are major factors.

Umbilical cord prolapse

Incidence: 3.7% in breech (Confino *et al.*, 1985).
   Umbilical cord prolapse is:

- More frequent in primigravidae than multigravidae (6% and 3%, respectively).
- More common in premature labour and incomplete presentations (Footling type of breech presentation).
- Also linked to artificial rupture of membranes (ARM) and increases the incidence of cord compression.

Prolapse does not always cause cord compression, where the cervix is fully dilated a vaginal birth may still be possible.

Entrapment of after coming head

Incidence: 0–8.5% at term (Cheng & Hannah, 1993).
   'If the frank or complete breech passes easily through the pelvis, the head can be expected to follow without difficulty' (Enkin *et al.*, 2000). In a term baby, if the head is

not going to pass through the cervix and pelvis, the buttocks also will be obstructed and labour will not progress (Hofmeyr, 2001 citing Gebbie, 1982).

Entrapment is more common in a preterm baby (Stevenson, 1993) and may be related to maternal pushing being encouraged prior to, or following, misdiagnosis of full dilatation.

Hyperextension of the baby's head (star gazing)

Incidence: 5% (Confino *et al.*, 1985).

Hyperextension of the baby's head may occur due to the following factors:

- Cord around baby's neck
- Placental location
- Muscle spasm in baby
- Abnormalities in either the uterus or the baby
- When detected by ultrasound scan (USS), at term, a caesarean section will be advised.
- May be caused in labour by unnecessary intervention of the carer. Spontaneous pushing, not traction, should be encouraged; traction may cause extension of the baby's arms and head (Hofmeyr, 2000).

Head and neck trauma

Forceful traction by the carer may cause iatrogenic brain and spinal injuries (Banks, 1998).

Premature placental separation

This may be linked to maternal position in the second stage of labour (Cronk, 1998).

Labour and birth

Preparation/birth planning

Preparation will demonstrate the process that the woman and the midwife have gone through to reach the decision to have a vaginal breech birth. Points to consider include:

- The baby is in a good position and not considered too large.
- A skilled and competent midwife will support the woman in a breech birth.
- The woman, her partner and the midwife are informed regarding the anticipated process and progress of a breech labour and birth. The woman has confidence in her body and her midwife.
- Good communication between the woman and the midwife.

The midwife's role

- To support the woman in her innate ability to birth her baby.
- Not to manage the woman's care or labour.

- To ensure that she has appropriate support for herself, another midwife experienced in physiological and non-medicalized labour and birth.
- To ensure and maintain a sound knowledge of skills and techniques to assist a breech birth, should it become necessary.
- The midwife is in tune with, and able to recognize, assess and respond to problems, should they occur.

The mechanism of a breech birth

Midwives should refer to a suitable textbook to familiarize themselves with this mechanism.

Onset of labour

- Midwifery care and support is the same as for any labour.
- With maternal consent, palpate the uterus to check that the presentation and position of the baby has not changed.
- Banks (1998) suggests that a vaginal assessment in early breech labour is important to determine the presenting part, and to exclude cord, foot, knee or compound presentation. This should be carried out with the woman's consent and awareness of the purpose of the examination. She should be advised that it is expected that cervical dilatation may be minimal, to avoid her feeling demotivated.
- Cooper (1992) suggests that the presenting part is often higher in the pelvis than the midwife would expect with a cephalic presentation, and that the station is likely to go up and down more, during labour.
- If the woman is examined in a semi-recumbent position, assist her into an upright position immediately afterwards to avoid problems such as postural hypotension, fetal heart rate (FHR) irregularities and slowing of labour progress (Sleep *et al.*, 2000; Gupta & Nikodem, 2002).

Pain management

- Encourage the woman to apply skills she may have learnt antenatally such as relaxation, visualization, noise and mobility. Use massage, transcutaneous electrical nerve stimulation (TENS), support and so on. Chapter 15 also deals with how to help.
- The use of a birthing pool is controversial and needs to be explored on an individual basis according to the wishes of the woman, the experience of the individual midwife and the place of birth.
- There is no evidence that the use of an epidural is appropriate in a vaginal breech birth. Its use may be associated with a longer second stage (Chadha *et al.*, 1992). It is also likely to restrict mobility and inhibit positions to facilitate a breech birth.

First stage

- Care and observations are the same as for a cephalic birth:
  - no routine vaginal examinations

    ○ food and drink as desired by the individual woman
    ○ encourage regular emptying of the bladder.

Also use midwifery skills to monitor the progress of labour. Chapter 1 also covers alternative methods of assessing progress in labour.

- There may be a long latent phase in the first stage of labour due to a lack of application of the presenting part to the cervix but progress may escalate rapidly once an active first stage is reached.
- The woman may feel out of breath, or breathless, during or after contractions due to the pressure of the baby's head against her diaphragm. She may also experience the pain more in her back than the front.
- Multigravidae may experience little or no discomfort in early labour (pre 4 cm).
- No artificial rupture of membranes (ARM). If membranes rupture spontaneously, do a vaginal examination to exclude cord prolapse, foot or knee presentation, and check the fetal heart for cord compression.
- No augmentation of labour.
- A woman may choose or decline to comply with unit policy on electronic fetal monitoring (EFM). If used, do so in a way to encourage mobility rather than restrict it.
- A premature urge to push is unlikely in the term breech baby. The hip size in an extended or flexed breech baby is likely to equal the head size (Stevenson, 1993).

Second stage of labour

A latent phase may occur, as with cephalic birth, between full dilatation and the spontaneous urge to push. The woman will often doze during this period. Second stage contractions are often less frequent, shorter and less powerful. Maternal anal dilatation and pressure may 'diagnose' the second stage or a vaginal examination may be used to confirm full dilatation. In principle remember 'hands off the breech'. Just watch, wait and support. For a baby requiring assistance techniques for assisted breech delivery are dealt with later in Table 5.2.

- Multigravidae may experience the sensation and 'feel' the descent of the baby as being different to a previous cephalic baby.
- Meconium is to be expected due to the pressure on the baby's buttocks. Its presence does not necessarily indicate that the baby is, or has been, distressed (Hulme, 1992). Its presence becomes significant should the FHR become abnormal (Baker *et al.*, 1992; Mahomed *et al.*, 1994).
- When the buttocks reach the perineum it may be necessary to do an episiotomy, if it is tight or rigid and not stretching, despite good contractions and maternal effort, or to expedite the birth for fetal compromise.
- Banks (1998) suggests that if the membranes are intact they should be broken when the buttocks reach the perineum to allow any meconium to drain from the vagina. The close fit of the baby's bottom in the vagina usually prevents meconium from getting to the liquor around the baby's head.

- A rocking or an up and down motion during the descent of the baby's bottom is evident ('rumping') and is the same process as that of 'crowning' (Stevenson, 1993).

The birth

- No touching unless absolutely necessary or there is a complication.
- Extended legs look never ending but usually flop out on their own, shortly followed by the arms (Cronk, 1998).
- When born to the umbilicus, the cord may be compressed between the baby's head and maternal pelvis (both bony). Wharton's jelly affords some protection but expect the FHR to be slower. The lower heart rate is also due to the reduction in the placental site and thought to be an automatic reflex to conserve oxygen in the baby (Stevenson, 1993).
- If there is tension, a loop of cord may be brought down, but handle gently to avoid stimulating constriction and thus reducing oxygen to the baby.
- Allow the baby's body to take some of the weight. This will bring the chin on to the perineum, followed by the birth of the head.
- The midwife can give gentle support by either placing her hand under the buttocks, the baby 'sitting' in her hand, or by supporting the baby by the hips. This may be necessary, in some situations, to slow the birth of the head, prevent sudden decompression and thus avoid a tentorial tear and trauma to the perineum.

Box 5.1   Maternal positions for labour and birth.

Squatting
  - Advocated by Odent (1984) as being 'mechanically efficient, reduces the likelihood of having to pull the baby out and reduces the delay between the delivery of the baby's umbilicus and the baby's head'.
  - Maximizes the pelvic capacity but supported and hanging squats need to be practised in pregnancy (Banks, 1998).

Standing
  - Believed by some to be a more physiological position.
  - Conversely, it may be suggested that squatting and standing positions are not to be recommended until evidence suggests otherwise (Cronk, 1998) because they:
    - may make birth faster than necessary leading to rapid head decompression
    - may encourage the baby's arms to be swept up over its head, making the birth more difficult, possibly leading to Erb's palsy
    - may increase traction on the cord and placenta, leading to a reduced oxygen supply to the baby and/or early or too rapid placental separation.
  - The baby's body hangs straight down; this may encourage a deflexed head, exert extra pressure on the base of the neck and increase the risk of spinal cord damage.
  - Increased perineal tearing.

Hands and knees (all fours)
  - Gravity assists the descent of the baby.
  - Complements the attitude and action of the uterus.
  - Does not put undue traction or pressure on the placenta or cord.
  - Facilitates the birth of the baby's head.
  - Allows the baby to manoeuvre.

Table 5.2 Techniques for an assisted breech birth.

Technique	Procedure
Burns Marshall manoeuvre	• Baby 'hangs' by its own weight to encourage descent and flexion of the head. Take care not to let the head deliver too quickly. • When the nape of the neck and the hairline are visible, grasp the baby's ankles in one hand and, with slight traction, bring the body in an arc, over the mother's abdomen (left). • The other hand can be used to support the perineum and to prevent sudden delivery of the head (right). • Once the baby's mouth is clear the baby is able to breathe. • Take your time in letting the rest of the head deliver. 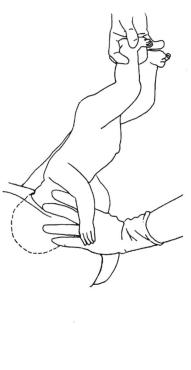 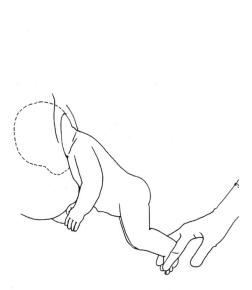
Mauriceau-Smellie-Veit manoeuvre	• Straddle the baby along one arm (usually the left in a right-handed individual) (see left image on next page). • Insert three fingers of that hand into the woman's vagina, placing the middle finger in the baby's mouth and the other on the cheekbones, to assist flexion, if necessary. • A second person can apply suprapubic pressure if necessary. • Two outer fingers of the other hand are now placed over the baby's shoulders with the middle finger on the occiput to assist and maintain flexion (see right image on next page). • Apply gentle traction and deliver the head following the curve of Carus.

Contd.

Table 5.2 Contd.

Technique	Procedure

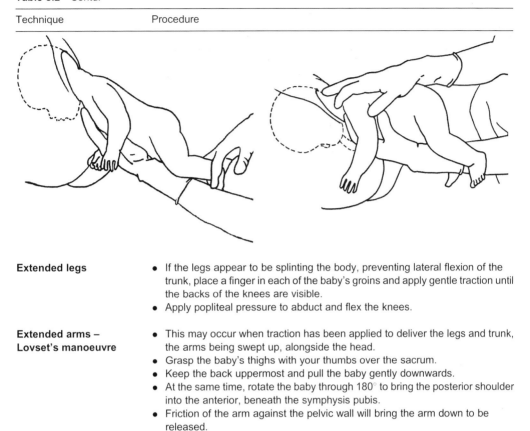

Extended legs	• If the legs appear to be splinting the body, preventing lateral flexion of the trunk, place a finger in each of the baby's groins and apply gentle traction until the backs of the knees are visible. • Apply popliteal pressure to abduct and flex the knees.
Extended arms – **Lovset's manoeuvre**	• This may occur when traction has been applied to deliver the legs and trunk, the arms being swept up, alongside the head. • Grasp the baby's thighs with your thumbs over the sacrum. • Keep the back uppermost and pull the baby gently downwards. • At the same time, rotate the baby through 180° to bring the posterior shoulder into the anterior, beneath the symphysis pubis. • Friction of the arm against the pelvic wall will bring the arm down to be released. • Repeat the manoeuvre in the opposite direction to release the other arm.
Extended head	• If the hairline does not become visible after the baby has been allowed to take its weight briefly, it is possible the head has extended. • Use the Mauriceau-Smellie-Veit manoeuvre

- When born to the nape of the neck, the heart rate can be felt or observed over the baby's chest.
- Flexion (chin to chest) of the baby's head may be assisted by gently placing an index finger in the baby's mouth and the other behind the back of the baby's head.
- Once the nose is free, any necessary suction of meconium or fluid can be done, by another midwife, whilst waiting for the rest of the head to birth.

The baby at birth

It is important to remember and discuss with parents that the mechanism of a breech birth is different to that of a cephalic baby and their appearance and response are likely to be different. This may be reflected in the initial 1-minute Apgar score being lower in breech babies born vaginally (Thorpe-Beeston *et al.*, 1992).

Remember that cephalic babies often 'rest' between the birth of the head and the body allowing adjustment from compression to decompression of the head. This does not occur with a breech birth and therefore may be a factor in the need to sometimes initiate resuscitation measures.

Breech babies may be slower to breathe spontaneously than cephalic babies and may initially have lax muscle tone and poor reflexes whilst having a good heart rate. A bag and mask or a resuscitaire should be on hand and ready to use if necessary. Whilst the baby is still on the pulsating cord, it is receiving oxygen from the mother if the placenta remains attached to the uterine wall.

The best place to give supportive measures, if required, is in the mothers' arms to enable her to stimulate the baby by voice and touch. If more extensive measures are required, they should be carried out close to the mother.

Third stage of labour

This should be conducted according to the woman's wishes, subject to events and discussion. The use of oxytocics should be withheld until the birth of the baby's head is completed.

Positions and techniques for breech birth

Although not researched within the vaginal breech birth scenario, empirical evidence suggests that views on the different positions for labour are divided in this area. Midwives should encourage and enable the woman to adopt whatever position is best for her. Box 5.1 summarizes the basic positions.

It is appropriate for midwives to familiarize themselves with, and practise, manoeuvres that may be necessary to assist a vaginal breech baby to be born. A brief outline is included in Table 5.2 but the midwife is strongly advised to consult an appropriate obstetric/midwifery text for more detail on these manoeuvres.

Summary

- *Hands off the breech* – damage is often a result of too much force being used.
- No 'routine' vaginal examinations.
- No 'routine' artificial rupture of membranes (ARM) – if spontaneous rupture of membranes occurs check there is no cord/foot presenting.
- Avoid epidurals.
- Enable women to adopt positions spontaneously.
- No augmentation – if there is poor progress, consider caesarean section.
- Check fetal heart rate (FHR) regularly and act appropriately.
- Enable women to push spontaneously, give guidance if necessary.
- Meconium is to be expected.
- Episiotomy should be conducted only if felt necessary by the attending midwife.
- Breech babies may be slower to breathe spontaneously than cephalic – be prepared.
- Placenta and membranes should be delivered according to the woman's wishes, unless contraindicated.

- Ensure you are well supported by like-minded people.
- Enjoy and celebrate the birth.

Useful contacts

Association for Improvements in the Maternity Services (AIMS) AIMS Helpline: 0870 765 1433. Website: www.aims.org.uk.

Birthspirit Ltd 15 Te Awa Road, RD 3, Hamilton, New Zealand. Telephone: 64 7 856 4612. www.birthspirit.co.nz

Independent Midwives Association (IMA) 1 The Great Quarry, Guildford, Surrey GU1 3XN. Telephone: 01483 821104. Website: www.independentmidwives.org.uk

National Childbirth Trust (NCT) Alexandra House, Oldham Terrace, Acton, London W3 6NH. Enquiry line: 0870 444 8707. Website: www.nct-online.org

References

Baker, P.N., Kilby, M.D. & Murray, H. (1992) An assessment of the use of meconium alone as an indication for fetal blood sampling. *Obstetrics and Gynecology* **80**, 792–6.

Banks, M. (1998) *Breech Birth Woman Wise*. Birthspirit Books, Hamilton, New Zealand.

Banks, M. (2001) *Breech Birth Beyond the 'Term Breech Trial'*. Birthspirit website: www.birthspirit.co.nz (accessed January 2002).

CESDI (2000) *Confidential Enquiry into Stillbirths and Deaths in Infancy*, 7th Annual Report. Maternal and Child Health Research Consortium, London.

Chadha, Y.C., Mahmood, T.A., Dick, M.J. *et al.* (1992) Breech delivery and epidural analgesia. *British Journal of Obstetrics and Gynaecology* **99**, 96–100.

Cheng, M., Hannah, M. (1993) Breech delivery at term: a critical review of the literature. *Obstetrics and Gynaecology*, **82** (4), 605–18.

Confino, E., Gleicher, N., Elrad, H., Isajovich, B. & David, M.P. (1985) The breech dilemma – a review. *Obstetrical and Gynaecological Survey* **40** (6), 330–37.

Cooper, M. (1992) *Twins, Breech and VBAC* (Audiotape). Midwifery Today, Eugene, Oregon.

Cronk, M. (1998) Birthing a baby by the breech. *AIMS Journal* **10** (3), 6–8.

Frye, A. (1998) *Holistic Midwifery. A Comprehensive Textbook for Midwives in Home Birth Practice*, Vol. 1. *Care During Pregnancy*. Labrys Press, Portland, Oregon.

Gupta, J.K. & Nikodem, V.C. (2002) Woman's position during the second stage of labour (Cochrane Review). *The Cochrane Library* Issue 4. Update software, Oxford.

Gyte, G. (2001) Planned caesarean section versus planned vaginal birth for breech presentation at term: a randomised multicentre trial. *MIDIRS Midwifery Digest* **11** (1), 80–83.

Hannah, M.E., Hannah, W.J., Hewison, S.A. *et al.* (2000) Planned caesarean section versus vaginal birth for breech presentation at term: a randomised multicentre trial. *The Lancet* **356**, 1375–83.

Hofmeyr, G.J. (2000) Suspected fetalpelvic disproportion and abnormal lie. In *A Guide to Effective Care in Pregnancy and Childbirth* (Enkin, M., Keirse, M.J.N.C., Neilson, J. *et al.*, eds), pp. 185–95. Oxford University Press, Oxford.

Hofmeyr, G.J. (2001) citing Gebbie, (1982) Abnormal fetal presentation and position. In *Turnbull's Obstetrics* (Chamberlain, G. & Steer, P. eds), p. 557. Churchill Livingstone, Edinburgh.

Hulme, H. (1992) Meconium aspiration syndrome: reflections on a midwifery subject. *MIDIRS Midwifery Digest* **2** (2), 177.

Lancet correspondence (2001) Term breech trial. *The Lancet* **357** (9251), 225–8.

Mahomed, K., Nyoni, R. & Masona, D. (1994) Meconium staining of liquor in a low-risk population. *Paediatric and Perinatal Epidemiology* **8** (3), 292–300.

MIDIRS (1997) *Breech Baby What Are Your Choices?* Informed Choice Leaflet. Midwives Information and Resource Service and the NHS Centre for Reviews and Dissemination.

Odent, M. (1984) *Birth Reborn*. Souvenir Press, London.

Robinson, J. (2000) Midwives need training in the lost art of breech birth. *British Journal of Midwifery* **8** (7), 447.

Robinson, J. (2000/2001) Breech babies – caesarean or vaginal birth? *AIMS Journal* **12** (4), 12–13.

RCOG (1997) *Effective Procedures in Maternity Care Suitable for Audit. 4.7 Breech Presentation at Term*. Royal College of Obstetricians and Gynaecologists: Clinical Audit Unit, RCOG Press, London.

RCOG (1999) *The Management of Breech Presentation*. Guideline No. 20. Royal College of Obstetricians and Gynaecologists, RCOG Press, London.

Sleep, J., Roberts, J. & Chalmers, I. (2000) The second stage of labor. In *A Guide to Effective Care in Pregnancy and Childbirth*, 3rd edn (Enkin, M., Keirse, M.J.N.C., Neilson, J. *et al.*, eds), pp. 289–99. Oxford University Press, Oxford.

Stables, D. (1999) *Physiology in Childbearing with Anatomy and Related Biosciences*. Baillière Tindall, London.

Stevenson, J. (1993) More thoughts on breech. *Midwifery Today*, No. 26, Summer, 24–5.

Sweet, B.R. & Tiran, D. (eds) (1997) *Mayes Midwifery*, 12th edn. Baillière Tindall, London.

Thorpe-Beeston, J.G., Blanfield, P.J. & Saunders, N.J.S. (1992) Outcome of breech delivery at term. *British Medical Journal* **305**, 746–7.

6   Labour and birth after a previous caesarean section

Introduction

Women who have had a previous caesarean section may request a vaginal birth in subsequent pregnancies because they want to experience the satisfaction of giving birth themselves. Additionally, many women dread the thought of caring for a new baby and other children when recovering from the major abdominal surgery that results from having a caesearean section. Women who opt for a vaginal birth after a previous caesarean section are usually advised to labour and birth in hospital because of the possibility of uterine rupture from the previous caesarean scar. However, some women will choose to give birth at home and some of those who choose hospital may decline certain aspects of their care (such as having a cannula *in situ* or remaining on continuous fetal monitoring).

The chance of achieving a vaginal birth after a caesarean (VBAC) is not significantly altered by the reason for the first caesarean which may include 'cephalopelvic disproportion', 'failure to progress' or having had more than one previous caesarean section (Enkin, 2000). Around 75% of VBAC women do give birth vaginally, but the remaining 25% who have repeat caesareans will do so for many reasons although rarely for uterine rupture (Horn, 2003).

In putting the rates into perspective Enkin (2000) states that the risk of having an emergency caesarean section for serious acute conditions in labour (such as for fetal distress, antepartum haemorrhage or cord prolapse) is 2.7%, or up to 30 times more likely than for a uterine rupture with a planned vaginal birth after a caesarean section.

Incidence

- Just over half of the cases of true rupture of the uterus are in women who have not had a previous caesarean section (Enkin, 2000).
- Women who have had a previous caesarean section, who subsequently opt for a vaginal delivery, have a between 0.09 and 0.8% chance of having a scar rupture (Enkin, 2000).
- Enkin (2000) states that women who have had three or more previous caesarean sections are only at a marginally increased risk of scar dehiscence (asymptomatic separartions of the uterine scar).

Facts

- There are several contraindications to a trial of labour. Factors that appear to carry a significant risk of rupture include if the incision is unknown, classical or a low vertical incision, or the woman has had a previous hysterotomy (Enkin, 2000), or the 'single-suture closure technique' (Gaskin, 2002) has been used (more commonly in the USA).
- Caesarean sections are associated with maternal morbidity and serious, potentially life-threatening, complications such as pulmonary embolism and deep vein thrombosis (Wagner, 2000). They also increase the chance in a subsequent pregnancy of placenta praevia and placenta accreta (Langdana *et al.*, 2001), both of which are linked to uncontrollable blood loss, hysterectomy and maternal death (Bakshi & Meyer, 2000).

- Vaginal deliveries have fewer complications, less risk of infection or haemorrhage (Wagner, 2000), shorter recovery times, and something that many women crave, the potential for a more fulfilling birth experience (NCT, 1999; Horn, 2003).

Midwifery care

Care at induction of labour

It is only wise to attempt to induce labour when there is a genuine, valid indication to do so.

Women hoping for a vaginal birth can need lots of extra support. This is an opportune time to discuss the woman's previous birth and for the midwife to offer positive information, explanation and reassurance.

Criteria and care at induction are otherwise the same as any woman undergoing an induction of labour. NICE (2001a) guidelines recommend that the induction should take place on the labour ward where more staff are available to monitor the woman. The *Report on Confidential Enquiries into Maternal Deaths* (DoH, 1998) recommend one low dose of the prostaglandin Prostin® in 24 hours for any woman with a scar on her uterus. Suspected hyperstimulation at induction has resulted in maternal death from a ruptured uterus (DoH, 1998).

Enkin (2000) suggests that the evidence supports selective, appropriate use of artificial rupture of the membranes (ARM) and/or oxytocin (see also the bullet point 'slow labour' under the heading 'Other procedures' on page 99).

Labour care in hospital

A woman who has had a previous caesarean is usually considered 'high risk'. Below are common guidelines for care in an obstetric unit. (Care at home or in a birthing centre is covered on pages 99–101.) However, their use is not all based on evidence of their effectiveness, more on routine and assumed advantages they may confer if something goes wrong. Bearing in mind that a ruptured uterus is infrequent, many women will have consented to interventions which are not benign in themselves and not without morbidity. Therefore, the midwife providing care can advise and give information but it must remain the woman's decision as to whether she wishes to consent to all or some of these 'procedures' or interventions.

Labour support and information sharing

Horn (2003) suggests women who have had a previous caesarean section often experience a great deal of trepidation when they consider a vaginal birth. They may have experienced an earlier arduous labour or a frightening emergency situation which will be hard for them to forget. Many women naturally dread the possibility of reliving the experience.

It is vital to give clear explanations and lots of reassurance and support to the woman in labour and her birthing partner(s). Discuss her birth plan, her expectations and discuss the likelihood of various scenarios. The indication for the previous caesarean should be discussed in relation to its relevance, if any, on the possible outcome of the current labour.

Wainer Cohen (1991) suggests that a woman needs more reassurance and support around the same time in her labour when she had the previous caesarean section.

Electronic fetal monitoring

There is no one specific fetal heart rate (FHR) or uterine activity pattern that indicates the onset of a uterine rupture, although retrospective review of casenotes/cardioto-cographs (CTGs) by Menihan (1999), identified that a significant number of women with uterine rupture exhibited variable and/or late decelerations commonly leading to the onset of an FHR bradycardia. Such information leads most obstetricians to recommend continuous fetal monitoring of the heart rate for any woman who has had a previous caesarean.

It is commonly assumed that having continuous fetal monitoring in high-risk cases confers benefits. However, robust randomized controlled trials (RCTs) suggest this is not the case (Grant, 2000). NICE (2001) draw on the more controversial 'expert opinions' to conclude that women deemed high risk should be 'offered' continuous EFM during labour. Continuous monitoring significantly increases obstetric intervention, including the caesarean section rate, something VBAC women are trying to avoid. The woman may decide to opt for intermittent auscultation (IA) in order to increase her chances of achieving a normal birth (Beech Lawrence, 2001). Chapter 17 provides more information on monitoring the fetal heart rate.

Other procedures

- **Siting a cannula**. This may not be required, but if an emergency occurs, it is hypothesized that a cannula already *in situ* will save time, especially if the woman has poor veins or if she becomes shocked and peripherally shut down. If the woman consents to a cannula in labour it will need to be flushed 4–6 hourly with 5 ml of normal saline to ensure it remains patent. Some women will not want a cannula as a 'just in case' measure, and would rather wait until a direct indication arises.
- **Bloods**. These are taken for a full blood count analysis (FBC) and cross matching, and are commonly sent to be stored in the Pathology Laboratory where they can be tested in the event of an emergency.
- **Fasting**. This has traditionally been enforced upon any woman at possible risk of an emergency caesarean section and general anaesthetic. Johnson *et al.* (2000) state that aspiration of gastric contents still occurs with general anaesthetics administered to women who have fasted, as gastric aspiration is a problem associated with poor anaesthetic technique when administering a general anaesthetic and not with having food in the stomach. Since fasting can lead to poor progress, the diagnosis of dystocia and a cascade of interventions, it should be avoided (Johnson *et al.*, 2000).
- **Regular antacids/hydrogen ion inhibitors** (such as ranitidine, cimetidine). These encourage rapid emptying of the stomach contents, as well as reducing the acidity of the stomach. Evidence supports their use as conferring possible benefit should an emergency anaesthetic be required (Johnson *et al.*, 2000).

- **Epidural**. Some clinicians recommend epidurals 'just in case' a caesarean is needed. Epidurals are not always advisable due to their various side effects and complications in someone aiming to attain a normal birth. However, some clinicians also recommend that a woman with a scar on her uterus should avoid an epidural for fear that it may mask the pain of a ruptured uterus which would then go unnoticed. Enkin (2000) claims that this is unlikely. Each case is individual. Women should have an epidural only if they want one for pain relief or because there is a direct benefit, such as an impending caesarean section.

- **Slow labour**. Enkin (2000) suggests that the evidence supports the appropriate use of artificial rupture of the membranes (ARM) and/or the use of oxytocics. It is not necessary to terminate a slow labour with a caesarean just because the obstetrician is fearful of using oxytocics in this scenario. Judicious use should be confined to women who genuinely require it and it must be used with caution to prevent hyperstimulation of the uterus. Close observation of the strength, frequency and duration of the contractions is required. Chapter 4 also deals with other methods to stimulate uterine contractions in Table 4.1.

- **Second and third stages**. Care should be as per a normal labour.

  A scar on the uterus is not a contraindication to a physiological third stage. Be aware that although rare, there is an increased chance of placenta accreta, following a previous caesarean section (Langdana *et al.*, 2001). This serious, and potentially life-threatening, condition can only be accurately predicted antenatally by magnetic resonance imaging (MRI) scanning, although the expense of MRI usually deters its routine use (Horn, 2003). Ultrasound may indicate a low, anterior placenta which suggests the possibility of placenta accreta, but it is not usually accurately diagnosed until manual removal is attempted (AAFP, 2000/2001). An adherent placenta is usually evidenced by not only its failure to deliver but also by bleeding (which may be concealed) if it has partially separated. The doctor should be informed promptly and the woman observed for signs of shock. Placental bleeding may be concealed behind the actual placenta. In such a case, the blood loss is impossible to assess as it may not 'come away' until the placenta is delivered.

Preparing for birth at home/birthing centre

While the majority of birthing centres do not usually encourage VBAC, a home birth after a caesarean is more of an option for women. It is up to each mother to make an informed choice about whether it is right for her. In order to make that choice she needs accurate information. She has a right to choose to stay at home and she also has a right to unemotive, unbiased information about the possible risks associated with VBAC. It is up to each woman to assess the information about the relative risks of hospital and home VBAC in her own individual circumstances and to make her own decision. Women who find they are not comfortable, or not supported by their community midwife, often turn to independent midwives who are usually experienced in attending VBACs at home and in hospital (Horn, 2003).

- **Support groups and information sharing**. The midwife can advise the woman about support groups for information, support and advice (see 'Useful contacts' at the end of this chapter).

- **Documentation**. During the antenatal period, the community/independent midwife should inform the supervisor of midwives (SOM) of the woman's decision to birth at home/birthing centre. Clear documentation of her decision and related conversations had with her, if appropriate, should be documented.
- **Weighing up the risks**. The midwife should put the risks into perspective, for example over half of all ruptured uteri are in women who have no scar on their uterus. Labour at home is physiological and not artificially stimulated. Any serious obstetric emergency at home/birthing centre poses significant delays (compared to a hospital) in receiving appropriate assistance. So although the risk of a ruptured uterus in labour is infrequent (a 0.09–0.8% chance of uterine rupture), if it was to occur, the woman must be aware that it is a potentially life-threatening emergency. The midwife will need to discuss with her client the estimated time it would take to transfer to hospital in any emergency and the possible implications of this delay for the woman and her baby.

Labour care at home/birthing centre

Care should proceed as per normal labour. Chapter 2 also covers the care of a woman having a home birth.

- **Transfer**. The transfer rate for a woman attempting a VBAC at home is thought to be higher than the national average as midwives and mothers tend to be cautious and transfer at the first sign of trouble. The *National Birthday Trust Report* found that 28% of its small sample of mothers planning home VBACs transferred for a variety of reasons although none was for a ruptured uterus (Chamberlain *et al.*, 1994).
- **Ruptured uterus**. Be aware of the signs and symptoms of a ruptured uterus (see Box 6.1). See page 201 for a description of the basic care for shock and maternal collapse.
- **Emergencies**. Midwives should plan in advance what would happen in the possible event of a serious obstetric emergency, such as a scar rupture.
- **Precautionary optional interventions**. The woman or midwife may wish to consider a cannula *in situ*, the taking of bloods, or the use of antacids/hydrogen ion inhibitors during labour.

Suspected ruptured uterus at home/birthing centre

- Call a paramedic ambulance.
- Ask them to inform the labour ward who should in turn inform relevant staff, theatres and blood bank, etc., so they can prepare for the woman's arrival.
- While awaiting the ambulance/and during transit:
  - treat for collapse/shock – two large cannula, commence intravenous (IV) fluids, run quickly and give oxygen
  - check the woman's pulse and the FHR. In a serious rupture, the woman may quickly become shocked. In a severe ruptured uterus, the outlook may be bleak for the baby and the fetal heart may not be audible

    ○ if at all possible, prepare as best as possible for theatre before arrival at hospital. Remove jewellery, ensure the woman has an identity/allergy bracelet and anything further the midwife may manage to achieve to expediate the process.

Chapter 2 also covers emergency transfer to hospital from a home birth.

Signs and symptoms of uterine scar rupture

Be vigilant. Although uncommon, the uterus can rupture in the antenatal period, at induction, during labour/birth, and even during the third stage of labour. Not all women have the clear scar pain by which diagnosis is obvious. Some women may simply become uncomfortable, quiet, even restless or agitated. It is this change in their behaviour that can be quite distinctive and indicative of a rupture. Box 6.1 provides a summary of signs and symptoms to watch out for.

Box 6.1 Signs and symptoms of uterine scar rupture.

Pain
- Sudden uterine or scar pain.
- A feeling of 'giving way' (Silverton, 1993).
- The lower abdominal pain may come with a contraction, or be a constant unrelenting pain.
- The woman may find it too painful to have her uterus touched or palpated.

Uterus/contractions
- Solid, tonic uterus, or
- Contractions may stop or dwindle.

Fetal heart rate
Abnormal fetal heart changes may occur such as a prolonged or variable decelerations, usually progressing to a serious bradycardia (Menihan, 1999).

Shock
- The woman may look:
  - ○ pale, cool and clammy
  - ○ restless, agitated or withdrawn
  - ○ she may say she is frightened and that something is wrong
  - ○ she may vomit.

- Changes in vital signs:
  - ○ tachycardia
  - ○ sometimes low blood pressure
  - ○ breathlessness, respirations > 24 breaths per minute.

Bleeding
- Bleeding may sometimes be evident from the vagina, as blood-stained amniotic fluid or as a fresh bleeding.
- Sometimes, such as after the baby is born, a ruptured uterus may start to rise, as it fills with blood
- Placenta accreta is undeliverable vaginally, as the placenta is imbedded into the myometrium. It is associated with a previous scar on the uterus. This serious complication can be life threatening for the woman and is associated with uncontrollable bleeding which may necessitate hysterectomy (Bakshi & Meyer, 2000; Langdana *et al.*, 2001).

If there is any doubt, an experienced obstetrician should be contacted immediately. If at home or a birthing centre then immediate transfer to hospital in a paramedic ambulance is indicated.

A ruptured uterus – a childbirth emergency

- Call for help – emergency obstetric team consisting of anaesthetist, obstetrician, paediatrician, midwifery staff.
- Proceed to immediate delivery.
- If an instrumental birth is indicated (during the second stage) the woman will need to go straight to theatre afterwards for uterine repair.
- Treat for shock – intravenous infusion (IVI), bloods for cross-matching, etc. (see also Chapter 12, including Box 12.6 for information on basic care for shock).
- For care at home/birthing centre see previous heading 'Suspected ruptured uterus at home/birthing centre'.

Summary

In hospital

- Care as per normal labour, but in addition:
  - ○ Cannula (flushed 4–6 hourly) is an optional precaution, advisable if the woman has poor veins
  - ○ Bloods taken (test only in an emergency)
  - ○ Eating and drinking is not contraindicated
  - ○ Regular use of antacids/hydrogen ion inhibitors.
- Cardiotocograph (CTG) may be recommended, but evidence suggests this does not necessarily confer benefits.
- Be vigilant for signs of uterine rupture.
- Prostaglandin/ARM/oxytocics can be used with caution and are not contra-indicated.
- Epidural is not contraindicated.

At home/birthing centre

- Clearly documented discussion(s) about home birth after a previous caesarean.
- Care as above.
- Be prepared for transfer if necessary.

Useful contacts

Association for Improvements in the Maternity Services (AIMS)   AIMS Helpline: 0870 765 1433. Website: www.aims.org.uk

Caesarean Support Network   55 Cooil Drive, Isle of Man IM2 2HF. Telephone: 01624 661269.

Home birth reference website   www.homebirth.org.uk [VBAC at home].

National Childbirth Trust (NCT)   Alexandra House, Oldham Terrace, Acton, London W3 6NH. Enquiry line: 0870 444 8707. Website: www.nct-online.org

References

AAFP (2000/2001) *Advanced Life Support in Obstetrics (ALSO). Course Syllabus Manual*, 4th edn. American Academy of Family Physicians, Leawood, Kansas.

Bakshi, S. & Meyer, B.A. (2000) Indications for and outcomes of peripartum hysterectomy: a five-year review. *Journal of Reproductive Medicine* **45** (9), 733–7.

Beech Lawrence, B. (2001) Electronic fetal monitoring: do NICE's new guidelines owe too much to the medical model of childbirth? *The Practising Midwife* **4** (7), 31–3.

Chamberlain, G., Wraight, A. & Crowley, P. (1994) *National Birthday Trust Report – Report of the Confidential Enquiry into Home Births*. Parthenon Publishing Group, London.

DoH (1998) *Why Mothers Die, 1994–1996. Report on Confidential Enquiries into Maternal Deaths in the United Kingdom*. Department of Health, The Stationery Office, London.

Enkin, M. (2000) Labor and birth after a previous caesarean section. In *A Guide to Effective Care in Pregnancy and Childbirth*, 3rd edn (Enkin, M., Keirse, M.J.N.C., Neilson, J. *et al.*, eds), pp. 359–71. Oxford University Press, Oxford.

Gaskin, I. (2002) An interview with Ina May Gaskin. Interviewer: Sarah Wickham. *The Practising Midwife* **5** (1), 38–9.

Grant, A. (2000) Care of the fetus during labor. In *A Guide to Effective Care in Pregnancy and Childbirth*, 3rd edn (Enkin, M., Keirse, M.J.N.C., Neilson, J. *et al.*, eds), pp. 267–80. Oxford University Press, Oxford.

Horn, A. (2003) VBAC at home. Website: www.homebirth.org.uk (accessed April 2003).

Johnson, C., Keirse, M.J.N.C., Enkin, M. & Chalmers, I. (2000) Hospital practices – nutrition and hydration in labor. In *A Guide to Effective Care in Pregnancy and Childbirth*, 3rd edn (Enkin, M., Keirse, M.J.N.C., Neilson, J. *et al.*, eds), pp. 255–66. Oxford University Press, Oxford.

Langdana, F., Geary, M., Haw, W. *et al.* (2001) Peripartum hysterectomy in the 1990s: any new lessons? *Journal of Obstetrics and Gynaecology* **21**, 121–3.

Menihan, C.A. (1999) The effect of uterine rupture on fetal heart rate patterns. *Journal of Nurse-Midwifery* **44** (1), 40–46.

NCT (1999) Caesarean Section – Extent of Choice, 2nd edn. National Childbirth Trust, London.

NICE (2001a) *Clinical Guideline D – Induction of Labour*. National Institute for Clinical Excellence, London.

NICE (2001b) *Clinical Guideline C – The Use of Electronic Fetal Monitoring*. National Institute for Clinical Excellence, London.

Silverton, L. (1993) *The Art and Science of Midwifery*. Prentice Hall International, London.

Wagner, M. (2000) Choosing caesarean section. *The Lancet* **356**, 1677–80.

Wainer Cohen, N. (1991) *Open Season: Survival Guide for Natural Childbirth and VBAC in the 90s*. Bergin and Gavery, New York.

7 Pre-eclampsia

Annette Briley

Introduction

The information given in this chapter is intended as background information and is based on currently available evidence. It is intended to increase the understanding of midwifery care and the management of women with pre-eclampsia.

Pre-eclampsia is a condition peculiar to pregnancy, characterized by raised blood pressure (BP) and proteinuria. It can be associated with seizures (eclampsia) and multi-organ failure in the mother, while fetal complications include growth restriction and placental abruption (Shennan & Chappell, 2001).

Increased maternal and fetal morbidity and mortality are the consequences of pre-eclampsia. In the developed world, this disease is a leading cause of maternal death, and in the UK most of these deaths are associated with suboptimal care, particularly by intrapartum carers (Kaunitz *et al.*, 1985; DoH, 1996).

Underlying pathophysiology of pre-eclampsia

Pre-eclampsia is associated with abnormal implantation of the placenta and concomitant shallow trophoblastic invasion (Pijnenborg,1994) leading to reduced placental perfusion. The maternal spiral arteries (also colloquially known as the uterine arteries) fail to undergo their normal physiological vasodilation; blood flow may be further impeded by atherotic changes causing obstruction within the vessels.

This pathology causes increased resistance in the uteroplacental circulation with impaired intervillus blood flow, and results in ischaemia and hypoxia which is manifested during the second half of pregnancy (Graham *et al.*, 2000).

A similar picture of inadequate trophoblastic invasion is also apparent in pregnancies complicated by fetal growth restriction in women with no pre-eclampsia. This suggests that the maternal syndrome of pre-eclampsia must be associated with additional factors.

Incidence

The prevalence of pre-eclampsia varies according to the characteristics of the population and the definitions used to describe it (Davey & MacGillivray, 1988; Chappell *et al.*, 1999).

- It occurs in less than 5% of most populations, and recent prospective studies have indicated an incidence as low as 2.2%, even in a primigravid population which is known to have a higher prevalence (Higgins *et al.*, 1997).
- Up to 20% of all pregnant women will be hypertensive during pregnancy, of these less than 10% will suffer serious disease.
- Pregnancy-induced hypertension (PIH) is elevated BP with no proteinuria and no pathology related to the pregnancy. Pregnancy-induced hypertension is approximately three times more common than pre-eclampsia (Shennan & Chappell, 2001).
- The International Society for the Study of Hypertension in Pregnancy (ISSHP) have adopted the term 'gestational hypertension' to describe all hypertensive women, with or without proteinurea, who were normotensive with no proteinuria previously.

- In the UK less than 10 women will die each year but in the less developed world 50 000 maternal deaths per year are attributed to eclampsia, and a similar number are estimated from pre-eclampsia (Duley, 1992).

Facts

- All midwives will see women with pre-eclampsia throughout their professional lives.
- Antenatal women with pre-eclampsia need close monitoring. Placental insufficiency is a common problem in early onset pre-eclampsia and this can lead to intrauterine growth restriction (IUGR), placental abruption or intrauterine death.
- Late onset hypertension (after 37 weeks) rarely results in serious morbidity for mother or baby. However, hypertension that presents early results in the majority of women developing the syndrome of pre-eclampsia (Shennan & Chappell, 2001).
- In severe pre-eclampsia the main causes of maternal death are cerebral haemorrhage and adult or acute respiratory distress syndrome (DoH, 2001). Therefore management during the intrapartum period concentrates on *blood pressure control* and *fluid balance*.

Associated risk factors

- There is a well-established genetic link; a family history of a mother or sister increases risk four- to eight-fold (Lie *et al.*, 1998).
- There is evidence of a paternal influence. Women have twice the risk if pregnant by a partner who has previously fathered an affected pregnancy (Need *et al.*, 1983).
- Pre-eclampsia is ten times more likely to occur in first pregnancies; miscarriages and terminations of pregnancy offer some protection against this disease in subsequent pregnancies (Strickland *et al.*, 1986).
- Multiple pregnancies have more than double the risk (Duley *et al.*, 2001).
- A new partner returns a woman's risk to that of a primigravida (McCowan *et al.*, 1996).
- Obesity (those with a body mass index of > 29) increases risk four-fold (Shennan *et al.*, 1996). The UK has the highest levels of obesity in Europe.
- Underlying maternal medical conditions increase risk: chronic hypertension (Kyle *et al.*, 1995), renal disease (Cheston, 1996), glucose intolerance including gestational diabetes (Duley *et al.*, 2001), previous pre-eclampsia (20% risk of recurrence) and underlying thrombotic tendency, particularly antiphospholipid syndrome (Brown *et al.*, 1998).

Signs and symptoms

Clinicians cannot rely on BP and proteinuria alone to diagnose pre-eclampsia as these are only clinical signs of end organ damage. Just under 50% of all women presenting with eclampsia will have had no previous hypertension or proteinuria (Douglas & Redman, 1994).

The diagnosis must be considered in women with fetal involvement or other signs such as:

- Epigastric pain.
- Headache/visual disturbances.
- Intrauterine growth restriction (IUGR).
- Note: Oedema is no longer considered an effective sign of pre-eclampsia, the only exception to this is rapid onset facial oedema.

Severe pre-eclampsia is considered in the presence of:

- Severe hypertension (greater than 160/110 mmHg), or
- Hypertension with additional symptoms, such as:
  - headache
  - visual disturbance
  - epigastric pain
  - clonus (brisk reflexes)
  - platelet count below 100 ($\times 10^9$ per litre)
  - aspartate transaminase (AST) more than 50 IU/l

All women presenting in the antenatal period with hypertension and proteinuria should have:

- A symphysis fundal height assessment.
- A cardiotocogram (CTG).
- Ultrasound assessment of fetal growth.
- Liquor volume assessment (ammotic fluid index – AFI).
- Umbilical artery Doppler analysis.
- In some units a uterine artery Doppler waveform assessment may also be carried out.

Maternal observations should include:

- Regular BP and proteinuria checks.
- Blood tests (see also 'Pre-eclampsia' under the heading 'Blood tests for specific conditions and blood pictures' on page 252).
  - Platelet count. Endothelial dysfunction results in platelet dysfunction. If the platelet count is greater than 50×10^9 per litre haemostasis is likely to be normal, but delivery is often considered if the platelet count falls below 100.
  - Clotting studies. Necessary because pre-eclampsia can cause disseminated intravascular coagulation.
  - Uric acid or urate levels. These are used to assess the severity of the disease and its progression. However, severe disease can occur in the presence of normal uric acid concentration.
  - Plasma urea and creatinine concentrations. Raised levels of these are generally associated with late renal involvement and serious disease. They are not a useful *early* indicator of disease severity, but should be obtained longitudinally to assess the progression of renal involvement.
  - Liver function tests. Pre-eclampsia can cause several problems in the liver, for example subcapsular haematoma, rupture and hepatic infarction.
- Some units undertake uterine artery Doppler waveform anaylsis. This is undertaken at 20–24 weeks gestation and is not repeated after 24 weeks because there is no variation after this time (Bower *et al.*, 1993).

Intrapartum care of a woman with pre-eclampsia

Assessing blood pressure and urine testing

Box 7.1 summarises the main points of assessing BP and urine testing.

Box 7.1   Assessing blood pressure (BP) and urine testing.

Diastolic
- Diastolic BP $\geq$ 90 mmHg on two or more consecutive occasions 4 or more hours apart, *or*
- Diastolic BP $\geq$ 110 mmHg on any one occasion.

Mean arterial pressure (MAP)
- MAP between 125 and 140 mmHg for more than 45 minutes will require medical referral and treatment.
- MAP $\pm$ 140 mmHg for more than 15 minutes, then urgent medical aid and treatment is required.
- MAPs over 150 mmHg represent serious risk of cerebral autoregulatory dysfunction and subsequent risk of cerebral haemorrhage.

Proteinuria
- One 24-hour collection with total protein excretion $\geq$ 300 mg per 24-hours, *or*
- Two 'clean-catch midstream' or catheter specimens of urine collected 4 or more hours apart measuring 2 or more ++ on reagent strip.

During labour/postnatally:
- The quality of the specimen is important during labour and postnatally, hence catheter specimens should be taken to reduce the risk of contamination from lochia and liquor.
- In borderline pre-eclampsia a clean-catch mid-stream specimen can be used, however, if the protein content appears high then a catheter specimen is advisable.

Severe hypertension (see also 'Signs and symptoms' in the 'Introduction')
- Systolic > 160 mmHg or diastolic $\geq$ 110 mmHg or a MAP > 125 mmHg (DoH, 2001).

If the woman is symptomatic:
- Inform clinical team (senior midwife/obstetricians and anaesthetists, SCBU/NICU, consultant obstetrician/anaesthetist and neonatologist are aware).
- Treatment – hydralazine infusion.

Blood pressure measurement

Care with blood pressure measurement is essential. There is plenty of evidence in the literature to suggest that this is often poorly performed, commonly impacting on practice. Factors to consider include:

- **Digit preference**. Rounding the final digit of the BP to 0 occurs in more than 80% of BP measurements in antenatal care and therefore lacks accuracy (Shennan & Shennan, 1996).
- **Correct cuff**. The midwife should always use the appropriately sized cuff. The standard bladder used (23 × 12 cm) is *too* small for approximately 25% of the pregnant population, and its incorrect use results in over diagnosis of hypertension because this 'undercuffing' commonly results in an overestimation of BP by more than 10 mmHg. Overcuffing has the opposite, although far smaller effect, by underestimating BP by less than 5 mmHg (Shennan & Shennan, 1996).

Measure the woman's arm circumference; if it is *greater than* 33 cm, and therefore the bladder size is less than two-thirds the circumference of the arm, you need a *large* adult cuff.

- **Maternal positioning**. Ensure the woman is positioned correctly with the mercury scale at the level of the heart.
- **Movement and concentration**. Avoid moving and talking during the procedure. This is especially important when using an automated device, as movement will mean the machine will be unable to record the BP accurately.
- **Check automated devices**. Make sure they have been validated for use in pregnancy. If not, or you are unsure, use mercury sphygmomanometry where possible. It is the 'gold standard'. Some automated devices will display 'ERR' or bleep to let the clinician know the BP needs repeating, others do not. Check which type you are using. Most automated devices have been found to under record BP in pre-eclampsia. Appendix A lists the machines that have been validated for use in pregnancy and pre-eclampsia.
- **Korotkoff's sounds**. During measurement keep the rate of cuff deflation at 2–3 mm/second. This prevents over diagnosis of diastolic hypertension. Korotkoff phase 4 (the fading or changing of the sound) is *no longer recommended*, due to problems with reproducibility. Several randomized controlled trials (RCTs) have shown it is both safe and appropriate to use Korotkoff phase 5 (the disappearance of sound) (Shennan *et al.*, 1996).

Urine testing

During urine testing discrepancies can arise with the interpretation of proteinuria. False negatives and positives are common when using dipstick urinalysis. So:

- Any previous 24-hour urine collections should be used to confirm diagnosis.
- Women with proteinuria greater than 300 mg in 24 hours should be considered at risk.
- New innovations in bedside automated devices relating proteinuria to creatinine, with proven accuracy, are likely to aid clinical practice in the near future.

Care during labour

Most units have developed a protocol for the management of the sick pre-eclamptic woman in labour. All midwives should know where it is and that it is updated as new evidence becomes available.

The decision to deliver will depend on maternal and fetal condition, and gestation. This will influence the place and mode of delivery, which ideally should take place in a consultant unit with neonatal care facilities (DoH, 1996). Multidisciplinary communication and documentation regarding management of labour, tests results and decisions is essential to ensure a high standard of care. It is important that the midwife caring for the woman should have experience of providing high-risk care and if not, should be supported and supervised by a more experienced colleague.

Preterm birth

Pre-eclampsia is a major cause of iatrogenic prematurity. Many pre-eclamptic women are induced or delivered preterm, and many babies will be admitted to the neonatal unit following delivery, accounting for 15% of all preterm deliveries. If less than 34 weeks, the administration of maternal corticosteroids has been shown to reduce respiratory problems in the newborn (Guinn *et al.*, 2001).

If time allows, liaise with the woman and her family and the neonatal unit. This may include a visit or meeting the staff. Some women may require transfer to a specialist neonatal unit and this is likely to be very frightening for the woman and her family. Taking time to explain what is happening and why may offer some reassurance.

Midwifery support

Due to the increased medicalization and surveillance during labour and delivery, it is easy for the midwife to focus on monitoring the woman to the neglect of the woman's psychological needs. Explanations regarding recommended interventions must be given in terms that the woman and her partner understand. Talking in a relaxed voice and providing appropriate lighting can help add to an atmosphere of calmness, which can communicate to all those involved in caring for the woman in labour.

Often women with pre-eclampsia can become very sick very quickly and they are often frightened by this. They need constant reassurance and explanation, as do other family members, in order to make sense of what is happening.

Monitoring maternal and fetal condition

- Blood pressure
  - Blood pressure should be recorded every 15 minutes (see Box 7.1).
  - Beware that the devices used, cuff size, positioning and technique are subject to inaccuracies (for more information see 'Blood pressure measurement', page 109).
  - Many labour ward protocols use mean arterial pressure (MAP) to influence management.
- Fluid balance
  - Maintain a strict fluid balance chart.
  - In moderate to severe pre-eclampsia, ensure the woman has intravenous (IV) access, with a suitable cannula for the administration of IV fluids or medication. This is particularly important if the woman has a fit.
  - Women who are severely ill will probably not want to eat or drink in labour. However, most women will want some oral fluids. Because fluid management can be critical in such women, local protocols may advise the restriction of fluids in labour to a predefined amount.
  - Antacids are usually recommended to pre-eclamptic women routinely during labour because they are at increased risk of operative delivery.

Monitoring the fetal heart rate

Continuous CTG is recommended (NICE, 2001) for monitoring the fetal heart rate (FHR) and any abnormality in the trace reported and action taken including fetal blood sampling (FBS), where appropriate (see also the algorithm given in Appendix E).

Analgesia

General comfort measures, including verbal reassurance, touch, massage and adopting comfortable positions (within the restrictions of monitoring equipment) should not be forgotten. These simple, non-invasive measures may help to promote a feeling of being supported and cared for which should help the woman to cope with the stressful experience of a closely monitored labour.

In severe pre-eclampsia epidural/spinal analgesia is the preferred method of pain relief both for labour and operative deliveries. Policies vary between units but if the woman's platelets are considered extremely low – around 80 or lower – an epidural may not be advisable. Epidurals are recommended because they cause vasodilation which can result in a reduction in the BP and attenuate any surges in BP. They are also advantageous should an operative delivery be indicated. Intubation (GA) is best avoided and is less likely to be needed if there is an effective epidural/spinal anaesthetic because it causes hypertension and laryngeal oedema, both of which can make the whole process hazardous. However, the ultimate choice is the woman's and if she declines epidural or spinal anaesthesia, once she knows the reasons why they are recommended, the midwife must support her in that decision.

Second stage

- Management of the second stage will depend on maternal and fetal well-being. If the condition of both allows, often a 'normal' second stage is conducted. In moderate to severe pre-eclampsia there tends to be a low threshold for instrumental delivery.
- Ensure experienced medical aid is nearby, and there are two midwives caring for the woman in the room at this time.
- Spontaneous pushing, while not discouraged, is not encouraged until the vertex is clearly visible on the perineum. The BP should be checked between contractions. Active pushing/Valsalva is contraindicated as it involves directed, prolonged breath holding and prolonged bearing down which alters heart rate and stroke volume.
- The supine position is associated with compression of the distal aorta and reduced blood flow to the uterus and lower extremities (Sleep *et al.*, 2000). It also prolongs the second stage, causes a reduction in circulating oxytocin and causes fewer contractions and FHR abnormalities (Gupta & Nikodem, 2002). Side lying or appropriate alternative postures are preferable.

Anaesthesia

General anaesthesia should be avoided wherever possible, as intubation can cause severe hypertension.

Drugs used in the treatment of severe hypertension

If the woman has not delivered, colloids are usually infused before treatment is initiated to maintain uteroplacental circulation and thus prevent hypotension and concomitant fetal distress.

Hydralazine

Hydralazine is commonly used in the acute management of women with hypertension and is titrated against the woman's blood pressure.

- 5 mg IV in fluid
- Repeated every 20 minutes at 5 mg IV
- With a maximum cumulative dose of 20 mg (DoH, 2001).

After repeated doses, if the BP remains *high* or the woman is tachycardic (> 120 bpm) labetalol can be added or used to replace hydralazine.

Labetalol

Labetalol is given as:

- 20 mg IV, at 10-minute intervals
- Increasing by 40 mg, 80 mg and 80 mg
- Up to a cumulative dose of 300 mg (DoH, 2001).

Oral Labetalol is also used in mild cases but this will depend on local protocols.

Glyceryl trinitrate

Glyceryl trinitrate may be infused postnatally as a third line of treatment for severe hypertension.

Care of a woman receiving drug treatment for severe hypertension

- Monitor closely, ensuring the BP reduces *gradually*.
- Monitor the FHR for signs of fetal compromise.
- Low threshold for CVP line.

Fluid balance management

Because women with pre-eclampsia have leaky capillary membranes and a predisposition to low albumin levels, they can be prone to pulmonary oedema if fluid administration is excessive or unmonitored. General guidelines include:

- Strict fluid balance charts should be maintained.
- These women are strongly advised to have a catheter *in situ*.
- A urometer is used to accurately record output each hour.
- 100 ml output over 4 hours is sufficient and most protocols limit colloid fluid intake to 85 ml per hour.

HELLP syndrome

HELLP syndrome (H = haemolysis, EL = elevated liver enzymes, LP = low platelets) is a severe complication of pre-eclampsia. The degree of severity of HELLP syndrome is *not dependent* on the severity of hypertension; it is also reported in normotensive women.

Underlying pathophysiology of HELLP

Impaired liver function is an element of HELLP syndrome.

Haemolysis

Haemolysis is the breakdown of red blood cells causing the release of haemoglobin into the blood plasma. This is a normal process at the end of the life span of each red blood cell (RBC) after around 120 days. Normally this haemolysis is slow enough for the RBC to be removed by the liver, spleen and bone marrow. When this process occurs more rapidly, and RBC production is unable to keep up the resultant decrease in the number of circulating RBCs, it causes microangiopathic haemolytic anaemia.

Elevated liver enzymes

HELLP syndrome impairs liver function. Women commonly complain of epigastric pain, which is caused by obstruction of blood flow in the hepatic sinusoids by intravascular fibrin deposition.

Low platelets

Platelets are the first line of defence against bleeding. They work by:

- Plugging holes in capillaries (primary haemostasis)
- Initiating coagulation
- As the blood escapes through bigger holes, eventually platelets become an integral part of most clots

Thrombocytopenia is due to the increased consumption or destruction of platelets.

Incidence

- Occurs in 0.2% of all pregnancies.
- It is more common in women with proteinuric hypertension (affecting 4–12% of women with pre-eclampsia or eclampsia).

Signs and symptoms

- HELLP syndrome is commonly diagnosed when the results of pre-eclampsia blood tests are reviewed.

- Women may complain of epigastric pain.
- Women may bleed excessively (for example at a cannula site) and the blood fail to clot.

Care of a woman with HELLP syndrome

Once HELLP syndrome is evident, *urgent delivery* is required. However, this is problematic due to:

- Problems with low platelets, therefore regional blocks are contraindicated.
- The woman is a poor candidate for general anaesthesia (GA) as intubation increases BP.
- The woman will bleed excessively at caesarean section.
- These women already have a coagulopathy, with reduced intravascular volume, therefore a postpartum haemorrhage is particularly problematic.

Consequently management includes:

- Low threshold for central venous pressure (CVP) line.
- It is imperative to accurately record fluid balance.

Management of eclampsia

When pregnant women fit, due to pre-eclampsia, it is known as eclampsia. This suggests it is different from many other sorts of convulsion, such as those due to epilepsy, but in fact this is not the case. In the event of a fit, it is important to stabilize the mother before the baby is delivered. Remember: *eclampsia is an absolute indication for urgent delivery* once the maternal condition is stabilized. It is extremely important that the midwife explains everything that is going on to the woman and her birth partners/ relatives.

Note: If a pregnant woman presents in a semi-conscious or drowsy state then *non-eclamptic convulsions* should be considered. Other conditions such as epilepsy are more likely to be the cause than eclampsia.

Incidence

Less than 1% of women with pre-eclampsia will have an eclamptic fit (Shennan & Chappell, 2001).

Facts

- Prophylactic use of anticonvulsants is controversial (Duley and The Magpie Collaborative Group, 2002).
- The Collaborative Eclampsia Study (Duley *et al.*, 1995) showed that the administration of magnesium sulphate following a convulsion, when compared to diazepam and phenytoin, resulted in significantly less maternal ventilation, pneumonia and fewer Intensive Therapy Unit admissions.

Signs and symptoms preceding an eclamptic fit

Sometimes eclampsia is preceded by the woman feeling:

- Unwell
- Headache
- Blurred vision
- Epigastric pain
- Nauseated, and she may vomit
- She may become confused and disorientated

Often there is *no* warning.

Care during/following an eclamptic fit

Immediate action

- **Keep calm!**
- **Summon help.**
  - ○ Get medical aid, and others to help.
  - ○ Pull the emergency bell if in hospital, dial 999 if at home.
- **Ensure the woman is in a safe environment.**
  - ○ Remove obvious dangers.
  - ○ Do not try to restrain the woman.
  - ○ Ensure that, once the fit has finished, the woman is in the left lateral position as this allows optimal uteroplacental blood flow.
- **Note the time and length of the fit.**

Subsequent action

- **Gain IV access**. This will enable IV drugs to be administered and blood to be taken.
- **Monitor the baby**. Use CTG *in situ*.
- **Maternal observations**
  - ○ BP.
  - ○ Proteinuria (via catheter specimen).
- **Catheterize**. This will mean that urinary output and urine can be accurately monitored.
- **Reassure**
  - ○ Talk camly and quietly to the woman throughout and afterwards reassure her constantly even though she may appear semi-conscious.
  - ○ Reassure the woman's partner and other relatives where possible, they will be very frightened by this.
- **Documentation**. Record all events accurately, including the details of the length/time of the actual fit.

Drugs used in the treatment of eclampsia

Magnesium sulphate anticonvulsant therapy

Check *local protocols* for the regime used where you work. These are updated as evidence emerges. A typical magnesium sulphate anticonvulsant therapy regime involves

- A loading dose of 4 g given slowly over 5–10 minutes.
- As a maintenance infusion of 1–2 g/hour, usually at the discretion of the consultant.
- Continue infusion for at least 24 hours following the last seizure.
- Recurrent seizures should be treated by a further bolus of 2 g magnesium sulphate (DoH, 2001).

Other drugs

'If repeated seizures occur despite the use of magnesium sulphate, options include diazepam (10 mg IV) or thiopentone (50 mg IV). Intubation may become necessary in such women in order to protect the airway and ensure adequate oxygenation. Further seizures should be managed by intermittent positive pressure ventilation and muscle relaxation' (RCOG, 2003).

Care of a woman receiving magnesium sulphate anticonvulsant therapy

Monitor the woman for:

- **Reflexes**. Conduct hourly clinical monitoring of the patella reflexes. If absent magnesium sulphate therapy should be stopped.
- **Respiration**. Monitor respiration rate hourly. If there is a respiration rate of less than 14 respirations a minute and/or a pulse oximetry of less than 95% O_2 saturation then magnesium sulphate therapy should be stopped.
- **Blood levels**. Blood samples may be taken to assess magnesium levels 1 hour after commencing the maintenance dose and repeated at 6-hourly intervals. The therapeutic range is 2–4 mmol/l
  - if the *serum urea* is > 10 mmol/l, *or*
  - if the magnesium level is > 4 mmol/l,
    then the dose needs to be *reduced*
  - if magnesium levels are < 1.7 mmol/l then the dose needs to be *increased*.
- **Fluid balance**. Observe urinary output hourly. Magnesium is excreted through the kidneys and therefore the dose will be need to be reduced if oliguria persists (output less than 100 ml/4 hr).

The midwife should also monitor that the woman is tolerating the treatment.
Signs of toxicity include:

- Reduced/absent patella reflexes.
- Weakness.
- Nausea.
- Hot flushes.

- Blurred vision.
- Slurred speech.

Summary

- Severe pre-eclampsia is typically BP $\geq 160/110$ mmHg or MAP ≥ 125 mmHg (DoH, 2001) or hypertension BP $\geq 140/90$ mmHg and proteinurea (≥ 0.3 g/day or $\geq 2+$) with symptom(s): headache/visual disturbances/epigastric pain/clonus.
- Blood picture including low platelets < 100.
- Clinicians should be alert to women who present with atypical symptoms (DoH, 2001).

Labour care

- BP should be recorded every 15–20 minutes.
- Check the automated devices are validated for use in pre-eclamptic women.
- Many labour ward protocols use mean arterial pressure (MAP) to influence management.
- Maintain a strict fluid balance chart.
- Ensure intravenous access, with a suitably sized cannula.
- In severe pre-eclampsia a catheter with a urometer is used to accurately record output each hour with a 100 ml per 4-hour output being sufficient. Most protocols limit fluid intake to 85 ml/hr.

Hydralazine infusion

- If administered during labour colloids may be infused before treatment is initiated.
- Monitor closely – ensure the BP reduces *gradually*.
- CTG.
- CVP line if oliguric or fluid overload.

Eclampsia

- When pregnant women fit due to pre-eclampsia it is called eclampsia.
- Eclampsia is an absolute indication for immediate delivery.

Magnesium sulphate anticonvulsant therapy

- Hourly patella reflexes/hourly O_2 saturation of $>95\%$ or magnesium sulphate therapy to be stopped.
- Observe for signs of toxicity.
- Blood magnesium levels 1 hour after commencing treatment, repeated 6 hourly. Therapeutic range is 2–4 mmol/l.
- Observe urinary output hourly for oliguria (output less than 100 ml/4hr).

Useful contacts

Action on Pre-eclampsia (APEC)   84–88 Pinner Road, Harrow, Middlesex, HA1 4HZ. Telephone: 020 8863 3271. Helpline: 020 8427 4217. Website: www.apec.org.uk

Confidential Enquiry into Stillbirths and Deaths in Infancy (CESDI) on 1 April 2003 changed to Confidential Enquiry into Maternal and Child Health (CEMACH)   CEMACH Central Office, Chiltern Court, 188 Baker Street, London NW1 5SD. Telephone: 020 7486 1191.

Tommy's, the baby charity 1 Kennington Road, London SE1 7RR. Telephone: 08707707070. Information line: 0870 777 3060. Website: www.tommys-campaign.org Research, education and information for parents and professionals.

References

Bower, S., Bewley, S. & Campbell, S. (1993) Improved prediction of pre-eclampsia by two stage screening of uterine arteries using the early diastolic notch color Doppler imaging. *Obstetrics and Gynecology* **82**, 78–83.

Brown, M.A., Buddle, M.L., Farrell, T., Davis, G. & Jones, M. (1998) Randomised trial of management of hypertensive pregnancies by Korotkoff phase IV or phase V. *The Lanchet* **352**, 777–81.

Chappell, L.C., Seed, P.T., Briley, A.L. *et al.* (1999) Prevention of pre-eclampsia by antioxidants: a randomised trial of vitamins C and E in women at increased risk of pre-eclampsia. *The Lancet* **347**, 810–16.

Cheston, T. (1996) Pre-eclampsia. In *Midwifery Practice: Core Topics I* (Alexander, J., Levy, V., Roch, S., eds), pp. 132–46. Macmillan, London.

Davey, D.A. & MacGillivray, I. (1988) The classification and definition of the hypertensive disorders of pregnancy. *American Journal of Obstetrics and Gynecology* **158**, 892–8.

DoH (1996) *Why Mothers Die, 1991–1993. Report on Confidential Enquiries into Maternal Deaths in the United Kingdom.* Department of Health, HMSO, London.

DoH (2001) *Why Mothers Die, 1997–1999. The fifth report of the Confidential Enquiries into Maternal Deaths in the United Kingdom.* Department of Health, RCOG Press, London.

Douglas, K.A. & Redman, C.W.G. (1994) Eclampsia in the United Kingdom. *British Medical Journal* **309**, 1395–400.

Duley, L. (1992) Maternal mortality associated with hypertensive disorders of pregnancy in Africa, Asia, Latin America and the Caribbean. *British Medical Journal* **99**, 547–53.

Duley, L., Carroli, G., Belizan, J. *et al.* (1995) Which anticonvulsant for women with pre-eclampsia – evidence from the collaborative eclampsia trial. *The Lancet* **345**, 1455–63.

Duley, L., Henderson-Smart, D., Knoght, M. & King, J. (2001) Antiplatelet drugs for prevention of pre-eclampsia and its consequences: systematic review. *British Medical Journal* **322**, 329–33.

Duley, L. & The Magpie Collaborative Group (2002) Do women with pre-eclampsia and their babies benefit from magnesium sulphate? The Magpie Trial: a randomised placebo-controlled trial. *The Lancet* **359**, 1877–90.

Graham, C.H., Postovit, L.M., Park, H., Canning, M.T., & Fitzpatrick, T.E. (2000) Adriana and Luisa Castellucci Award Lecture 1999: The role of oxygen in the regulation of trophoblast gene expression and invasion. *Placenta* **21**, 443–50.

Guinn, D.A., Atkinson, W., Sullivan, L. *et al.* (2001) Single vs weekly courses of antenatal steroids for women at risk of preterm delivery. *Journal of the American Medical Association* **286**, 1581–7.

Gupta, J.K. & Nikodem, V.C. (2002) Woman's position during the second stage of labour (Cochrane Review). *The Cochrane Library* Issue 4. Update software, Oxford.

Higgins, J.R., Walshe, J.J., Halligan, A., O'Brien, E., Conroy, R. & Darling, M.R. (1997) Can 24-hour ambulatory blood pressure measurement predict the development of hypertension in primigravidae. *British Journal of Obstetrics and Gynaecology* **104**, 356–62.

Kaunitz, A.M., Hughes, J.M., Grimes, D.A., Smith, J.C., Rochat, R.W. & Kafrissen, M.E. (1985) Causes of maternity mortality in the United States. *Obstetrics and Gynecology* **65**, 605–12.

Kyle, P.M., Buckley, D., Kissane, J., de Swiet, M. & Redman, C.W. (1995) The angiotensin sensitivity test and low-dose asprin are ineffective methods to predict and prevent hypertensive disorders in nulliparous pregnancy. *American Journal of Obstetrics and Gynecology* **173**, 865–72.

Lie, R.T., Rasmussen, S., Brunborg, H. *et al.* (1998) Fetal and maternal contributions to risk of pre-eclampsia: population based study. *British Medical Journal* **316**, 1343–7.

McCowan, L.M., Buist, R.G., North, R.A. & Gamble, G. (1996) Perinatal morbidity in chronic hypertension. *British Journal of Obstetrics and Gynaecology* **103**, 123–9.

Need, J.A., Bell, B., Meffin, E. & Jones, W.R. (1983) Pre-eclampsia in pregnancies from donor insemination. *Journal of Reproductive Immunology* **5**, 329–38.

NICE (2001) *Clinical Guideline C – The Use of Electronic Fetal Monitoring.* National Institute for Clinical Excellence, London.

Pijnenborg, R. (1994) Trophoblastic invasion. *Reproductive Medicine Review* **3**, 53–73.

RCOG (2003) *Clinical Green Top Guidelines: Management of Eclampsia (10).* Royal College of Obstetricians and Gynaecologists website: www.rcog.org.uk (accessed May 2003).

Shennan, A., Gupta, M., Halligan, A., Taylor, D.J. & de Swiet, M. (1996) Lack of reproducibility in pregnancy of Korotkoff phase IV by mercury sphygmomanometry. *The Lancet* **347**, 139–42.

Shennan, A.H. & Chappell, L.C. (2001) Pre-eclampsia. *Contemporary Clinical Gynaecology and Obstetrics* **1**, 353–64.

Shennan, C. & Shennan, A. (1996) Blood pressure in pregnancy: the need for accurate measurement. *British Journal of Midwifery* **4** (2), 102–108.

Sleep, J., Roberts, J. & Chalmers, L. (2000) The second stage of labor. In *A Guide to Effective Care in Pregnancy and Childbirth*, 3rd edn (Enkin, M., Keirse, M.J.N.C., Neilson, J. *et al.*, eds), pp. 289–99. Oxford University Press, Oxford.

Strickland, D.M., Guzick, D.S., Cox, K., Grant, N.F., & Rosenfeld, C.R. (1986) The relationship between abortion in the first pregnancy and development of pregnancy-induced hypertension in the subsequent pregnancy. *American Journal of Obstetrics and Gynecology* **154**, 146–8.

8 Preterm labour and birth

'The birth of a baby should be one of the most special and joyful experiences a family can have and yet every year thousands of families experience the pain of losing a baby or seeing a tiny child fight for life.' (Briley *et al.*, 2002)

Introduction

'Preterm labour is defined as the occurrence of regular uterine activity which produces either effacement or dilatation prior to 37 completed weeks of pregnancy . . . The term threatened preterm labour is often used to describe pregnancies complicated by clinically significant uterine activity but without cervical change' (WHO, 1975)

The birth of a preterm baby can have devastating effects on the parents and family who are usually totally unprepared for such an event. Preterm labour can occur for a variety of reasons. Preterm births are more commonly associated with babies presenting in a malpresentation or an abnormal lie, and are more prevalent in multiple pregnancy and among babies with congenital malformations (Keirse, 2000).

In comparison to term births, preterm deliveries are more often associated with pre-existing conditions such as:

- Infection.
- Pre-eclampsia.
- Antepartum haemorrhage.
- Placenta praevia.
- Inadequate fetal growth.
- Severe disease in the mother.

Incidence

- 6.7% of births in the UK are preterm, i.e. under 37 weeks gestation (DoH, 1997).
- A significant number of babies are delivered preterm due to iatrogenesis, such as pre-eclampsia/eclampsia, placental abruption.
- Less than a quarter of preterm births occur before 32 weeks gestation (Atalla *et al.*, 2000; Keirse, 2000).

Facts

- Identifying women at risk of preterm labour remains imprecise, and prediction does not equate to prevention. Although there are various promising prediction methods, including cervical scanning and biochemical markers (fetal fibronectin, salivary oestriols, interleukins), as yet, there is no *one* totally reliable means of predicting preterm delivery (Briley *et al.*, 2002).
- As survival rates in babies increase so does the level of disability, relative to gestation (Costeloe *et al.*, 2000; CESDI, 2001).
- Higher survival rates in preterm infants have been attributed to (CESDI, 2001):
  - cephalic babies born vaginally
  - singleton deliveries
  - babies with a higher weight for gestation

○ sex of the baby – female babies have a 90.1% chance of survival and male babies a 86.3% chance.

- Risks of preterm birth include fetal death, intraventricular haemorrhage (70% for babies under 26 weeks, 30% at 26 weeks and rare after 33 weeks gestation [Atalla *et al.*, 2000]). Respiratory distress syndrome (RDS) affects 90% of babies born at 26 weeks and is virtually non-existent by term (Atalla *et al.*, 2000). Other complications include cerebral palsy, blindness and deafness, infection, hypoglycaemia, hypothermia, jaundice, necrotizing enterocolitis, and retinopathy of prematurity (Steer & Flint, 1999; Atalla *et al.*, 2000; Keirse, 2000; Keynon, 2001a).

Place of birth

In order to determine the best place for the baby to be born, clinicians first need to establish an accurate gestation. This will be most accurate if based on an early ultrasound scan (Neilson & Grant, 2000). The gestation for transfer varies between facilities but generally:

- Babies less than 32 weeks gestation may benefit from specialist neonatal facilities.
- Evidence suggests that extremely preterm infants (24–28 weeks gestation) should be born in a unit with specialist neonatal facilities.
- Some preterm babies are born unplanned at home. Such babies may require prompt transfer to a hospital with the appropriate facilities. Unplanned preterm delivery at home is considered later in this chapter.

Transfer guidelines

For some women, transfer to a hospital with specialist neonatal facilities may be indicated. In an estimated 50% of preterm transfers, the woman's condition makes transportation hazardous (Atalla *et al.*, 2000) and 17% of mothers transferred in preterm labour, end their transfer in adult intensive care (Steer & Flint, 1999).

If the decision is made to transfer then photocopy the woman's notes to take on transfer.

- The midwife and a trained paramedic should always accompany the woman during transfer (CESDI, 2003).
- Staff involved in transfers should be trained in transfer arrangement (CESDI, 2003).

Do not transfer a woman if:

- The birth is approaching rapidly (usually evident by strong contractions, every 2 or so minutes, and the woman's heavy breathing or increasing 'distress').
- The woman's condition appears unstable – such as a woman who is actively haemorrhaging (such as from a placenta praevia) or she has severe pre-eclampsia.

Use of antibiotics

There is increasing evidence that infection is a major causative factor in preterm labour (Kenyon *et al.*, 2001a). In suspected or diagnosed infection, intravenous (IV) antibiotics should be commenced (Kenyon *et al.*, 2001a) even before a diagnosis of infection can be confirmed by blood tests, cultures and swabs (DoH, 2001).

If the woman's membranes have ruptured, broad-spectrum antibiotics (such as erythromycin) should be recommended, as these appear to hold benefits for the baby including a possible reduction in childhood disability (Kenyon *et al.*, 2001a).

In preterm labour, if there is no evidence of infection and no ruptured membranes, the ORACLE II trial found that antibiotics were not of benefit and, therefore, not indicated (Kenyon *et al.*, 2001b).

Prophylactic corticosteriods

Women should be aware that antenatal corticosteriods appear to benefit the preterm baby because they encourage the release of pulmonary surfactant in the fetal lungs.

- *Every effort should be made to administer a corticosteroid regime* (CESDI, 2003), as this is the single most effective intervention in reducing respiratory complications, necrotising enterocolitis, intraventricular haemorrhage and mortality in preterm infants (Crowley, 2002; CESDI, 2003).
- Corticosteroids reduce RDS by 40–60% (Crowley, 2002).
- Following the first course of steroids babies get the maximum benefit after 24 hours and for up to 7 days (Crowley, 2002).

Currently controversy exists over whether single or multiple doses of corticosteroids are the most beneficial in women undelivered but still at risk. Repeat doses of antenatal corticosteroids should not be routinely administered as multiple doses may be associated with possible increased morbidity in infants (Guinn, 2001; SPCERH, 2002).

The use of corticosteroids such as betamethasone is covered in Chapter 23.

Diagnosing labour

Threatened preterm labour and actual preterm labour are not necessarily distinguishable at the onset. Various tests, including biochemical tests such as detecting fetal fibronectin (arising from changes in the membranes and uterine wall) and cervical ultrasound, are not yet widely available (Walkinshaw, 2001).

Every unit should have clear guidelines for the diagnosis of preterm labour and its subsequent management.

Preterm, prelabour rupture of the membranes (PPROM)

Preterm, prelabour rupture of the membranes (PPROM) is the most common event preceding preterm delivery and is present in 30–40% of cases. PPROM has a high association with maternal infection (Kenyon *et al.*, 2001a). The use of antibiotics was dealt with above.

- If PPROM occurs between 24 and 34 weeks, half of the women will deliver within 4 days, 70–80% within 1 week (Walkinshaw, 2001).
- Survival rates in PPROM are directly linked to gestation at membrane rupture rather than duration of membrane rupture, with a high risk of chorioamnionitis and pulmonary hypoplasia in very preterm infants (Walkinshaw, 2001).

- Maternal sepsis is estimated at around 2% in women with PPROM, and is a rare but significant danger to the mother's health (Walkinshaw, 2001) Mild maternal pyrexia and fetal tachycardia are the most common signs of infection/chorionitis (Wang & Smaill, 2000). Maternal infection is covered further in Chapter 9.

Regular contractions

Opinions vary, but Walkinshaw (2001) suggests 8 contractions in 60 minutes. Painful contractions coming regularly should be monitored.

Cervical dilatation

A speculum examination should be performed, *in preference to a digital examination*, in order to visualise the cervix, or take swabs. CESDI (2003) found that too many inappropriate digital examinations were performed in preterm labour.

- Digital examination should be avoided in preterm labour, as it may introduce organisms into the os, and may augment labour (Atalla *et al.*, 2000. CESDI, 2003).

Digital examination is *contraindicated* in suspected infection or PPROM (CESDI, 2003).

Mode of delivery

The mode of delivery remains controversial. The CESDI (2001) report examining data on babies born at 27–28 weeks gestation found that of those of cephalic presentation 53% were delivered by caesarean section, 44.1% were spontaneous vaginal and 2.7% had an instrumental vaginal delivery. Survival rates for babies with cephalic presentation were significantly higher for those babies born by spontaneous vaginal birth and forceps delivery (91.7% and 91.2%, respectively) than those born by caesarean (87.3%). It is speculated that perhaps those born by caesarean are more compromised, hence the poorer results. Keirse (2000) found that there is no evidence to support any advantage to a caesarean birth over a vaginal birth for:

- An uncompromised, preterm infant.
- The extremely preterm infant.
- A preterm breech infant.
- A severely malformed baby.

Undertaking a caesarean section on a poorly formed, lower-uterine segment carries significant risks of complications for the woman (Atalla *et al.*, 2000). Caesarean should also be avoided in the presence of suspected chorioamnionitis (Atalla *et al.*, 2000).

Delaying delivery by drug use

A group of drugs known as tocolytics is often used to attempt to delay delivery. These include betamimetics (such as ritodrine, terbutaline and salbutamol), prostaglandin synthetase inhibitors (such as Indomethicine) and oxytocin antagonists (such as Astoban). These drugs are used in the hope of allowing time to:

- Administer a corticosteroids regime.
- Commence antibiotics.

- Allow for time for transfer to a specialist neonatal unit, if necessary.
- To delay severe prematurity at around 24 weeks. At this stage of gestation 24–48 hours may make a difference to the baby's survival.
- Once the steroid course and/or transfer to a specialist unit have been completed, there is no benefit in the betamimetic infusion continuing (Joint Formulary Committee, 2003).

Betamimetics are the most commonly used drugs to delay preterm delivery but can have serious side effects. Details on the care of a client with a ritodrine infusion are covered in Chapter 23.

The use of betamimetics does not appear to improve perinatal mortality (Keirse, 2000).

Tocolytics should be avoided in women with:

- A fetal death or a fetal abnormality that is incompatible with life (Walkinshaw, 2001).
- A fetal or maternal condition requiring urgent delivery (Walkinshaw, 2001).
- Active bleeding (as tocolytics relax the uterus).
- Preterm rupture of the membranes (PROM) and/or infection. Here there is probably no benefit in stopping labour (Keirse, 2000).

Care related to specific causes of preterm labour

Listed below are some specific types of preterm labour, in addition see later in this chapter under the heading 'Midwifery care during a non-complicated preterm labour and birth'.

Very preterm infants (22–26 weeks) and babies with lethal malformations

In 10–15% of all preterm births the baby has died before the onset of labour or has lethal malformations that are incompatible with life (see also Chapter 13). Fetal death, or a baby with abnormalities incompatible with life, will come as a shock to the parents and this can be a deeply distressing time. Keirse (2000) recommends that care in such cases should be directed at maternal, rather than the baby's, interests.

The increasing survival rates of very preterm infants are compounded by an increasing level of disability (CESDI, 2001). The EPICure study in 1995 found that of babies born at 25–26 weeks gestation, half of the survivors had either mental and psychomotor development disabilities, neuromotor function disabilities, sensory and communication function disabilities (Costeloe *et al.*, 2000).

Specific care

- Due to heightened emotions and anxiety, many parents cannot take in information given to them at such a stressful time (Calam *et al.*, 1999). Carers must be prepared to repeat explanations and talk sensitively, in understandable terms, about the possible outlook, however bleak, for the baby. Ballard *et al.* (2002) found that neonatologists tend to defer to the parental requests rather than adhering to their best judgement. This was particularly marked if parents were considered litigious.

This, Ballard *et al.* suggest, may increase the resuscitation of infants born near the limits of viability.

- An ultrasound scan should be available at this time to exclude serious abnormalities and to confirm presentation (Keirse, 2000).
- There is unlikely to be any direct benefit for the baby in performing a caesarean section. The lower segment is poorly formed and maternal morbidity is higher (Keirse, 2000).
- Staff trained in neonatal resuscitation and thermal care of neonates and *at least one experienced clinician* experienced in tracheal intubation should attend the birth of any infant less than 28 weeks' gestation (CESDI, 2003).
- Paediatrician(s)/neonatologist(s) should document and discuss with the woman and her partner prior to the birth:
  - the approximate outlook/possible prognosis for their baby
  - the likely events that will follow at birth
  - whether to commence or withhold treatment/resuscitation in a very preterm or seriously malformed baby.

Breech presentation

Breech presentation is more common among preterm infants and is associated with higher antepartum stillbirth and neonatal mortality rates than cephalic preterm babies (Keirse, 2000). This is in part due to the increased incidence of congenital abnormalities associated with preterm breech presentations and not necessarily with the mode of delivery (Atalla *et al.*, 2000; Keirse, 2000).

Specific care

- Midwives working in all environments are likely to be the only professional available when faced with an unplanned breech delivery (Robinson, 2000). Midwives must ensure they have the training, knowledge and skills to deal with such an occurrence (CESDI, 2000).

Delivery of breech babies is also covered in Chapter 5.

Twins

Twins have a prevalence towards being born preterm. CESDI (2001) suggest that the assumed higher mortality rate of twins (compared to singletons) was not evident in their study of 27–28-week gestation deliveries.

Specific care

- Ultrasound scanning should be available to confirm the presentations of both twins.
- Avoid causing complications, encourage upright positions, especially for the birth. Avoid lithotomy, unless genuinely required, because it is likely that the second twin will have problems descending. Avoid inappropriate interventions, such as

artificial rupture of the membranes (ARM) for a second twin, with the potential to cause serious problems. Patience is needed.

- Extra staff and resuscitation equipment should be prepared in advance to receive both babies.
- Despite the extra people in the room, try to preserve the woman's privacy and maintain a calm atmosphere.

Preterm birth at home

Preterm birth at home, sometimes without any clinician present, has a high mortality and these, usually unplanned deliveries, affect the statistics for home birth in general.

Specific care

- **Care cannot be very prescriptive** as preterm births at home occur in a variety of situations. They are frequently unplanned, quick deliveries, which may present the midwife with the problems of a compromised preterm baby and, occasionally, an acutely ill mother. However, they may be very straightforward.
- **Hypothermia** is a very real risk to the preterm infant (CESDI, 2003). It is *vital* to dry the baby well at birth and initiate skin-to-skin contact, as this has a stabilising effect on preterm infants (Christensson *et al.*, 1992). Keep the room warm (25°C or above) and the baby dry.
- **Delay cord clamping** (Keirse, 2000; Mercer, 2001). Clamp and cut the cord leaving it long and encourage early feeding (Whitelaw *et al.*, 1998) providing the baby's condition is satisfactory.
- **Transferring to hospital** is probably advisable in any baby pre 35–36 weeks. Bear in mind that many preterm babies can appear well at delivery but can develop difficulties in the hours following birth.
- Unless requiring active resuscitation, to keep the baby warm tuck the baby skin-to-skin with mum for the transfer (Christensson *et al.*, 1998). Box 8.1 deals with the advantages of skin-to-skin contact and resuscitation is covered in Chapter 21.

Midwifery care during a non-complicated preterm labour and birth

'From the parents' point of view, a premature baby raises a multitude of difficulties, especially since the outcome for any individual baby is never certain. Their experience is, by definition, too early and is often shrouded in the trappings of emergency, panic and heightened medical intervention. Irrespective of infant outcome the experience itself is often highly stressful and long-term ramifications have been noted'. (Sherr, 1995)

Maternal anxiety and stress

In addition to addressing the parent's fears about their preterm baby, try reducing external stressful stimuli caused by bright lights, noise, interruptions and lack of privacy. This is not just about being 'thoughtful', it is about reducing the psychological

Box 8.1   Advantages of skin-to-skin contact (not just cuddled or held).

Stabilizing affect on preterm infants
- The stress of separation from the mother can have serious, negative, physical consequences. The newborn even has a separation distress cry (Christensson *et al.*, 1992).
- Separation increases the baby's stress response, respiratory effort and oxygen requirements.

Maternal-infant attachment enhanced
Skin-to-skin contact enhances maternal-infant attachment (De Chateau & Wilbert, 1997) this can be particularly important for preterm babies due to the later separations, which can occur if the baby is admitted to SCBU/NICU.

Superior thermoregulation
Thermoregulation provides warmth which, even in babies weighing 1500 g, is a superior form of warming when compared to radiant overhead heaters or incubators (Christensson *et al.*, 1998).

Enhanced father-infant attachment
- One study of preterm infants found that the earlier fathers held their preterm babies, the sooner they reported positive feelings towards them (Sullivan, 1999).
- While prolonged skin-to-skin contact is essential for the mother and baby, midwives can be proactive in involving the father in giving skin-to-skin contact.

Breastfeeding benefits
Improved duration of breastfeeding, compared to preterm infants who were merely held but were denied direct skin-to-skin contact (Whitelaw *et al.*, 1998). Breastfeeding is particularly important for preterm infants.

---

stress for the woman with all its very physical side effects. Stress hormones, among other effects, do reduce pain tolerance, inhibit contractions, affect progress and decrease the flow of oxygen to the placenta and baby (Ginesi & Niescierowicz, 1998a, b); Ockenden, 2001). In creating a calm room, others who enter it will also be notably more relaxed!

Preparation for a baby born early – parental fears

- As for any woman in labour, the woman in preterm labour needs one-to-one midwifery support in order to help her cope with pain and to enable her, despite her concerns for her tiny baby, to have a positive birth experience (see also Boxes 1.4 and 1.5 and Chapter 15 for further details on helping women cope with labour).
- Due to the heightened parental anxiety, staff may need to repeat explanations several times and talk in more understandable terms (Calam *et al.*, 1999).
- Discuss with the woman/couple the likely events that will follow in labour and at the birth: who will be present; if resuscitation is anticipated, to what level; and the likelihood of their baby requiring special care.
- Ideally, the parents should visit the SCBU/NICU (Neonatal Intensive Care Unit) prior to birth. If labour is advancing, suggest that her partner visit. It is also potentially beneficial for a member of the neonatal team to come and talk to the parents (CESDI, 2003).

FIRST STAGE OF LABOUR

A woman in preterm labour can be supported and monitored much as anyone in labour. In the absence of medical complications, vital signs and contractions should be monitored as per normal labour. The woman should be supported to eat and drink, ambulate and so on.

Checklist

- Establish an accurate gestation.
- Administer a corticosteroids regime.
- Are antibiotics indicated?
- Are the relevant people aware? Liaise with the midwife in charge/paediatrician/ SCBU/Neonatal Unit/confirm a cot is available.
- Theatre staff including the anaesthetic team should be informed.
- Prepare the birth environment/resuscitation equipment.

Care in the first stage of labour

- **Remain mobile and upright**. This will aid optimal fetal positioning (essential to enhance the normal progress and safe descent of the small baby). Lying in the supine position should be avoided as it increases fetal heart rate (FHR) abnormalities (Gupta & Nikodem, 2002) which are more likely to occur in a preterm birth (Atalla *et al.*, 2000).
- **Eating and drinking** is not contraindicated (Johnson *et al.*, 2000).
- **Regular antacids/hydrogen ion inhibitors** (such as ranitidine, cimetidine) may confer benefits should an emergency anaesthetic be required (Johnson *et al.*, 2000).
- **Comfort and pain relief**. The 'safest' form of pain relief is continuous, supportive one-to-one midwifery care in labour, as this is proven to reduce interventions and improves both maternal and fetal outcomes (Hodnett, 2002). Avoid narcotic analgesics such as pethidine which can cause respiratory depression, drowsiness and depressed reflexes – including suppressing the reflex to suck (Joint Formulary Committee, 2003).

Iatrogenic interventions

As a midwife, it can be difficult to challenge routine-based care when clinicians assume the advantages outweigh the disadvantages. However, iatrogenic, invasive, interventions should be avoided unless deemed absolutely essential.

- Digital vaginal examination may increase the rate of ascending infection and has been shown to shorten the preterm prelabour rupture of the membranes (PPROM) delivery interval (CESDI, 2003).
- Discuss alternative ways of monitoring progress with the obstetric team. Avoid performing vaginal examinations without a valid indication and certainly not for the sake of 'routine'. Midwives should ask themselves, 'what information will be gained by performing a vaginal examination?', particularly since preterm labour is unlikely to need augmenting (see also 'Assessing progress in labour' in Chapter 1).

- Artificial rupture of the membranes is not advisable with any baby at increased susceptibility of cord compression (such as growth-restricted babies or oligohy-dramnios [Moore, 1996] preterm babies) or cord prolapse (in 50% of cases of cord prolapse ARM is a direct cause [Prabulos & Philipson, 1998]). Artificial rupture of the membranes increases the risk of severe variable FHR decelerations (Goffinet *et al.*, 1997) and is not advisable in maternal infection (including Group B Strepto-coccus and HIV).

Monitoring fetal well-being

Evidence suggests that in preterm infants electronic fetal monitoring (EFM) confers no advantage over intermittent auscultation (IA) and significantly increases obstetric interventions and maternal morbidity (Atalla *et al.*, 2000; Grant, 2000). It should be considered that preterm infants have different heart patterns to term infants as the baby's immature autonomic nervous system responds to stress (Atalla *et al.*, 2000). An abnormal trace may require the assessment of fetal acidosis via blood sampling. This should be considered in the absence of maternal infection from 34 weeks gestation (NICE, 2001).

Preterm infant heart rate patterns:

- Higher baselines, sometimes 170 bpm (Davis, 1997).
- More prone to reduced variability, tachycardia and bradycardia (Atalla *et al.*, 2000; Walkinshaw, 2001).
- Variable decelerations occur in more than 75% of preterm labours (Atalla *et al.*, 2000).
- Very preterm babies can be difficult to continuously monitor and, therefore, can only be monitored intermittently.
- Despite worrying features on the preterm cardiotecograph (CTG), the majority of babies will not be acidotic (Atalla *et al.*, 2000).

SECOND STAGE OF LABOUR

Some preterm infants may be born quicker than anticipated. Be ready to deliver the baby into a warm, relaxed atmosphere with the appropriate people present and resuscitation equipment pre-prepared. Give the baby straight to the mother for important skin-to-skin contact while you assess the baby's condition (see Box 8.1).

- **Full dilatation**. Consider are the signs there? Give it a little time. Avoid a vaginal examination to confirm what may be evident.
- **Avoid arbitrary time limits**. Time limits should not be placed on the duration of the second stage as there is no link between time per se and poor neonatal outcome. 'If the mother's condition is satisfactory, the baby's condition is satisfactory, and there is evidence that progress is occurring with descent of the presenting part there are no grounds for intervention' (Sleep *et al.*, 2000).
- **Non-active pushing is vital** to avoid fetal compromise, lower Apgars, and forceps intervention (Keirse, 2000; Gupta & Nikodem, 2002). So do not allow directed prolonged breath holding and bearing down (Sleep *et al.*, 2000). Reassure the woman that she is doing well when pushing at her own pace.

- **No benefit from using an episiotomy and/or forceps** to protect the preterm baby's delivering head. A forceps delivery is only justifiable in cases of diagnosed fetal compromise as forceps may confer more harm than good. (Keirse, 2000; Sleep *et al.*, 2000). Episiotomy has only two indications, primarily for acute fetal compromise and occasionally for an unyielding perineum. Due to the preterm baby's smaller head, an unyielding/rigid perineum is unlikely to be a problem.
- **Ventouse** is not recommended in births before 34 weeks gestation, due to the soft skull of the baby (Atalla *et al.*, 2000).

Care at/immediately after birth

- Skin-to-skin contact and delayed cord clamping should be considered a safe way of giving optimum care to low-risk preterm babies and not a 'luxury'. Always deliver the baby straight into the mother's arms (see Box 8.1).
- If the paediatrician is flexible, and the baby requires just basic suction and oxygen, it can be a bonus if this can be completed with the baby still attached to its umbilical cord and in mum's arms. If administering oxygen via a funnel, ensure this does not waft and cool the baby.
- For resuscitation that is more intensive, the baby will need to be taken to the heated resuscitaire.

THIRD STAGE OF LABOUR

Delayed cord clamping is very important for preterm infants. However, many staff are unaware that simple resuscitation measures can take place with the baby still attached to its cord.

- Even in active management delayed cord clamping is associated with great advantages including a 50% increase in red cell volume, which reduces the duration of supplemental oxygen dependence and reduces the red cell transfusion requirements due to anaemia in preterm babies (Keirse, 2000).
- Large studies have supported the theory that delayed clamping appears to be 'disadvantage free' for preterm babies. Despite the higher haematocrit levels in late clamped preterm infants, there is no increase in symptomatic polycythemia or jaundice (Mercer, 2001).
- Transfusion via the cord is 'quicker' if the baby is held below the level of the uterus for 30–60 seconds, which may be important in distressed or hypovolaemic (pale/mottled skin) infants in need of early separating from the cord for resuscitation purposes (Mercer, 2001).
- Keirse (2000) summarizes by stating that there is no justification for rushing to clamp and cut the cord unless intensive paediatric resuscitation is required. When eventually clamping the cord prior to cutting it, leave the baby's end long in case the baby later requires umbilical catheterization.

Preparation of the environment for the birth

Liaise with colleagues before the birth is imminent. The delivery suite co-ordinator may well keep other clinicians up to date so that the midwife can remain with the woman. The co-ordinator can then contact other staff on the midwife's behalf, for example when she rings the buzzer.

Very preterm babies, babies with suspected abnormalities, or severely compromised babies will require a consultant paediatrician/neonatologist present for the birth. In such births, the paediatrician will probably require assistance from a dedicated midwife or SCBU/NICU nurse to assist solely in resuscitation. It will remain the paediatrician's decision to commence or withhold treatment and this is normally discussed with the woman and her partner prior to the birth. This should not be the responsibility of junior staff (Keirse, 2000).

Preparations should include:

- The room should be 25°C or above (WHO, 1997), the windows shut and fans switched off.
- The resuscitaire should be checked, stocked and switched on in the birthing room.
- Warm towels should be available to dry the baby and a warm hat and clothing for the baby to wear available.
- The paediatrician/neonatologist experienced in intubation should be aware and present.

Resuscitation

- Keep newborns warm, dry and draught free during resuscitation.
- Even if the baby is very unwell, let the mother hold her baby or at least look at his or her face and touch the baby before he/she is taken to the SCBU/NICU.
- If the baby requires transfer to the SCBU, encourage the woman's birth partner to go too. The partner may be 'sent back' but at least they will have seen where the baby is going and, once the baby has been stabilized, can return to visit.
- Ensure, where possible, that the baby is labelled and has up-to-date notes to take to SCBU/NICU.

Neonatal resuscitation is covered further in Chapter 21.

Summary

- Identifying women at risk of preterm labour remains imprecise. A previous preterm birth is the single best predictor of preterm delivery.
- As survival rates in babies increase so does the level of disability, relative to gestation.
- Parents may be extremely worried and unable to retain information. Explanations may need repeating, with sensitivity and in simple terms.
- If a specific maternal, or fetal, complication occurs treat with the appropriate care.

Evidence supports:

- Administration of a corticosteroid regime.
- Appropriate cot available for gestation.
- Antibiotics in PPROM or if infection thought present in the woman.
- Appropriately skilled persons available and dedicated to providing resuscitation.

- Keep the birthing room warm, minimize draughts and dry the baby at birth.
- Skin-to-skin contact for the baby at birth for thermoregulation, stabilization of respiration, heart rate and reduced stress response. (Minor care, suction and funnel oxygen should be administered with the baby still attached via the umbilical cord.)
- Delay clamping of the cord and leave the baby's cord long.

Evidence supports *avoiding*:

- ARM/or 'routine' vaginal examinations.
- Narcotic analgesia.
- Active pushing.
- Prone maternal position.
- Non-indicated episiotomy/forceps.
- Early clamping of the umbilical cord.

Useful contacts

BLISS The Premature Baby Charity   68 South Lambeth Road, London SW8 1RL. Telephone: 0870 7700 337. Helpline: 0500 618 140. Website: www.bliss.org.uk
Parent support telephone network by parents, for parents, with babies in SCBU/NICU.

Confidential Enquiry into Stillbirths and Deaths in Infancy (CESDI) on 1 April 2003 changed to Confidential Enquiry into Maternal and Child Health (CEMACH)   CEMACH Central Office, Chiltern Court, 188 Baker Street, London NW1 5SD. Telephone: 020 7486 1191. Website: www.cemach.org.uk

Tommy's the baby charity   1 Kennington Road, London SE1 7RR. Telephone: 0870 770 7070. Information line: 0870 777 3060. Website: www.tommys-campaign.org
Research, education and information for parents and professionals.

Twins and Multiple Births Association (TAMBA)   2 The Willows, Gardener Road, Guildford, Surrey GU1 4PG. Telephone: 0870 770 3305. Website: www.tamba.org.uk

References

Atalla, R., Kean, L. & McParland, P. (2000) Preterm labor and prelabor rupture of the membranes. In *Best Practice in Labor Ward Management* (Kean, L.H., Baker, P.N. & Edelstone, D.I., eds), pp. 111–39. WB Saunders, Edinburgh.

Ballard, D.W., Li, Y., Evans, J. *et al.* (2002) Fear of litigation may increase resuscitation of infants born near the limits of viability. *Journal of Pediatrics* **140** (6), 713–18.

Briley, A., Crawshaw, S. & Hughes, J. (2002) *Premature Labour – Information for Parents.* Tommy's the baby charity, London.

Calam, R.M., Lambrenos, K. & Cox, A.D. (1999) Maternal appraisal of information given around the time of preterm delivery. *Journal of Reproductive and Infant Psychology* **17** (3), 267–80.

CESDI (2000) *Confidential Enquiry into Stillbirths and Deaths in Infancy*, 7th Annual Report. Maternal and Child Health Research Consortium, London.

CESDI (2001) *Confidential Enquiry into Stillbirths and Deaths in Infancy*, 8th Annual Report. Maternal and Child Health Research Consortium, London.

CESDI (2003) *Project 27/28: An Enquiry into Quality and Care and its Effect on Survival of Babies Born at 27/28 Weeks.* Stationery Office, London.

Christensson, K., Bhat, G.J., Amadi, B.C. *et al.* (1998) A randomised study of skin-to-skin versus incubator care for rewarming low risk hypothermic neonates. *The Lancet* **352**, 1115.

Christensson, K., Siles, C., Moreno, L. *et al.* (1992) Temperature, metabolic adaption and crying in healthy full-term newborns cared for skin-to-skin or in a cot. *Acta Paediatrica* **91**, 488–93.

Costeloe, K. Hennessy, E., Gibson, A.T. *et al.* (2000) EPICure study: outcomes to discharge from hospitals for infants born at the threshhold of viability. *Pediatrics* **106**, 659–71.

Crowley, P. (2002) Prophylactic corticosteriods for preterm birth (Cochrane Review). *The Cochrane Library* Issue 4. Update software, Oxford.

Davis, E. (1997) *Hearts and Hands – A Midwife's Guide to Pregnancy and Birth*, 3rd edn. Celestial Arts, Berkeley, California.

De Chateau, P. & Wilbert, B. (1997) Longterm effect on mother infant behaviour of extra contact during the first hour postpartum. II. A follow up at three months. *Acta Paediatrica* **66**, 145–51.

DoH (1997) *NHS Statistical Bulletin, 1997/28.* Department of Health, London.

DoH (2001) *Why Mothers Die, 1997–1999. The fifth report of the Confidential Enquiries into Maternal Deaths in the United Kingdom.* Department of Health, RCOG Press, London.

Ginesi, L. & Niescierowicz, R. (1998a) Neuroendocrinology and birth. 1: Stress. *British Journal of Midwifery* **6** (10), 659–63.

Ginesi, L. & Niescierowicz, R. (1998b) Neuroendocrinology and birth. 2: The role of oxytocin. *British Journal of Midwifery* **6** (12), 791–6.

Goffinet, F., Fraser, W., Marcoux, S. *et al.* (1997) Early amniotomy increases the frequency of fetal heart rate abnormalities. *British Journal of Obstetrics and Gynaecology* **104**, 548–53.

Grant, A. (2000) Care of the fetus during labor. In *A Guide to Effective Care in Pregnancy and Childbirth*, 3rd edn (Enkin, M., Keirse, M.J.N.C., Neilson, J. *et al.*, eds), pp. 267–80. Oxford University Press, Oxford.

Guinn, D.A., Atkinon, W., Sullivan, L. *et al.* (2001) Single vs weekly courses of antenatal steroids for women at risk of preterm delivery. *Journal of the American Medical Association* **286**, 1581–7.

Gupta, J.K. & Nikodem, V.C. (2002) Woman's position during the second stage of labour (Cochrane Review). *The Cochrane Library* Issue 4. Update software, Oxford.

Hodnett, E.D. (2002) Caregiver support for women during childbirth (Cochrane Review). *The Cochrane Library* Issue 4. Update software, Oxford.

Johnson, C., Keirse, M.J.N.C., Enkin, M. & Chalmers, I. (2000) Hospital practices – nutrition and hydration in labor. In *A Guide to Effective Care in Pregnancy and Childbirth*, 3rd edn (Enkin, M., Keirse, M.J.N.C., Neilson, J. *et al.*, eds), pp. 255–66. Oxford University Press, Oxford.

Joint Formulary Committee (2003) *British National Formulary.* 45th edn. British Medical Association and Royal Pharmaceutical Society of Great Britain, London.

Kenyon, S.L., Taylor, D.J., Tarnow-Mordi, W. *et al.* (2001a) Broad spectrum antibiotics for preterm, prelabour rupture of the membranes: the ORACLE I randomised trial. *The Lancet* **375**, 979–88.

Kenyon, S.L., Taylor, D.J., Tarnow-Mordi, W. *et al.* (2001b) Broad spectrum antibiotics for spontaneous preterm labour: the ORACLE II randomised trial. *The Lancet* **375**, 989–94.

Keirse, M.J.N.C. (2000) Preterm birth. In *A Guide to Effective Care in Pregnancy and Childbirth*, 3rd edn. (Enkin, M., Keirse, M.J.N.C., Neilson, J. *et al.*, eds), pp. 347–58. Oxford University Press, Oxford.

Mercer, J.C. (2001) Current best evidence: a review of the literature on umbilical cord clamping. *Journal of Midwifery and Women's Health* **46** (6), 402–14.

Moore, T.R. (1996) Oligohydramnios. In *Protocols for High Risk Pregnancies*, 3rd edn (Queenan, J.T. & Hobbins, J.C., eds), pp. 488–95. Blackwell Science, Oxford.

Neilson, J. & Grant, A. (2000) Imaging ultrasound in pregnancy. In *A Guide to Effective Care in Pregnancy and Childbirth*, 3rd edn (Enkin, M., Keirse, M.J.N.C., Neilson, J., eds), pp. 53–9. Oxford University Press, Oxford.

NICE (2001) *Clinical Guideline C – The Use of Electronic Fetal Monitoring*. National Institute for Clinical Excellence, London.

Ockenden, J. (2001) The hormonal dance of labour. *The Practising Midwife* **4** (6), 16–17.

Prabulos, A.M. & Philipson, E.H. (1998) Umbilical cord prolapse. Is time from diagnosis to delivery critical? *Journal of Reproductive Medicine* **43** (2), 129–32.

Robinson, J. (2000) Breech babies – caesarean or vaginal birth? *AIMS Journal* **12** (4), 12–13.

Sheer, L. (1995) *The Psychology of Childbirth*. Blackwell Science, Oxford.

Sleep, J., Roberts, J. & Chalmers, L. (2000) The second stage of labor. In *A Guide to Effective Care in Pregnancy and Childbirth*, 3rd edn (Enkin, M., Keirse, M.J.N.C., Neilson, J. *et al.*, eds), pp. 289–99. Oxford University Press, Oxford.

SPCERH (2002) *Scottish Obstetric Guidelines and Audit Project. The Preparation of the Fetus for Preterm Delivery*. SPCERH 1 Guideline Update. Scottish Programme for Clinical Effectiveness in Reproductive Health, Aberdeen Maternity Hospital, Aberdeen.

Steer, P. & Flint, C. (1999) Pre-term labour and preterm rupture of membranes. In *ABC of Labour care* (Chamberlain, G., Steer, P. & Zander, L., eds), pp. 20–23. BMJ Books, London.

Sullivan, J.R. (1999) Development of father-infant attachment in fathers of preterm infants. *Neonatal Network* **18** (7), 33–9.

Walkinshaw, S.A. (2001) Preterm labour and delivery of the preterm infant. In *Turnbull's Obstetrics*, 3rd edn (Chamberlin, G. & Steer, P., eds), pp. 493–520. Churchill Livingstone, Edinburgh.

Walsh, D. (2000a) Evidence-based care. Part 3: Assessing women's progress in labour. *British Journal of Midwifery* **8** (7), 449–57.

Walsh, D. (2000b) Evidence-based care. Part 6: Limits on pushing and time in the second stage. *British Journal of Midwifery* **8** (10), 604–608.

Wang, E. & Smaill, F. (2000) Infection in pregnancy. In *A Guide to Effective Care in Pregnancy and Childbirth*, 3rd edn (Enkin, M., Keirse, M.J.N.C., Neilson, J. *et al*, eds), pp. 154–68. Oxford University Press, Oxford.

Whitelaw, A., Heisterkamp, G., Sleath, K. *et al.* (1998) Skin to skin contact for very low birthweight infants and their mothers. *Archives of Disease in Childhood* **63**, 1377–81.

WHO (1975) *International Classification of Diseases*, Vol. 1. World Health Organization, Geneva.

WHO (1997) *Thermal Protection of the Newborn*. WHO/RHT/MSN/97.2. World Health Organisation, Geneva.

9 Maternal infection around the time of birth

This chapter focuses on infections which require specific care during the intrapartum period and/or immediately following birth.

Introduction

Infections during pregnancy can adversely affect the health of both mother and baby. Some acute infections present a risk of cross-infection to anyone who may come into contact with the woman, including her family, staff and other mothers and their babies. Infections can vary from chronic conditions, such as herpes or human immunodeficiency virus (HIV), to an acute infection presenting with a seriously unwell woman, such as with pyelonephritis. Other infections, such as Chlamydia or Group B Haemolytic Streptococcus, may be symptomless in the mother but be serious for the baby.

Facts: acute and chronic infections

Acute infections

- Maternal sepsis is not a disease of the past. Acute infection can spread quickly and, on rare occasions, if untreated, can tragically cause the death of the woman (DoH, 2001c).
- In the Confidential Enquiries into Maternal Deaths in the United Kingdom (DoH, 2001c) 14 women were identified as dying from sepsis. The report recommended that any woman who appears systemically unwell with a pyrexia and tachycardia requires thorough screening and prompt treatment.
- Urinary tract infection (UTI) is the most common infection affecting pregnant women and is often a causative factor in preterm birth and low birthweight babies (Smaill, 2002a).
- Preterm prelabour rupture of the membranes (PPROM) can be associated with maternal infection. Some 30% of preterm labours are caused by, and complicated by, infection (Atalla *et al.*, 2000; Kenyon *et al.*, 2001).
- Clinicians need to avoid spreading infections in the mother from one part of the woman's body to another and also to her baby. This includes avoiding (unless essential) vaginal examinations, artificial rupture of the membranes (ARM), use of a fetal scalp electrode (FSE), epidural (Swanson & Madej, 1997) and even caesarean section, particularly in an acute infection with possible chorioamnionitis (Atalla *et al.*, 2000).

Chronic infections

- Sexually transmitted infections (STIs) are on the increase; the most common conditions are Chlamydia, non-specific urethritis and wart virus infections (DoH, 2001b). STIs can be transmitted to the baby *in utero* or during birth.
- Women infected with HIV or hepatitis are not always identified preconceptually or antenatally. These women pose a risk of transmitting infection to their baby as well as to health professionals exposed to infected blood and other bodily fluids.
- Midwives should institute basic standards for preventing cross-infection and take

universal precautions when dealing with body fluids, regardless of a client's HIV or hepatitis status.

Signs and symptoms

A woman with an acute infection will usually present with general signs of infection, commonly a pyrexia and feeling unwell. In addition, she may well have several symptoms specific to a particular infection. Box 9.1 examines the signs and symptoms of a maternal infection.

Box 9.1 Signs and symptoms of maternal infection.

Early signs of infection
- Slight rise in maternal temperature (Atalla *et al.*, 2000).
- Fetal tachycardia (Atalla *et al.*, 2000; Keirse *et al.*, 2000).
- Feeling unwell.

Advanced signs of infection
- Feeling unwell.
- High temperature.
- Maternal and/or fetal tachycardia.
- Intrauterine death.
- A baby who is unwell at birth (see also Box 9.3).
- Non-specific features of *acute infection* include: feeling generally unwell, fever, headache, malaise, or myalgia.
- Uterine tenderness and an offensive smelling vaginal discharge/liquor – while very serious for the mother can be a huge risk for the baby (Keirse *et al.*, 2000).
- Other specific symptoms of infection can include: vomiting, diarrhoea, a vaginal discharge, a rash, a cough, or cystitis with lower back/flank pain (Irving & Humphreys, 2000).

Screening and assessment
- Referral to the obstetric team.
- Assessment: maternal temperature, pulse rate and urine tested. Fetal heart rate (FHR) monitored.
- Two sets of blood cultures (in serious infection) (Irving & Humphreys, 2000).
- Depending on the woman's history and clinical features, send *urgent* and repeated bacterial specimens (DoH, 2001c) such as:
  - vaginal/cervical swabs
  - urine specimen
  - a throat swab
  - sputum specimen
  - faeces for culture

Care in labour

- If the mother has a contagious infection, such as an enterovirus infection or gastroenteritis, she should have her own room and bathroom facilities and infection control measures should be instituted. The infection control team/nurse specialist should also be contacted.
- The obstetric team should liaise with the microbiologist regarding appropriate treatment/antibiotics, which should commence pending the results of bacterial specimens and blood culture results (DoH, 2001c).

- Closely monitor maternal temperature, pulse and fetal heart rate (FHR) as well as how the mother is feeling.
- Be aware of the signs of shock, indicating possible sepsis (see also Chapter 12, page 201, for signs and symptoms of shock).
- Iatrogenic, invasive, risk-inducing interventions, such as ARM and vaginal examinations, should be avoided. Studies with preterm infants suggest that the rate of ascending infection is linked to the number of vaginal examinations (Atalla *et al.*, 2000).
- In acute infection, an epidural may be contraindicated due to the risk of abscess formation and/or of causing meningitis in the woman (Swanson & Madej, 1997).
- If the woman has an acute infection with possible chorioamnionitis, caesarean section is usually avoided unless essential (Atalla *et al.*, 2000).

Care following birth

- If the source of the mother's infection is unknown, or thought to involve the genital/uterine area, a set of observations (temperature, heart rate and respirations) should be taken on the mother and baby even if the baby appears well at birth. See also Box 9.3, given later, for typical symptoms of infection in the newborn.
- The paediatrician may request swabs, bloods and antibiotics for the baby, pending culture results.
- The baby born to a mother who is unwell should be observed for 48 hours following birth. Parents should be aware of what to look for in a baby that is unwell. This is particularly important for babies born at home, discharged home early or born to a mother deemed a high infection risk. Parents should not hesitate to contact their general practitioner if they are concerned about their baby.

Infection control/prevention of cross-infection

Some infections pose a risk not only to the mother and baby but to other newborns and staff alike (such as gastroenteritis). Cross-infection must be considered in any febrile woman, particularly if the baby is born unwell. Liaise with the infection control nurse specialist, the neonatal intensive care unit/special care baby unit (NICU/SCBU) and institute infection control and barrier nursing procedures to protect other neonates until the results of cultures are known.

Hand cleansing/decontamination (DoH, 2001a)

- Effective hand washing decontaminates the hands from physical soiling and microorganisms and is important to reduce cross-infection. Preparation of the hands by wetting under tepid water then applying soap thoroughly over all the surfaces of the hands and rubbing together vigorously for 10–15 seconds, should be followed by thorough rinsing and then drying of both hands with paper towels.
- The use of alcohol-based handrubs is effective in destroying microorganisms and should be used after each and every direct client contact.

Protection when carrying out invasive procedures

- Cover any cuts or abrasions with a waterproof dressing.
- Wear gloves when there is the potential for exposure to blood, body fluids, secretions and excretions.
- Aprons should be worn as a *single use* item for any one procedure that carries the risk of exposure to blood, body fluids, secretions and excretions.
- Eye protection should be worn if there is a risk of exposure to blood, body fluids, secretions and excretions, such as when attending a birth.

The use and disposal of sharps

- The handling of sharps should be kept to a minimum and not passed directly from hand to hand.
- Used needles should not be recapped but should be disposed of into a sharps container at the point of use.
- The main causes of sharps injuries are by needles associated with certain procedures including venepuncture, administration of medication via intravenous (IV) lines and recapping of needles following use. The DoH (2001a) considers all sharps injuries preventable and estimates that the average risk of transmission of blood-borne pathogens following a single percutaneous exposure to be:
  - hepatitis B virus (HBV) = 33.3% (1 in 3)
  - hepatitis C virus (HCV) = 3.3% (1 in 30)
  - human immunodeficiency virus (HIV) = 0.31% (1 in 319).

Urinary tract infection – asymptomatic bacteriuria/pyelonephritis

Bacteriuria, a sign of urinary tract infection (UTI), affects between 1 and 2% of pregnant women. Urine testing and screening for asymptomatic bacteriuria in pregnancy results in a reduction in pyelonephritis, preterm birth and low birthweight babies (Smaill, 2002a).

Signs and symptoms

- Urinalysis/dipstick urine test is successful in detecting most asymptomatic UTI. The findings of nitrates, blood and protein can all be suggestive of infection.
- A clean catch, mid-stream specimen of urine (MSU) tested for culture, sensitivity and colony count.

Screening and treatment

- Bacteriuria may be asymptomatic.
- Frequency, nocturia and dysuria suggest an acute infection. In addition, fever, flank pain, nausea and vomiting all indicate severe infection and probable acute pyelonephritis which can lead to life-threatening sepsis in the woman (Irving & Humphreys, 2000).
- Treatment is with broad-spectrum antibiotics, while awaiting the results of culture and sensitivity, which can then be tailored to antibiotic sensitivity (DoH, 2001c).

Care in labour

- A woman in labour with an acute UTI is likely to feel very unwell and to be suffering from lower back/flank pain due to the spread of infection to her kidneys. In order to ease the back discomfort, the midwife can help the woman find comfortable positions. Apply warm (such as microwave wheatgerm packs) or cool packs as a soothing compress on the woman's back.
- Mild maternal pyrexia and fetal tachycardia are the most common signs of infection/chorioamnioitis (Atalla *et al.*, 2000). Depending on maternal well-being, check the woman's temperature 1–4 hourly and pulse hourly.
- Analgesia should be discussed in advance and reviewed as the need arises. If the woman would like an epidural, discuss this in advance with the anaesthetist. In acute and severe maternal infection, an epidural is usually contraindicated (Swanson & Madej, 1997).
- Keep a fluid balance chart and ensure the woman has a reasonable fluid intake (IV fluids may be recommended if the woman feels nauseous and/or is unable to tolerate oral fluids).

See also 'Care in labour' on pages 139–40.

Care following birth

- IV antibiotics and maternal observations should continue post-birth and any concerns reported promptly.
- The woman may feel weak and unwell and she is likely to require extra rest and help in caring for her baby.

See also 'Care following birth' on page 140. Box 9.3 (page 145) lists the typical symptoms of infection in the newborn.

Group B Streptococcus/beta haemolytic Strep (GBS)

Group B Streptococcus (GBS) is the commonest cause of life-threatening infection in newborns in the UK, affecting 1:1000 live births or approximately 700 babies a year (GBSS, 2003). Some 90% of GBS infection is early onset, which means it is usually acquired *in utero* where it has crossed broken or intact membranes and reached the baby (Feldman, 2001). The likelihood of the baby acquiring the disease is directly related to the density of maternal colonization and the immaturity of the infant, with infants weighing < 2.500 kg having the highest overall rate of infection (Smaill, 2002b).

Group B Streptococcus can be found on the hands and in the respiratory tract of a colonized person and may be passed to the baby from repeated exposure 48 hours to 3 months after birth; this is known as late onset GBS. The risk of a baby developing late onset GBS decreases with age, GBS infection in babies is rare after 1 month of age and virtually unknown after 3 months. Everyone, whether they know they're colonized or not, should wash their hands and carefully dry them for the first 3 months of a baby's life.

Signs and symptoms

- Group B Streptococcus is present in 30% of the adult population's gut; it can harmlessly colonize the vaginal tract and is not normally associated with symptoms in the woman (Feldman, 2001).
- 60–70% of babies with early onset GBS are symptomatic at birth, and 90% are symptomatic in the first 2 days of life (Feldman, 2001) (see also Box 9.3 later for symptoms of infection in the newborn).

Screening and treatment

The Public Health Laboratory Service (PHLS) GBS Working Group suggests there is insufficient evidence to recommend routine screening for GBS carriage (PHLS, 2001). However, one large US study has suggested that a 'screening based approach' (taking cultures) prevents more cases of early onset disease GBS than the commonly used 'risk based approach' (Schrag *et al.*, 2002).

Screening-based approach (cultures)

The gold standard 'enriched broth' method for culturing is the most effective technique for detecting GBS (Yancey *et al.*, 1996) but is not routinely available in the UK. The results take over 36 hours to obtain, by which time many women deemed 'at risk' may have delivered.

Standard culture tests performed in the UK have a low predictive value in identifying women who are actually colonized with GBS at term, even when tested in the late antenatal period (Yancey *et al.*, 1996). Standard vaginal swabs will only detect 50% of cases of women colonized with a GBS infection (Feldman, 2001).

Risk-based approach

There are seven situations where GBS is a significant risk factor for the newborn baby, and these are classified in Box 9.2. Women considered high risk should be offered a course of antibiotics in labour to reduce the dangers of GBS for the newborn baby.

To prevent the majority of cases of GBS infection in the newborn, women with *any* risk factor would need IV antibiotics from the time of rupturing their membranes and/ or from the start of labour and for, ideally, at least 4 hours before the birth (GBSS, 2003).

Care in labour (including antibiotic regime)

- The risk of a GBS infection in the baby must be balanced against the wishes and beliefs of the woman in labour and against her personal risk of a rare but significant adverse reaction to the antibiotics.
- If the membranes rupture, or the woman starts to labour, IV antibiotic prophylaxis is recommended to prevent most GBS infections in babies. Treating a baby with antibiotics after delivery may be too late (GBSS, 2003).
- Avoid iatrogenic, invasive, risk-inducing interventions, such as ARM and vaginal examinations, which may increase the risk of ascending infection.

Box 9.2 Risk factors for group B streptococcus (GBS) (GBSS, 2003). Reproduced with kind permission from Group B Strep Support.

High risk This scenario multiplies the risk by ten times
- Where the pregnant woman has previously had a baby who developed a GBS infection.

High to moderately high risk A mother who carries GBS multiplies the risk by at least four times
- Where the pregnant woman is found to carry GBS during the present pregnancy.
- Where the pregnant woman has had GBS detected in a urine sample at any time in pregnancy (which should have been treated at the time of diagnosis).

Reduced risk Each of these individual factors increases the risk of GBS three times:
- Where labour or membrane rupture is preterm (pre-37 completed weeks of pregnancy).
- When the membranes have been ruptured for more than 18–24 hours.
- When the woman has a pyrexia of 37.8°C or higher.

The PHLS (2001) advises that women in the moderate to high-risk groups (described above) should receive intravenous (IV) antibiotic prophylaxis and those women in the reduced-risk group should consider receiving IV antibiotics.

According to the GBSS (2003) the antibiotic regime for use with ruptured membranes and/or in labour for women who tolerate penicillin is:

- Initially IV penicillin G 3 g (or 5 mU) at least 4 hours prior to delivery where possible.
- Followed by 1.5 g (or 2.5 mU) at 4-hourly intervals until delivery.

For women who are allergic to penicillin use:

- Clindamycin 900 mg intravenously every 8 hours until delivery (GBSS, 2003).

Care following birth

- If the baby appears well, encourage skin-to-skin contact and early breastfeeding.
- Carry out baseline observations while the baby nestles with its mother. These should include temperature, heart rate and respirations, as well as observing for grunting or other symptoms, which may not have been present at birth but may develop in the hours following birth.
- The baby should be assessed regularly and observed for 48 hours following birth. The parents of babies born at home or mothers 'at risk' of GBS transmission should be made aware of what to look for in a baby that is unwell.

Paediatric assessment following birth

- If the mother received IV antibiotics less than at least 4 hours before the birth, the paediatrician should investigate and initially commence the baby on antibiotics until it has been established that the baby is not infected (GBSS, 2003).
- At birth, a baby with any symptoms, see Box 9.3, requires prompt assessment for treatment with a pro-active view to giving IV antibiotic therapy.

Box 9.3 Typical symptoms of infection in the newborn.

- Grunting
- Lethargy
- Irritability/constant crying
- Tachycardia or bradycardia
- Hypothermia or pyrexia
- Abnormal (fast or slow) breathing rates with cyanosis of the skin
- Poor feeding
- High or low blood pressure

Treating GBS infection in the newborn baby

The recommended minimum length of in-patient IV antibiotic treatment for babies who actually develop GBS infection is 10 days (or 14 days if the baby develops meningitis). Treatment should also be given to an infected baby's twin or triplet even if that baby appears to be well at the time, since infection of the second twin is common (GBSS, 2003).

Sexually transmitted infections

Many women will not know that they have a sexually transmitted infection (STI). Those who do know may carry with them the burden of guilt that their baby is 'at risk' of exposure to the infection. There are various agencies and groups that can offer women information, screening, and emotional and personal support, some of which are given at the end of this chapter.

Clinicians can help the woman by discussing openly the issues concerning the specific infection and the risks related to transmission in a non-judgemental and supportive way. Midwives must be aware of the importance of maintaining confidentiality. Sexual partners (past and present) may need to be contacted and treated.

HIV AND AIDS

The number of human immunodeficiency virus (HIV) infections newly diagnosed in 2000 was the highest since reporting began and the numbers of newly acquired infections were through heterosexual sex. An estimated 30 000 people are living with HIV in the UK, a third of whom are undiagnosed (DoH, 2001b).

For an HIV positive woman, the pregnancy and the baby's birth can both be highly emotionally charged events. The woman will be only too aware of her own serious illness and that her baby may be born HIV positive. Intrauterine transmission can occur during pregnancy, birth or from breastfeeding. It is thought that a woman who has recently been infected, or a woman who has acquired immunodeficiency syndrome (AIDS), is more likely to have an infected baby (AVERT, 2003). HIV positive women need sensitive care from all staff, specific counselling and time to talk. Women may request a side room but many mothers will wish to be among other new parents and not segregated. Confidentiality is vital.

Signs and symptoms

AIDS is a late manifestation of HIV. During the HIV stage people can feel well and not suspect they have the disease. In the later stages, the person's immune system is unable to cope with opportunistic infection and they can eventually continually contract minor or major illnesses for which their body can offer no defence. At present, there is no cure (AVERT, 2003).

The infection rate in babies is approximately 1 in 6 babies (DoH, 2001b).

Screening and treatment

Screening is increasingly offered pro-actively to pregnant women as part of the government's national objectives to decrease the number of mother-to-infant transmissions by 80% (DoH, 2001b). HIV is diagnosed by means of an antibody blood test. However, there can remain a window of 3 months from contracting HIV, to the detection of antibodies in the blood (AVERT, 2003).

While the condition is not curable, drug treatments, such as antiretroviral therapies, appear successful in delaying or reducing the severity of infections and reducing the risk of HIV vertical transmission from mother to baby (Shaffer *et al.*, 1999; Brocklehurst, 2002a).

Care in labour

- Clinicians should take universal barrier precautions whatever the client's HIV status, see 'Infection control/prevention of cross-infection' earlier in this chapter.
- An elective caesarean will reduce the transmission risk to the baby by 50% and, therefore, is the recommended mode of delivery.
- If the woman decides to labour or her HIV risk status is high, but unknown, the following should be considered:
  - Shaffer *et al.* (1999) found that when zidovudine was administered orally, 3 hourly in labour, this resulted in a 37–50% efficacy in the prevention of vertical transmission rates
  - Antepartum/intrapartum haemorrhage, instrumental delivery or severe genital tract trauma is thought to increase the risk of transmission (Irving & Humphreys, 2000)
  - Avoid invasive procedures including episiotomy, fetal scalp electrode (FSE) and ARM
  - The risk of vertical transmission is increased if the membranes rupture, longer than 4 hours significantly increases this risk (Wang & Smaill, 2000).

Care following birth

- Breastfeeding doubles the transmission risk so artificial milk feeding is strongly recommended (Dunn *et al.*, 1992).
- A baby who is HIV positive will not necessarily have symptoms until several months or years old. However, the mother/parents will probably wish their baby to have a special type of blood test known as a PCR (polymerase chain reaction)

test. This sensitive test detects the HIV virus itself and the baby can usually be tested by the age of 3 months, sometimes earlier (AVERT, 2003).

- Parents should be advised of the potential benefits of the baby commencing anti-retroviral therapy after birth (AVERT, 2003).

SYPHILIS

Syphilis has recently increased in line with the rise of HIV (DoH, 2001b). Due to routine antenatal screening and treatment, the tragic effects of this disease for the baby are now rare (Wang & Smaill, 2000).

Syphilis, which has 'minor' initial symptoms, can often go unreported. If the disease is left untreated, transmission can occur during pregnancy usually during the third trimester or during birth. Risks to the baby can be devastating and include abortion, stillbirth, preterm birth and there is a perinatal death rate of 20% (Wang & Smaill, 2000).

Signs and symptoms

- Primary – a painless sore (chancre) appears in addition to enlarged lymph glands.
- Secondary – rashes around the vulva/anus and enlarged lymph glands.
- Tertiary syphilis affects the central nervous system and the cardiovascular system.

Screening and treatment

- Syphilis is screened for via a blood test, which is usually offered to women routinely at booking.
- Treatment includes large doses of penicillin (or erythromycin) for 14–21 days (Walker, 2002).
- Any past sexual partners should be contacted and treated (Enkin, 2000).

Care following birth

- If the adequacy of the mother's treatment is unknown, or if the mother did not have penicillin, the baby should receive treatment (Walker, 2002).
- Of those babies who survive, many will have acquired congenital syphilis, which can cause physical disabilities and mental retardation (Enkin, 2000).

GONORRHOEA

Gonorrhoea can be transmitted to the baby via the genital tract during birth. Risks to the baby include gonococcal ophthalmia neonatorum and systemic neonatal infection. Risks to the mother include endometritis and pelvic sepsis (Brocklehurst, 2002b).

Signs and symptoms

Gonorrhoea can cause a purulent discharge from the vagina and urethra, and burning pain on passing urine *but* it is usually symptomless.

Screening and treatment

- Screening is not usually routine but in any woman with a history of high-risk sexual activity, or of having any other sexually transmitted disease, screening should be offered (Wang & Smaill, 2000).
- The 'gold standard' for testing is by cervical swab sent for culture, preferably taken at booking (Wang & Smaill, 2000).
- Treatment: penicillin, or if resistant, third generation cephalosporins (Brocklehurst, 2002b).

Care following birth

- Gonococcal ophthalmia presents as severe conjunctivitis or sticky eyes, and is usually evident in the newborn baby 2–5 days following birth. This can lead to corneal adhesions leading to blindness if untreated (Silverton, 1993).
- Treatment of the baby with penicillin, tetracycline, or erythromycin is preferable to silver nitrate and is also effective against Chlamydia (Brocklehurst, 2002b).

CHLAMYDIA TRACHOMATIS

Chlamydia is present in up to 12% of women. Left untreated it can result in pelvic inflammatory disease, which can lead to infertility and ectopic pregnancy. It can also be associated with cervical cancer (DoH, 2001b). The risks to the baby include abortion, preterm birth and transmission through contact with infected vaginal secretions at birth.

Signs and symptoms

Chlamydia is usually asymptomatic, although some women experience pain and discomfort from cervicitis, salpingitis or urethral syndrome (DoH, 2001b).

Screening and treatment

- Screening involves a cervical Chlamydia swab.
- Treatment is by erythromycin or amoxicillin in pregnancy. Tetracycline is effective but contraindicated during pregnancy (Brocklehurst & Rooney, 2000).

Care following birth

- Chlamydia is the most common cause of neonatal conjunctivitis and can lead to blindness if untreated (Brocklehurst & Rooney, 2000).
- The newborn baby can acquire the infection through the birth canal with an 18–50% chance of developing conjunctivitis and a 3–18% chance of developing Chlamydia pneumonia (Brocklehurst & Rooney, 2000).

HERPES SIMPLEX II

Herpes simplex II is a sexually transmitted virus that can remain dormant until the person becomes stressed or unwell. It is usually a chronic, reoccurring ulcerative condition which if active at the time of birth carries serous risks if transmitted to the newborn.

Signs and symptoms

- Primary herpes infection causes a mild fever and a general feeling of being unwell.
- The development of painful lesions around the internal and external genitalia/ cervix, which ulcerate, usually healing within 3 weeks.

Screening and treatment

- Viral shedding cannot be diagnosed by blood tests or cultures, only by the visualization of lesions (Enkin, 2000).
- Women with recurrent herpes may be offered acyclovir, one week prior to their expected date of delivery in order to reduce the risk of a subsequent herpes outbreak at the time of birth (Enkin, 2000).

Care in labour

- Active herpes should be diagnosed by clinical inspection of the genital area for visible lesions (internally and externally) at the onset of labour or spontaneous rupture of the membranes (Irving & Humphreys, 2000).
- Transmission risk to the baby is thought to be 50% if the mother has a primary herpes attack at the time of delivery.
- Caesarean section is only indicated if the infection is active and therefore lesion(s) have been visualized (Enkin, 2000).

Care following birth

- The baby should be screened for infection and treated if necessary.
- In infected babies, there is a 50% mortality rate (Irving & Humphreys, 2000).
- Central nervous system damage and eye damage can occur (Enkin, 2000).

HEPATITIS B

Hepatitis B is a blood-borne virus that causes inflammation of the liver. Women can acquire hepatitis from exposure to infected blood such as by IV drug use or from a blood transfusion. Some strains of hepatitis are endemic in certain countries including southeast Asia. Around 25% of carriers will suffer from life-threatening complications including chronic liver disease, cirrhosis, and primary hepatocellular carcinoma (Irving & Humphreys, 2000).

Signs and symptoms

Hepatitis B is characterized by jaundice, malaise, low fever, vomiting and anorexia.

Screening and treatment

- Anyone with a history of jaundice, or from a high-risk group, should be offered screening.
- As yet there is no cure for this condition.
- Prevention is by vaccination of those persons at possible risk, such as babies born to women who have hepatitis and carers such as midwives and obstetricians.

Care in labour

- Infectious hepatitis can trigger preterm labour.
- Clinicians should take universal barrier precautions whatever the client's hepatitis status. See 'Infection control/prevention of cross-infection' earlier in this chapter.
- Avoid invasive procedures including ARM, FSE and episiotomy.

Care following birth

- Any baby born to a mother who has hepatitis B should be offered vaccination immediately after birth and no later than 24 hours following delivery.
- The paediatrician should discuss vaccination with the parents prior to birth. If the parents give consent for their baby to receive the vaccination, the paediatrician can prescribe it in advance, to prevent any delay in its administration following delivery.
- For optimum protection of the newborn, vaccination should be repeated at 1 and at 6 months of age. Irving & Humphreys (2000) note how the uptake of follow-up vaccinations remains very poor.

Summary

- Basic standards of universal precautions should be instituted, not just with those women whose infection status is known.
- Liaise with the infection control specialist.

Acute infection

- Refer the woman to the obstetric team if there is any sign of infection.
- A slight raise in maternal temperature and tachycardia are usually the earliest clinical signs of infection.
- Any woman with a fever and offensive discharge requires prompt screening and commencement of parenteral antibiotics. Appropriate bloods, swabs, etc., should be taken for screening.
- Observe the baby at birth for signs of infection. A baby with any symptoms (Box 9.3) requires prompt assessment for treatment.

- Institute standard infection control procedures to prevent cross-infection to staff and other women and their babies.
- Parents should be aware of what to look for in a baby that is unwell and who to contact. This is particularly important for babies born at home, discharged home early or born to a mother posing a potential infection risk.

Chronic infection

- Many clients with HIV or hepatitis are of unknown infection status and, as such, may pose an infection risk to others, particularly their unborn baby.
- Parents will require emotional support and explanations if their baby is born unwell with an infection.

Useful contacts

AVERT   4 Brighton Road, Horsham, West Sussex, RH13 5BA. Telephone: 01403 210202. Website: www.avert.org
AIDS and HIV Information Service.

Department of Health (DoH)   Richmond House, 79 Whitehall, London SW1A 2NS. Telephone: 020 7210 4850.
The National Strategy for Sexual Health and HIV is available free. Also on website: doh.gov.uk/nshs

Group B Strep Support (GBSS)   PO Box 203, Haywards Heath, West Sussex RH16 1GF. Telephone: 01444 416176. Website: www.gbss.org.uk
GBSS is affiliated to Contact a Family.

National AIDS Helpline   Telephone: 0800 567 123
A UK only, free helpline operating 24 hours a day.

NHS Direct   Telephone: 0845 46 47.
Provides information and advice, 24 hours a day, including comprehensive information on local services and specialist helplines.

Public Health Laboratory Service (PHLS)   61 Colindale Avenue, London NW9 5DF. Telephone: 20 8200 1295. Website: www.phls.org.uk

Sexwise   Telephone: 0800 282930.
A support helpline providing services specifically for young people.

References

Atalla, R., Kean, L. & McParland, P. (2000) Preterm labor and prelabor rupture of the membranes. In *Best Practice in Labor Ward Management* (Kean, L.H., Baker, P.N. & Edelstone, D.I., eds), pp. 111–39. W.B. Saunders, Edinburgh.

AVERT (2003) Data from AIDS & HIV Information Service. Website: www.avert.org (accessed May 2003).

Brocklehurst, P. (2002a) Interventions for reducing mother-to-child transmission of HIV infection (Cochrane Review). *The Cochrane Library*, Issue 4. Update software, Oxford.

Brocklehurst, P. (2002b) Interventions for treating gonorrhoea in pregnancy (Cochrane Review). *The Cochrane Library*, Issue 4. Update software, Oxford.

Brocklehurst, P. & Rooney, G. (2000) Interventions for treating genital Chlamydia trachomatis infection in pregnancy (Chochrane Review) *The Cochrane Library*, Issue 4. Update Software, Oxford.

DoH (2001a) The Epic Project: Developing national evidence-based guidelines for preventing healthcare associated infections. Phase 1: Guidelines for preventing hospital acquired infections. *Journal of Hospital Infection* Supplement 47, S21–S37.

DoH (2001b) *The National Strategy for Sexual Health and HIV*. Department of Health, London.

DoH (2001c) *Why Mothers Die, 1997–1999. The fifth report of the Confidential Enquiries into Maternal Deaths in the United Kingdom*. Department of Health, RCOG Press, London.

Enkin, M. (2000) Infection in pregnancy. In *A Guide to Effective Care in Pregnancy and Childbirth*, 3rd edn (Enkin, M., Keirse, M.J.N.C., Neilson, J. *et al.*, eds), pp. 154–68. Oxford University Press, Oxford.

Feldman, R. (2001) Group B Streptococcus prevention of infection in the newborn. *Modern Midwife* **4** (3), 16–18.

GBSS (2003) *Group B Streptococcus Support Group Medical Advisory Panel Recommendations*. Copy available on website: www.gbss.org.uk (accessed April 2003).

Irving, W. & Humphreys, H. (2000) Management of women with infective problems In *Best Practice in Labor Ward Management* (Kean, L.H., Baker, P. & Edelstone, D.I., eds), pp. 493–6. WB Saunders, Edinburgh.

Keirse, M.J.N.C., Ohlsson, A., Treffers, P. *et al.* (2000) Prelabor rupture of the membranes. In *A Guide to Effective Care in Pregnancy and Childbirth*, 3rd edn (Enkin, M., Keirse, M.J.N.C., Neilson, J. *et al.*, eds), pp. 197–210. Oxford University Press, Oxford.

Kenyon, S.L., Taylor, D.J., Tarnow-Mordi, W. *et al.* (2001) Broad spectrum antibiotics for preterm, prelabour rupture of the membranes: the ORACLE I randomised trial. *The Lancet* **375**, 979–88.

PHLS (Group B Streptococcus Working Party) (2001) *Interim 'Good Practice' Recommendations for the Prevention of Early Onset Neonatal Group B Streptococcal GBS Infection in the UK*. Central Public Health Laboratory/Public Health Laboratory Service, London.

Schrag, S.J., Zell, E.R., Lynfield, R. *et al.* (2002) Early onset neonatal group B streptococcal disease, a population based comparison of strategies to prevent early onset group B streptococcal disease in neonates. *The New England Journal of Medicine* **347** (4), 233–9.

Shaffer, N., Chuachoowong, R., Mock, P.A. *et al.* (1999) Short course zidovine for perinatal HIV-1 transmission in Bangkok, Thailand: a randomised control trial. *The Lancet* **353**, 773–80.

Silverton, L. (1993) *The Art and Science of Midwifery*. Prentice Hall International, London.

Smaill, F. (2002a) Antibiotics for asymptomatic bacteriuria in pregnancy (Cochrane Review). *The Cochrane Library*, Issue 4. Update Software, Oxford.

Smaill, F. (2002b) Intrapartum antibiotics for Group B streptococcal colonisation (Cochrane Review). *The Cochrane Library*, Issue 4. Update Software, Oxford.

Swanson, L. & Madej, T.H. (1997) The febrile obstetric patient. In *Clinical Problems in Obstetric Anaesthesia*. (Russell, I.F. & Lyons, G., eds), pp. 123–31. Chapman & Hall, London.

Walker, G. (2002) Antibiotics for syphilis diagnosed during pregnancy (Cochrane Review). *The Cochrane Library*, Issue 4. Update Software, Oxford.

Wang, E. & Smaill, F. (2000) Infection in pregnancy. In *A Guide to Effective Care in Pregnancy and Childbirth*, 3rd edn (Enkin, M., Keirse, M.J.N.C., Neilson, J. *et al.*, eds), pp. 154–68.

Yancey, M.K., Schuchat, A., Brown, L.K., Ventura, V.L. & Markenson, G.R. (1996) The accuracy of late antenatal screening cultures in predicting genital group B strepcococcal colonisation at delivery. *Obstetrics and Gynecology* **88**, 811–15.

10 Assisted delivery: forceps and midwife ventouse delivery

Cathy Charles

Introduction

With good labour support, most women will experience a spontaneous vaginal delivery. Some women, however, for a variety of reasons, will not. For those women the options are either an instrumental delivery or a caesarean section. An instrumental delivery carried out competently, in a supportive atmosphere, can still be a triumph for a woman, and a source of celebration. However, there is an increased risk of reduced maternal satisfaction with assisted delivery, particularly with a forceps delivery (Morgan *et al.*, 1982). Clinical competence is of course vital, but emotional support through assisted delivery is equally important.

Incidence and facts

The incidence of a forceps or a ventouse delivery varies widely in different settings. Good labour practice is likely to reduce the incidence of instrumental delivery and will include:

- Psychological support in labour (Hodnett, 2002).
- Appropriate food and drink in labour (Johnson *et al.*, 2000).
- Encouraging mobilization/upright position (Gupta & Nikodem, 2002).
- Avoidance of continuous cardiotocograph (CTG) monitoring for low-risk women (NICE, 2001).
- Avoidance of arbitrary second stage time limits if progress is being made (Sleep *et al.*, 2000).
- Use of intravenous (IV) oxytocics if necessary in a slow second stage.

Johanson & Menon (2002) concluded that ventouse is the method of choice for assisted delivery because:

- A ventouse delivery is less likely to end in a caesarean section, possibly due to the higher effectiveness of ventouse in, for example, the deflexed occipitoposterior (OP) position. However, some attempted ventouse deliveries will end in a forceps delivery.
- Forceps are more likely to succeed than ventouse, mainly because it is possible to pull harder.
- A ventouse birth causes fewer serious maternal injuries and fewer neonatal facial and cranial injuries. There are more reports of cephalohaematoma and retinal haemorrhage in ventouse births, but these do not appear to have long-term complications.
- No difference in 1-minute Apgar score with a trend towards a lower 5-minute Apgar score in ventouse births.
- A ventouse delivery may be difficult if there is marked caput, as suction may be hard to maintain. Following repeated fetal blood sampling attempts, ventouse may be inadvisable, due to the risk of scalp trauma.
- Ventouse requires maternal effort. Some clinicians prefer forceps, or resort to them, when ventouse fails.

Indications for an instrumental delivery

- Failure to progress/maternal exhaustion in second stage.
- Fetal distress (non-reassuring CTG, possibly in conjunction with fetal blood sample pH <7.20).
- Elective shortening of the second stage for fetal or maternal benefit (there are few absolute indications here as obstetricians differ in their views on this subject).

Care of a woman undergoing instrumental delivery

A calm and sensitive manner towards a woman undergoing instrumental delivery is *crucial*. Explanations need to be clear and informative, with plenty of support given to the woman and her birth partner(s), for whom such an experience may be a frightening ordeal.

Communication

Debating options at this stage of labour is not always easy. Some women may be feeling very much in control. Others may be exhausted, in extreme pain, and not receptive to discussion. If there are concerns about the condition of the baby, staff may feel under pressure to press on with an assisted delivery, and limit debate. It is easy to talk glibly of 'informed choice'; many stressed women in labour will consent to almost anything that offers them a way out.

Birth partners can feel extremely stressed and tired; they may display anger or aggression, as they try to cope with their own and the woman's distress. It may be the partner, rather than the woman, who asks questions at this point. Conversely they may block discussion, saying 'Just get on with it, she's been through enough'.

Ensure a woman is prepared for the possibility of caesarean section, should the instrumental attempt fail.

Client support

'As fluorescent lights go on, the room fills with people, she hears the metallic clang of lithotomy poles, the sound of tearing paper as instrument packs are opened, the loud voices of people issuing instructions. She may feel disorientated, as the bed is pumped higher, she is tilted back, moved down the bed, legs uncomfortably suspended. As well as these sounds and sensations, she senses the anxiety levels of her attendants (there is something very dramatic about to happen here, so no matter how much pain I'm in now, it is about to get a whole lot worse)'. (Charles, 2002)

One obvious fact about instrumental deliveries is that they are frightening for women. Preferably one staff member should focus solely on the emotional needs of the woman and her birth partner(s). If another midwife is not available, this might be a maternity auxiliary/health care assistant.

Resist the urge to put all the lights on: a sudden flood of fluorescent light is frightening, increases the atmosphere of drama, and may make a woman feel naked and vulnerable. Perineal illumination and 'spot' areas of lighting, where necessary, are quite sufficient.

The two most painful moments for the mother, apart from the birth itself, are the forceps blades/ventouse cup insertion and subsequent checking of the instrument's position. Ensure someone is there to prepare and support her through these painful procedures.

Analgesia

This is the woman's decision, guided by professional advice. Theoretically, ventouse delivery pain is not significantly greater than from spontaneous birth, since the cup, unlike forceps, takes up no space alongside the head. Pain mainly results from initial cup insertion, followed by the usual delivery sensations. However, fear may increase pain perception.

- Epidural analgesia may be advisable for a forceps delivery. Ensure it is adequately 'topped up' prior to delivery. Some doctors may instead administer a pudendal block.
- Some women may prefer to use entonox instead of, or in addition to, other methods of analgesia. Ensure that sufficient entonox has been inhaled prior to commencing the procedure.
- Perineal lignocaine infiltration prior to ventouse cup insertion may help; there may also be a placebo effect from having given 'something' prior to the procedure.
- It is helpful to explain to a woman undergoing ventouse delivery that her urge to push is important, as this birth will be a collaboration.

Positioning

- Following explanations and consent, the woman's legs should be gently and symmetrically lifted and supported in an adducted hip position. Lithotomy is not essential although some women may be comfortable in this position, particularly if staff experiment with pole height and adjust the position of the woman's buttocks relative to the poles.
- It is quite possible to carry out a instrumental delivery with two helpers supporting the heels (Charles, 2002).
- For ventouse, other positions such as left lateral or squatting have been suggested (Johanson, 2001). Most professionals will prefer to apply the cup with the woman in a semi-recumbent position. Once applied, there is no reason why a woman should not take up a lateral or squatting position. Squatting is known to increase the pelvic outlet diameter. Having said this, many professionals are more comfortable working with the method they are accustomed to and may resist alternative suggestions.
- Think aortocaval occlusion. Often this is forgotten during instrumental delivery. Create a small lateral tilt from a wedge or pillow.

Bladder care

Most women produce little urine in the second stage, and/or have difficulty micturating. Catheterization was once 'routine' prior to instrumental delivery. Vacca (1997) however states, 'A catheter need only be passed if the woman is unable to void or if the bladder is visibly or palpably distended'. In the absence of substantial research, professionals should use clinical judgement, or adhere to local protocol.

Episiotomy

This should not be a routine intervention performed with every instrumental delivery (Vacca, 1997; AAFP, 2000/2001), or done simply to prevent a tear. An episiotomy is only usually indicated for severe fetal distress or for a truly rigid perineum (Sleep *et al.*, 2000), although as forceps take up space alongside the head there may be an increased indication during a forceps delivery.

If indicated it should only be performed when the perineum has been stretched thin by the descending head. Clinical judgement should be exercised, taking into account the flexibility of the perineum. Early episiotomy increases maternal morbidity, blood loss and haematoma formation, extension to the anal sphincter or rectum, and post-partum pain (Sleep *et al.*, 2000).

Consent for instrumental delivery should not imply that consent is given for episiotomy without further discussion.

Assisting at an instrumental delivery procedure

Mutual staff support

Instrumental deliveries are stressful for everyone. Staff are often intimidated by the 'medicalized' atmosphere, but should try to avoid appearing rushed. Usually there is reasonable time to prepare. Even if the intervention is for fetal distress, remember that if this were a caesarean section the time from problem diagnosis to delivery would be longer.

The doctor or midwife delivering the baby may appear calm but will be under pressure. Rudeness and roughness towards the woman, however, should not be tolerated. Positive attitudes and efficiency in opening packs, preparing equipment and communicating information will help ensure a safe birth, and give the mother confidence in her helpers.

Equipment preparation

- To an extent, this will depend on local practice.
- The vulva is cleansed and, usually, draped.
- Relevant sterile instrument packs are opened, and the delivering professional assisted, as requested.
- Incidence of shoulder dystocia and postpartum haemorrhage increases with instrumental delivery. Anticipate this, and be prepared.
- For a ventouse birth, an assistant may need to attach the suction tubing to the machine, and control the pressure. Leaks are usually due to poor tubing attachment, or the release pedal having been left depressed following a previous delivery. There are single-use complete hand-held ventouse systems available

which do not require a separate vacuum machine and can be operated by one person. Their size may make them appear less intimidating to the woman.

Instrumental procedure

Once packs are opened, a doctor normally performs a forceps delivery without further direct help.

For a ventouse delivery using a freestanding machine, the delivering professional gives instructions. Normally pressure starts at 0.2 (kg/cm^2), then increases to 0.8 in one step. There is no evidence that slowly increased pressure is of any benefit (Vacca, 1997).

Advocacy/accountability

Whilst the delivering professional is responsible for their own practice, midwives continue to have a duty of care towards their client, and continue to be accountable for their practice. If a midwife feels that further analgesia is required, or that the delivering professional is having difficulties, they must speak out, acting as an advocate for the client. This is not always an easy position to be in.

Post-procedure care

- A midwife should record any aspects of the birth, for example start of procedure, fetal heart auscultation, etc., to ensure an optimal written record of events.
- Once the baby is born, if all is well, events should follow just as if the woman had delivered unaided: skin-to-skin contact and early breastfeeding should be encouraged in the normal way. Parents should be aware that the baby's head may appear marked or moulded, but that this should disappear within hours.
- An anti-inflammatory such as diclofenac 100 mg given rectally (PR) following delivery/suturing may help the pain once any epidural or local anaesthetic has worn off.

A midwife ventouse delivery

Some midwives now carry out instrumental deliveries, following formal training and assessment, under specified criteria. Please read the previous section for general comments on instrumental delivery. The following section describes aspects specific to midwife ventouse (MV) delivery.

Criteria for a midwife ventous delivery

The criteria may vary according to local protocol.

- Fully dilated cervix.
- Occipitoanterior (OA) position (but not necessarily direct OA), well flexed.
- No acynclitism (head tilted to one side).
- Head no longer palpable (i.e. fully engaged) abdominally.

- Head below the level of the ischial spines
- Minimal caput or moulding only.
- Good contractions.
- Verbal maternal consent obtained.

If fetal distress occurs in a stand-alone midwife-only unit, and a ventouse midwife is called in, it is sensible to call an ambulance as well. If the circumstances are inappropriate for a MV delivery, immediate transfer is necessary.

Preparation

History

Review the antenatal and labour history, note parity, length of labour and fetal position during labour. Always beware of a slow 7–10 cm cervical dilatation interval. Slow second stage progress, particularly in multigravidae, may indicate dispropor-tion.

Assessment

A ventouse delivery should not be attempted unless the MV criteria given above are met.

It is important to remain focused and analytical throughout, and not be swayed by the enthusiasm of other staff or parents to achieve delivery. It is hard, particularly in stand-alone midwife-only units to decline a ventouse delivery because this means transfer to another unit. However, transfer following failed ventouse delivery, with the fetal distress that sometimes results, is worse.

An abdominal and a vaginal examination should be performed, with consent. Do not rely on the opinion of others, even if several staff reassure you that 'it's definitely OA...'. Check for yourself.

Monitor the contractions, if poor strength and/or frequency then IV oxytocic augmentation may be advisable.

Communication

Prior to physical examination, the midwife should introduce him/herself to the woman and partner. Attitude at this time is extremely important, and gaining a woman's confidence is crucial. In cases of presumed fetal distress, this discussion may have to be brief, but most clients understand, and under such circumstances will want actions rather than words.

It is important to acknowledge the woman's hard work so far. Explain the situation, and confirm the woman's (and her partner's) understanding. Try to present options, for example 'If I confirm that the baby is in the right position for ventouse delivery, then we can either do it now, or see how your pushing goes over the next 15 minutes...', giving the woman the choice. Some women, however, may be too dis-tressed to make such choices, or may perceive this as indecision. Midwifery judgement should be used, as with all women in labour, to decide the level of information given.

Remember that most post-birth emotional trauma appears to be associated with poor information giving and perceived loss of control (Green, 1990). Never under-estimate a woman's capacity to make choices, however distraught she may appear.

Analgesia, positioning and bladder care

This was covered in the preceding section entitled 'Care of a woman undergoing instrumental delivery'.

Equipment preparation

Midwife ventouse deliveries are normally performed using rubber or hand-held plastic cups. Check the suction by applying the cup to your hand. See also the section entitled 'Assisting at an instrumental delivery procedure' above.

The ventouse procedure

Performing a ventouse delivery

- Cup insertion is often painful, but with increasing experience, it can be performed smoothly and gently. Entonox may help.
- Immediately following a contraction (warn the woman what is about to happen), insert the squeezed, externally lubricated cup by gently slipping two fingers of the other hand into the introitus, retracting the perineum, and sliding the cup into the space created.
- The cup is manoeuvred into the optimal position. Vacca (1997) describes the flexion point which, in a well-flexed OA position, is typically around 3 cm from the posterior fontanelle. This is the point of the vertex where the cup should be applied (see Fig. 10.1).
- If the cup is correctly applied so that it lies over the flexion point, with the sagittal suture running centrally down, then traction will result in the smallest diameter of the fetal head (the suboccipitobregmatic and biparietal) being drawn through the birth canal (see also Fig. 4.5 for diameters of the fetal skull). This minimizes traction, thus increasing the likelihood of a successful birth and reducing trauma to mother and baby. In practice maternal tissue often inhibits cup positioning, so then the cup is simply placed as near as possible to the posterior fontanelle.
- The woman is often distressed following cup application, so reassure and congratulate her that the cup is now in place, and she has got through an unpleasant moment.
- Apply 0.2 (kg/cm^2) pressure, then check the position and ensure no maternal tissue is trapped in the cup. The process of feeling round the cup is another painful moment, especially anteriorly where space is tight, so warn the woman and proceed gently. If satisfactory, increase to 0.8 in one step.
- Await the next contraction. Encourage the woman to get her breath back, and focus on the coming need to push. Sometimes it helps to smile, get eye contact, and encourage an atmosphere of calm excitement, 'It really won't be long now ...'. This may recharge the atmosphere, giving the woman more energy. Beware though: a 'high adrenaline' environment may scare some women.

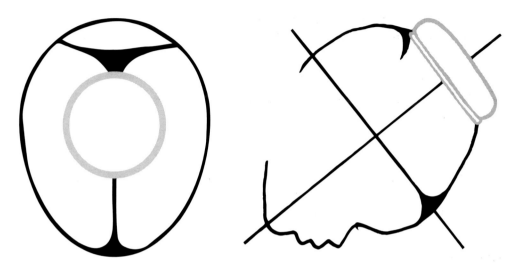

Fig. 10.1 Application of the ventouse cup. The cup is manoeuvred into the optimal position. In an occipitoanterior position the flexion point is typically around 3 cm from the posterior fontanelle with the sagittal suture running centrally down

- With the contraction, encourage the woman to push, and apply steady traction perpendicular to the cup. As the head comes under the symphysis and extends, the cup will rise from horizontal to almost vertical.
- The head should descend with each pull. Local policies dictate the number of pulls/cup detachments that are acceptable: the AAFP course (2000/2001) suggests the procedure should be abandoned following three cup detachments or if there is no progress for three consecutive pulls. Experienced midwives often recognize when a head will not deliver after just one pull, and will abandon the attempt immediately.
- As already discussed, it is not essential to perform an episiotomy for a ventouse delivery (Vacca, 1997; AAFP, 2000/2001); clinical judgement should be exercised, and appropriate consent obtained, as with any birth.
- Over-excited staff may be tempted to deliver the head quickly. Unless there is good reason to hurry, resist this urge! Remember how slowly a primigravid woman normally delivers: fast perineal stretching will cause increased pain and tissue trauma. Once the head is guided to the perineum, the woman's expulsive urge may do most of the rest of the work. Some midwives will hardly pull at all, as the perineum slowly distends. Such births can be true collaborations between midwife and mother. There are reports of women who believe they had only minimal help (Charles, 1999) and deny they have truly had an assisted delivery.

Advocacy/accountability

See also the earlier section 'Care of a woman undergoing instrumental delivery'. Remember: you are a ventouse midwife, not an obstetrician. Do not be drawn into making decisions outside your remit.

Post-birth discussion and care

Most ventouse midwives discuss the birth with the parents afterwards, congratulating the mother, and giving an opportunity for questions and explanations. Sometimes this is practicable only immediately following the birth. It is helpful to inform a woman that any subsequent birth is unlikely to require another assisted delivery. Some women and partners may find discussion supportive and reassuring. Others may be too shocked by events to be ready to 'revisit' them, or too preoccupied by their new baby to care. Sensitivity should be shown in this, as in all, birth matters.

Records

Indications and assessment for ventouse delivery should be recorded, as well as procedure and outcome. Ventouse midwives may wish to keep a 'log book' of deliveries (see Appendix B) and periodically review their practice, e.g. numbers of failed deliveries and shoulder dystocias.

It is helpful to log any ventouse deliveries that, after assessment, the midwife decides not to perform, and the subsequent outcome. These 'declined deliveries' may indicate a ventouse midwife's skill as much as the successful births achieved (see Appendix C).

Logbooks may form part of an overall audit of MV deliveries in some locations.

Summary

Role of the midwife in assisting at instrumental delivery

- Evidence suggests that ventouse is the mode of choice for most instrumental deliveries (Johanson & Menon, 2002).
- Instrumental birth can be frightening for the woman and her partner(s); communication and sensitivity are critical.
- Instrumental deliveries are stressful for staff too; they should make every effort to work well together.
- This is a difficult time for a woman to make choices. However, consent should always be sought before any intervention.
- Warn a woman of the possibility of caesarean section if instrumental delivery fails.
- Think aortocaval occlusion.
- The need for 'routine' catheterization/episiotomy is unsupported by evidence.
- Prepare a woman for the pain of ventouse cup/forceps insertion.
- A midwife remains accountable for her own practice, even though another professional has taken over the delivery.
- The midwife should act as an advocate for the woman, ensuring she has adequate analgesia, and voicing concerns about any suboptimal care.
- Be aware of the increased risk of shoulder dystocia and postpartum haemorrhage. Be prepared.

Performing a midwife ventouse (MV) delivery

- Midwife ventouse deliveries may be carried out under specified criteria.
- Midwives are not obstetricians – refer deviations from normality.
- Encourage slow head delivery to minimize perineal trauma.
- Plan ahead with post-delivery analgesia (e.g. diclofenac 100 mg PR).
- Record keeping: ensure accurate description of events. Ventouse midwives may keep logbooks of deliveries achieved, declined and failed.
- A post-birth discussion may be helpful for a woman and her partner, where possible. This is an ideal opportunity to congratulate a woman on her courage and endurance.

Useful contact

Baby Lifeline   Empathy Enterprise Building, Bramston Crescent, Tile Hill, Coventry CV4 9SW. Telephone: 02476 422135.
Website: www.babylifeline.org.uk

References

AAFP (2000/2001) *Advanced Life Support in Obstetrics (ALSO). Course Syllabus Manual*, 4th edn. American Academy of Family Physicians, Leawood, Kansas.

Charles, C. (1999) How it feels to be a midwife ventouse practitioner. *British Journal of Midwifery* **7** (6), 380–82.

Charles, C. (2002) Practising as a midwife ventouse practioner in an isolated midwife-led unit setting. *MIDIRS Midwifery Digest* **12** (1), 75–7.

Green, J.M. (1990) Expectations, experiences and psychological outcomes of childbirth: a prospective study of 825 women. *Birth* **17** (1), 15–23.

Gupta, J.K. & Nikodem, V.C. (2002) Woman's position during the second stage of labour (Cochrane Review). *The Cochrane Library* Issue 4. Update Software, Oxford.

Hodnett, E.D. (2002) Caregiver support for women during childbirth (Cochrane Review). *The Cochrane Library* Issue 4. Update Software, Oxford.

Johanson, R. (2001) *The Baby Lifeline B.I.R.T.H. Series*. Interactive Educational Video Series. Baby Lifeline Trading, Coventry. Reviewed by V. Tinsley *Midwifery Digest* **11** (2), 284–5.

Johanson, R.B. & Menon, V.J. (2002) Vacuum extraction vs forceps for assisted vaginal delivery (Cochrane Review). *The Cochrane Library* Issue 4. Update Software, Oxford.

Johnson, C., Keirse, M.J.N.C., Enkin, M. & Chalmers, I. (2000) Hospital practices – nutrition and hydration in labor. In *A Guide to Effective Care in Pregnancy and Childbirth*, 3rd edn (Enkin, M., Keirse, M.J.N.C., Neilson, J. *et al.*, eds), pp. 255–66. Oxford University Press, Oxford.

Morgan, B.M., Bulpitt, C.J., Clifton, P. & Lewish, P.J. (1982) Analgesia and satisfaction in childbirth (The Queen Charlotte's One Thousand Mother Survey). *The Lancet* **2**, 808–10.

NICE (2001) *Clinical Guideline C – The Use of Electronic Fetal Monitoring*. National Institute for Clinical Excellence, London.

Sleep, J., Roberts, J., & Chalmers, I. (2000) The second stage of labor. In *A Guide to Effective Care in Pregnancy and Childbirth*, 3rd edn (Enkin, M., Keirse, M.J.N.C., Neilson, J. *et al.*, eds), pp. 289–99. Oxford University Press, Oxford.

Vacca, A. (1997) *Handbook of Vacuum Extraction in Obstetric Practice*. Vacca Research, Albion, Queensland, Australia.

11 Haemorrhage and hypovolaemic shock around the time of birth

'Every unit should have a protocol for the management of haemorrhage and this should be reviewed and rehearsed on a regular basis. It should also be included as part of life support training. All members of staff, including those in the blood bank, must know exactly what to do to ensure that large quantities of cross-matched blood can be delivered without delay.' (DoH, 2001)

Introduction

Clinically, haemorrhage may be defined as significant blood loss sufficient to cause haemodynamic instability (AAFP, 2000/2001). Haemorrhage can occur prior to, during or following birth; it can be dramatic and sudden or slow and incipient. The Confidential Enquiries into Maternal Deaths (DoH, 2001) suggest that because obstetric haemorrhage is life-threatening and can occur rapidly, each unit should have a multidisciplinary massive haemorrhage protocol which is rehearsed regularly.

Incidence and facts

- As with any emergency situation, the woman will require explanations, ongoing reassurances and appropriate analgesia. The latter is often forgotten if clinicians are attempting to ascertain or control the source of the bleeding. Yet such interventions can be frightening and painful for the woman.
- Women at higher risk of haemorrhage should be advised to have their babies in a consultant unit with an on-site blood bank (DoH, 2001).
- The midwife should assess her client for any risk factors which predispose her to problematic haemorrhage. Higher risk groups include: women with placenta praevia (especially those with a previous caesarean or myomectomy scar), uterine fibroids, placental abruption, or previous third stage complications (DoH, 2001).
- It is often the slow, continuous bleeding that goes unnoticed; this type of bleeding can lead to maternal death (AAFP, 2000/2001).
- Clinicians tend to dramatically underestimate blood loss (AAFP, 2000/2001).

Signs and symptoms

The woman

- Depending on the type of haemorrhage, the woman may have symptoms such as pain and visible loss, and may become shocked (see Box 11.1). For specific signs and symptoms of antepartum/intrapartum haemorrhage see Table 11.1.
- During significant haemorrhage, blood is directed to the woman's vital organs. The woman becomes peripherally shut down, looking pale, feeling cold and clammy as she becomes shocked (Box 11.1). For details of basic care for shock see Chapter 12. Emergency bloods are dealt with in Box 11.2.
- The woman will develop a tachycardia and may become progressively more agitated and, in extreme cases, even gasp for air.
- If the woman becomes drowsy, even unconscious, collapse and cardiac arrest can rapidly follow.

The baby

- If the baby is undelivered, consider aortocaval occlusion. This is often forgotten during resuscitation. Create a firm lateral tilt from a wedge.
- In complete cardiac arrest *deliver the baby* within 5 minutes. Obstetricians do not need to prepare a sterile field and should go for the quickest incision possible (Bobrowski, 1994).

Box 11.1 Signs and symptoms of shock.

Physical symptoms in the woman
- Pale.
- Cold extremities, clammy.
- Weak.
- Agitated/frightened/irritated.
- May vomit.

Serious signs
- Breathless/bluey/gasping for air.
- Drowsy/semi-conscious/unconscious.

Measurable observations and vital signs

Serious signs
- Pulse > 100 beats per minute. Increasing tachycardia – rapid, thready or weak pulse
- Blood pressure systolic < 100 mmHg and diastolic < 50 mmHg. A drop in blood pressure is usually a late and ominous sign of severe compromise.
- Oxygen saturation – increasing breathlessness or peripherally blue around the mouth, fingers and feet.
- Cardiac/respiratory arrest.

Monitoring
- Use a valid automated blood pressure device (see Appendix A) to record the woman's observations every few minutes during an acute collapse.
- Monitor oxygen saturation.

Assessing blood loss – if a possible causative factor
- Evaluate slow, continuous bleeding.
- Suspect concealed blood loss if the mother develops incipient shock (palour, tachycardia, etc.) (AAFP, 2000/2001).

Antepartum/intrapartum haemorrhage

PLACENTA PRAEVIA

Placenta praevia is the abnormal location of the placenta in the lower uterine segment, which partially or completely covers the cervical os. As the pregnancy advances the woman is prone to haemorrhage, particularly if the cervix dilates, and the bleeding can be profuse.

Incidence and facts

- 0.5% of pregnancies, (AAFP, 2000/2001) of which 15% of placenta praevia are complicated by placenta accreta (McDonald, 1999).

- The only safe mode of delivery for complete placenta praevia is by caesarean section because the placenta is literally obstructing the baby's exit via the cervix.
- Placenta praevia is more common in women with a uterine scar and may be associated with uncontrollable uterine haemorrhage at delivery. Both an obstetric and an anaesthetic consultant should be available as a caesarean hysterectomy may become necessary (DoH, 2001).

For associated risk factors see Box 11.3.

Table 11.1   Signs, symptoms and diagnosis of placenta praevia and placental abruption.

	Placenta praevia	Placental abruption
Pain	• Usually painless	• Usually *severe* uterine pain
Uterus	• Soft • The woman's uterus is usually relaxed although around 25% of women will present with varying degrees of contractions (Lockwood, 1996)	• Tense/tender uterus • Uterine hypertonia is more common in severe cases and when the baby has died (Fraser & Watson, 2000)
Bleeding	• Usually visible	• Usually visible although in 20% of cases it may be concealed in the uterus (Fraser & Watson, 2000; AAFP, 2000/2001)
Baby	• Commonly non-engaged and ballotable, due to the placental location • 35% of babies present as unstable lie (Lockwood, 1996)	• Commonly normal lie and presentation
Vaginal examination	• Vaginal examinations are contraindicated in placenta praevia (as they can exacerbate bleeding, Fraser & Watson, 2000)	• Vaginal examinations are not contraindicated
Ultrasound scan	• Previous ultrasound scan reports to identify the location of the placenta and confirm fetal gestation	• Ultrasound scan to exclude placenta praevia • Ultrasound scanning is sometimes used to confirm a possible abruption if a retroplacental clot can be visualized

Box 11.2   Blood tests (see also Chapter 18).

Emergency bloods
Samples of blood are taken for:

- Group and cross-matching
- Full blood count (FBC)
- Clotting studies – fibrinogen levels, prothrombin time (international normalized radio) (PT/INR)/ activated partial thromboplastin time (APTT).

Kleihauer testing
This detects if fetal cells have crossed into the maternal circulation and is routinely tested in women who are Rh negative following a sensitizing event in pregnancy or following delivery.

Box 11.3 Risk factors associated with placenta praevia and placental abruption.

Placenta praevia
- Previous caesarean section (Langdana *et al.*, 2001).
- Multi-parity (McDonald, 1999).

Placental abruption
- Hypertension occurs in 25–50% of cases (Lockwood, 1996).
- Abdominal trauma – including domestic violence.
- High parity.
- Growth restriction (Lockwood, 1996).
- Uterine over-distension – including polyhydramnios (McDonald, 1999).
- Smoking.
- Some thrombophilias (McGeown, 2001).

PLACENTAL ABRUPTION

Placental abruption is the partial or total separation of the placenta from the uterus during pregnancy or labour.

Incidence and facts

- 1–2% of pregnancies (AAFP, 2000/2001).
- Fraser & Watson (2000) recommend that abruption should be considered in any woman with abdominal pain, with or without bleeding.
- Placental abruption is the most common obstetric emergency and a major cause of perinatal mortality (McGeown, 2001). For more information on loss of a baby, see Chapter 13.
- Half of moderate to severe cases of placental abruption develop clotting problems (Lockwood, 1996) as thromboplastins from the placental site are released and the bleeding behind the placenta uses up clotting factors.
- While many cases can be mild and the woman's pregnancy continues uneventfully, severe cases will require the co-ordinated care of obstetricians, midwives, anaesthetists and the haematology team (McGeown, 2001).

For associated risk factors see Box 11.3.

Care of a woman with placenta praevia/placental abruption

For associated risk factors see Box 11.3 and for signs, symptoms and diagnosis see Table 11.1.

- Check recent haemoglobin (Hb) levels.
- Have ready cross-matched blood (4 units).
- Ensure intravenous (IV) access with large cannula.
- Inform the anaesthetist, paediatrician, special care baby unit (SCBU)/neonatal itensive care unit (NICU), theatres.

In serious or anticipated ongoing haemorrhage the Confidential Enquiries into Maternal Deaths (DoH, 2001) recommend:

- A second large gauge cannula.
- A central venous pressure (CVP) line to accurately monitor fluid volume.
- Make sure the intensive care unit (ICU) is aware.

Reassure and explain to the woman and her partner what is happening. Discuss the possible outcomes, and if a caesarean section is likely, prepare them for this possibility. Any bleeding is in itself very frightening for the woman who naturally fears for her own and her baby's welfare. Her birth partner may be experiencing feelings of helplessness and concern. These fears may manifest as quiet anxiety or asking many, many questions or occasionally showing panic or aggression.

Maternal comfort and analgesia

- Women with placenta praevia can experience contractions (this happening in 25% of cases [Lockwood, 1996]) but in general, these are irregular, of varying strengths and uncomfortable rather than painful.
- Placental abruption can be very painful for some women. Support and reassurance are essential analgesia. In addition, try helping the woman get comfortable, use bean bags/pillows, massage, touch and pharmacological analgesia. Monitor the fetal heart rate (FHR) closely following any position changes.
- While an epidural may be possible, any maternal risk factors, such as low platelets and clotting problems, may preclude its safe use.

Monitoring maternal well-being

- **Vital signs**. Closely monitor the woman's vital signs – tachycardia is usually the first sign of maternal compromise associated with blood loss.
- **Intravenous infusion (IVI)**. To replace fluid loss ensure that IV fluids are in progress. Doctors should consider giving blood products.
- **Measuring blood loss**. Discreetly change and save soaked sanitary pads/incos but ensure the woman's privacy when doing this. Keep updated comparisons of estimated and measured ongoing blood loss on a fluid chart.
- **Possible anaesthetic required**. Ensure the anaesthetist is informed and can assess the woman's situation well in advance of a potential emergency anaesthetic being required (DoH, 2001). Also give regular antacids/hydrogen ion inhibitors as an emergency anaesthetic may be required (Johnson *et al.*, 2000).
- **Fetal heart rate (FHR) monitoring**. Sudden or abnormal FHR changes (such as an increasing tachycardia) could be an indication of compromise caused by severe

blood loss, which could quickly become fatal for the baby. Respond to any abnormal pattern promptly. See Appendix E for assessment of FHR.

Labour care and placental abruption

Where the bleeding is small or settling, and the maternal and fetal condition is satisfactory, the decision to labour and birth without intervention may well be appropriate (see Box 11.4). Evidence suggests that an attempt to deliver vaginally, inducing or augmenting with IV oxytocics, and using continuous electronic monitoring, may result in a 50% reduction in the caesarean rate without any significant affect on perinatal mortality (Fraser & Watson, 2000).

Box 11.4 Management of antepartum/intrapartum haemorrhage.

Wait and see/expectant management may be appropriate for:
- Mild to moderate bleeding.
- If the bleeding appears to have settled.
- If the baby is very preterm and the mother is stable (Fraser & Watson, 2000).

Immediate delivery is indicated if:
- Bleeding is thought to be heavy or ongoing.
- There is evidence of compromise to mother or baby (Hayashi, 2000).

- If the woman's condition is thought to be stable and she is labouring, then a partogram, fluid chart and observation chart should be commenced. Vital signs and blood loss will need regular observation and documenting to ensure the woman's condition remains stable.
- Note the frequency, regularity and strength of her contractions. As with any labour, they should increase in frequency, strength, and length. Contractions can present differently in such circumstances and birth can sometimes happen very rapidly. With some contractions small trickles of blood may be evident, which in conjunction with the woman's vital signs, and FHR, will require close monitoring.
- See also 'Care of a woman with placental bleeding – placenta praevia or placental abruption' described above.

For the birth preparations should 'include:

- Alerting the SCBU/NICU and theatre; make sure the paediatrician is aware. Only have the necessary clinicians present for the birth.
- The room should be warm and draught-free with warm towels available to dry the baby.
- The resuscitaire should be checked and the overhead heater on.

Third stage management:

- Delay cord clamping by at least 30+ seconds as this may have important clinical benefits for the hypovolaemic baby. Delayed clamping increases blood volume that is transfused to the baby by 20–50%, which increases the baby's haemoglobin and haematocrits (Prendiville & Elbourne, 2000). Babies who have suffered from placental abruption can be born pale and anaemic and may require a transfusion. The extra blood they receive via the cord may be vital for them (Mercer, 2001).

- Cord care. When eventually cutting the cord leave it long in case the baby later requires umbilical cord catheterization.
- Take cord blood for pH testing.
- Postpartum haemorrhage may pose a problem, therefore active management is recommended and a Syntocinon infusion should be pre-prepared.
- Finally, remember estimated blood loss is frequently *underestimated* (AAFP, 2000/2001).

Postpartum haemorrhage

Postpartum haemorrhage (PPH) can occur up to 24 hours after birth and usually involves significant blood loss via the genital tract. It has three causes, the 3Ts: *tone (uterine atony), tissue trauma* and, rarely, *thrombophilias* (clotting problems). The woman who suffers a PPH will usually find the whole experience frightening and traumatic. The fear, pain and discomfort experienced at the time of the incident is in itself a frightening experience which is likely to affect her future anxiety levels in any subsequent birth.

Clinicians should have awareness of predisposing risk factors to haemorrhage and anyone at 'high risk'. The midwife should ensure that the appropriate clinicians are aware (including a senior anaesthetist) and that the woman has an up-to-date haemaglobin result, blood cross-matched and that the woman is advised to have a large gauge cannula *in situ* (DoH, 2001).

Incidence and facts

- Postpartum haemorrhage occurs in 5% of all births, with 70% of those being caused by uterine atony (AAFP, 2000/2001).
- Life-threatening haemorrhage is estimated to occur in 6.7 per 1000 deliveries (DoH, 2001).
- The DoH (2001) suggests that the low number of deaths indicates that in general this condition is being well treated. However, there are still avoidable deaths from haemorrhage.
- Studies indicate that women die from postpartum haemorrhage an average of more than 5 hours following delivery. Such women have usually continued to bleed continuously, 'unalarming' amounts that have tragically gone unnoticed (AAFP, 2000/2001).
- The AAFP (2000/2001) recommends that following the completion of delivery paperwork, clinicians return to reassess the women's vaginal loss and vital signs in order to identify steady bleeding that may be ongoing. Midwives in the UK tend to check this as a matter of routine, including palpating the uterus and ensuring the mother has passed urine prior to transfer to the postnatal ward, or at a home birth prior to leaving the woman.

UTERINE ATONY (TONE)

Postpartum haemorrhage can be caused when the uterus is atonic and unable to reliably contract following birth. The aim of care is to deliver the placenta, if *in situ*, and ensure the uterus is well contracted. Predisposing risk factors include poly-hydramnios, multiple pregnancy, high parity, prolonged/induced/augmented labours, instrumental delivery, pregnancy induced hypertension (PIH), placental abruption, placenta praevia, previous postpartum haemorrhage.

Skills drill for postpartum haemorrhage

Box 11.5 describes the procedure to follow for postpartum haemorrhage.

TISSUE TRAUMA

The majority of women sustain some degree of trauma to the perineum following birth; occasionally such trauma will include large blood vessels. Predisposing risk factors include enforced expulsive pushing, macrosomia, instrumental delivery, and early/large episiotomy.

Types of tissue trauma

- **Tears**. Internal to the cervix or vagina, or external to the genitalia/perineum/anus.
- **Episiotomy**. If large or performed too early (such as before the perineum has thinned) episiotomies can cut through blood vessels resulting in uncontrolled bleeding. Episiotomy also increases the risk of third-degree tear (Sleep *et al.*, 2000).
- **Haematoma**. An acute haematoma is rare, approximately 1:1000 births. The bleeding is usually concealed and the volume of blood is often underestimated (Kean, 2000). Episiotomy is usually a related factor in 85–90% of haematomas (Kean, 2000).

TEARS/EPISIOTOMY

Signs and symptoms

Despite heavy blood loss, the uterus usually feels well contracted and does not gush blood from the vagina when pressed. Many midwives choose to give a precautionary dose of an oxytocic if they remain unsure of the source of the bleeding.

Treatment

External bleeding

- Locating the source of the bleeding can be very painful for the woman. Breathing some entonox may help here.
- The midwife should continuously talk through what she is doing and suggest the woman tells her if she needs the midwife to stop at any time.

Box 11.5   Skills drill for postpartum haemorrhage.

Deliver the placenta if *in situ*
- If the placenta is *truly* adherent, there is usually no bleeding.
- If separation is partial, the placenta may be difficult to remove completely and haemorrhage can be difficult to control.

↓

Rub up a contraction
- Rub the fundus in a firm circular motion – keep rubbing as required for up to a minute . . . The uterus should feel hard, not boggy or soft.
- Regularly re-assess – re-rub if the uterus starts to relax under the fingers.

↓

Give oxytocics/site IV
- Administer *oxytocic agents* (see Chapter 23).
- Warn the woman she may feel sick/vomit.
- Site a cannula (take routine emergency bloods – as per Box 11.2) and commence intravenous (IV) *Syntocinon 5–30 IU in 500 ml of fluids* (Hartmanns or normal saline).
- Run quickly initially, then slowly as the uterus responds.

↓

Catheterization
- This is important if the bladder is palpable or visible.

↓

By this point, most bleeding is controlled and responding to the oxytocics.

If it is not more help is needed and the obstetric team and anaesthetist should be called immediately, if they have not already been contacted.

At home call for a paramedic ambulance and follow the guidelines in the section 'Transfer of a woman with a retained placenta' on page 180.

↓

Re-assess
- Bleeding settling?
- Another cause?

'problems can arise because clinicians fail to move onto the next step . . . a more detailed examination of the genital tract is indicated.' (Campbell & Lees, 2000)

↓

Ongoing haemorrhage/replace blood loss
  According to the severity of the loss:
- Site a second large gauge cannula.
- Set up intravenous (IV) fluids.
- Use blood products as necessary.
- *Carboprost/Hemabate* (kept in the fridge) injected intramuscularly (IM) (warn the woman that this drug will make her feel very unwell).

↓

If haemorrhage is ongoing and severe:
- In hospital, transfer the woman to theatre for manual removal of the placenta and bi-manual compression.
- At home the midwife is faced with performing urgent manual removal and bi-manual compression (see Box 11.6 for a description of the procedure).

- A bleeding vessel can be hidden behind clots or oozing blood loss. So methodically check the area – the clitoris, labia, and perineum – dabbing firmly then wiping away the blood with gauze.
- Once located, a bleeding vessel is obvious as when dabbed clean, it instantly oozes or pumps blood, obscuring the view.
- Simply apply pressure to the bleeding point using some sterile gauze, or similar material, and hold firmly over the bleeding point for 5 or so minutes. This may be all that is required but keep a check on the area in the following hours.
- If still oozing, the bleeding vessel should be clamped and will require tying off (see Fig. 11.1). If at home, or a birthing centre, the midwife should do this promptly herself.
- If the bleeding is internal, or excessive, an obstetrician should be contacted.

Internal bleeding

- If the bleeding is thought to be internal, an experienced obstetrician should be contacted to carry out this uncomfortable examination.
- If at a home birth or birthing centre, the midwife will have to undertake this examination herself, as prompt arrest of the bleeding is essential.
- Bleeding from the cervix or deep in the vagina will require a speculum examination using a good light source and plenty of gauze. Open up a suture pack or line up some sponge holder forceps wrapped in gauze for dabbing the blood away to allow a view of the bleeding point.

(a)   (b)

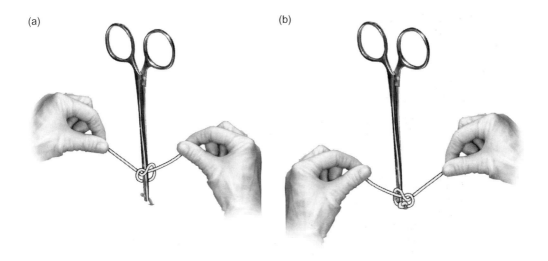

Fig. 11.1 Tying off a bleeding vessel. Bleeding vessels can be awkward to reach and tying them off may be painful for the woman. Grasp the vessel with a pair of forceps, then loop some thread around the forceps (this may require the aid of an assistant). Tie one throw of a knot – left thread over right (a) and slip the knot down past the end of the forceps to encircle the vessel. Pull the knot tight and then tie a second throw – right thread over left (b). The knot should be square and not slip. Trim the thread and then release the forceps carefully.

- If the bleeding is high up, packing or direct pressure should be applied and the woman transferred into hospital urgently for suturing under anaesthetic. Sutures should not be placed blind, deep in the vaginal fornix as they can cause uterine injury. Occasionally, bleeding tears of this kind need repairing via the abdomen (Kean, 2000).

Note: Keep a *count of gauze swabs* used 'before and after', as one could easily become 'lost'.

HAEMATOMAS

Signs and symptoms

Haematomas are not always visible and may even lie beneath sutures, but the signs/symptoms are usually:

- Severe vaginal/vulval/rectal pain.
- Unrelenting vaginal/vulval/rectal pressure.
- A visible mass deviating the vagina and rectum (AAFP, 2000/2001).
- Internal examination may not be tolerable as it may cause unbearable pain for the woman, which in itself should help assist the diagnosis of haematoma.
- Other signs include: discoloured swelling and blood-filled, oedematous tissues; signs of hypovolaemic shock.

Treatment

- For small haematomas of less than 3 cm, observation and analgesia are the course of action (Kean, 2000).
- For larger haematomas, analgesia and prompt treatment are essential.
- Most haematomas require surgical intervention: incision, drainage, and stemming of any bleeding vessel(s), followed by packing or suturing if the tissues are not too friable and damaged (Kean, 2000). This should preferably take place in sterile conditions and using a suitable anaesthesia. Antibiotic cover may be prescribed.
- Treat hypovolaemia if present.

Haematomas at home/birthing centre

- Prompt diagnosis (see above) is necessary.
- Stabilize, treat for hypovolaemia.
- Transfer to hospital via a paramedic ambulance.
- Entonox should be offered and additional, more effective analgesia should be discussed on arrival in hospital.

THROMBOPHILIAS/CLOTTING PROBLEMS

Some pregnancy-related conditions can give rise to clotting problems: a large placental abruption (usually in this case the baby will have died), severe pre-eclampsia/eclampsia, intrauterine death, amniotic fluid embolism and sepsis (AAFP, 2000/2001).

Some uncommon conditions, such as thrombocytopenia and von Willebrand's disease amongst others, can also affect clotting. Clotting problems are directly accountable for only 1% of postpartum haemorrhages (AAFP, 2000/2001).

Signs and symptoms

- Continued bleeding.
- Oozing from puncture sites.
- Predisposing factors as mentioned above.

Treatment

- Care should involve senior anaesthetic, obstetric, midwifery and haematology staff.
- Blood testing for immediate full blood count (FBC) and clotting studies (AAFP, 2000/2001) and cross-matching.
- Urgent fluid and blood product replacement, depending on the diagnosed coagulopathy (AAFP, 2000/2001).

Snapped cord and retained placenta

SNAPPED CORD

The cord can snap if it is short or friable, at or following birth. If the cord snaps, or the midwife can feel it tearing away on applying traction, then providing there is no haemorrhage it can wait. A snapped cord means that the placenta must be delivered by good maternal pushing efforts, in an upright position. Unless the placenta is truly adherent, this should be successful. Ensure the placenta is separated then follow 'Delivering a retained placenta', covered below.

Incidence

A snapped cord occurs at 3% of vaginal births (Prendiville & Elbourne, 2000).

RETAINED PLACENTA

A retained placenta and subsequent management (manual removal) can have a negative effect on the quality of contact the woman has with her newborn as well as her postpartum health. A retained placenta reduces time spent bonding, feeding and getting to know the new baby and in the longer term can leave the woman anaemic, tender and sore. In more severe cases it can result in acute haemorrhage, infection, secondary postpartum haemorrhage, hysterectomy and even maternal death (AAFP, 2000/2001).

The placenta is termed 'retained' if it is not delivered within a particular time limit, following the birth of the baby:

- Within 30 minutes following active management (AAFP, 2000/2001).
- Within 1 hour following expectant management (physiological third stage).

Incidence

- A retained placenta occurs in 3% of vaginal births (AAFP, 2000/2001).
- 15% of retained placentas are in women who have had a previous retained placenta (AAFP, 2000/2001).

Facts

- Injecting an oxytocic into the umbilical vein has been shown to increase the chance of delivering an otherwise retained placenta (Carroli & Bergel, 2002).
- There is no clear data to rule out the possibility that administering a routine oxyctocic for the third stage can increase the risk of retained placenta (Prendiville & Elbourne, 2000).
- Rarely, the placenta is truly adherent and imbedded into the uterus. Placenta accreta or percreta is usually discovered when attempting manual removal and, unfortunately, a hysterectomy is usually necessary to control emergency post-partum bleeding (AAFP, 2000/2001).

Midwifery role

- Despite attempts to deliver the placenta, if it remains retained the midwife will need to refer the woman to the obstetric team.
- Providing there is no urgency the conventional treatment for retained placenta is digital manual removal under anaesthetic in theatre. This is commonly in the form of a regional block but occasionally by general anaesthesia.
- In the absence of medical aid and in an emergency manual removal of the placenta can be undertaken by a midwife (UKCC, 1998) (see Box 11.6).

Delivering a retained placenta

Provided the woman's blood loss is normal/minimal the midwife can try the following:

- **Breastfeeding**. This stimulates natural oxytocin, which should help the uterus contract.
- **Controlled cord traction**. If an oxytocic has been administered, the midwife should make several attempts to deliver the placenta by applying traction on the cord and counter support/guard the uterus. Caution: if any 'gushing'/active bleeding occurs, stop any cord traction.
- **Maternal position**. Assist the mother to remain upright, such as squatting/kneeling or sitting on the toilet or a bedpan.
- **Encourage active pushing**. The woman may experience her contractions as 'period-type pains' at this stage and they may be infrequent. Encourage her to push with these 'pains'. Anecdotally, midwives who recommend this active pushing suggest that pushing may take a while and require many, many attempts but that it is often successful.
- **Palpable bladder**. Most women are unable to pass urine unaided at this stage. If the bladder is palpable, discuss with the woman the possibility of passing a

Box 11.6   Manual removal of the placenta and bi-manual compression (only to be undertaken by the midwife in an emergency).

Manual removal

While manual removal is fairly simple, it is likely to be very painful for the woman and carries the risk of infection and uterine rupture if performed too roughly. The woman should be offered entonox or anything else that is available. The procedure should be explained to her and her birth partner, who should then be offered the opportunity to leave the room perhaps to care for the baby or other children (Crafter, 2002).

- Observe aseptic technique and wear sterile, elbow length gloves.
- The external hand rests on the fundus, to prevent it moving away.
- Insert the fingers, then the hand into the vagina, through the os and trace the cord to locate the placenta.
- Locate the edge of the placenta and using a side-to-side movement gently coax the placenta away from the uterus (Crafter, 2002), cupping the separated cotyledons in the palm of the hand (AAFP, 2000/2001).
- Aim to deliver the placenta complete/intact (AAFP, 2000/2001).
- Once it has separated the placenta can be delivered by traction on the cord.
- The hand still inside the uterus should remain to 'brush' gently over the placental site, to dislodge any possible fragments left behind (Crafter, 2002).

Bi-manual compression

This is an extremely painful procedure and should only be performed if the bleeding continues and medical assistance is not available.

To perform internal bi-manual compression the midwife rubs up a contraction with the external hand on the fundus and keeps the other hand in a clenched fist shape pushed up against the anterior fornix of the vagina, thereby pressing the walls of the uterus together (Crafter, 2002).

---

catheter to empty the bladder (suggest to the woman she can use entonox during any catheterization) but do try sitting on a bedpan as a first option. A full bladder usually causes the uterus to be displaced.

- **Umbilical vein injection**. Evidence from a Cochrane Review suggests that injecting an oxytocic solution into the umbilical vein reduces the need for manual removal (Carroli & Bergel, 2002). In response to this AAFP (2000/2001) recommended:
  - ○ 20 IU Syntocinon diluted in 20 ml of normal saline.
  - ○ The cord has one vein and two arteries. Inject directly into the umbilical vein of the clamped and cut cord.
  - ○ *Caution*: Ensure the baby is separated from the mother's cord before attempting this.

If by this stage the placenta has not delivered vaginally, the obstetrician should be informed and he/she will probably decide to:

- Perform a vaginal examination. This is to ensure that the placenta is not simply separated and lying in the vagina/cervix and, if not, to assess if it is partially separated.
- Attempt removal by fundal pressure and/or cord traction.
- Proceed to manual removal of the placenta (MROP), ideally under anaesthetic,

followed by IV oxytocin infusion and prophylactic antibiotics.

- Bleeding and retained placenta. If the placenta is truly adherent (placenta accreta) there is usually no bleeding. If separation is partial, the placenta may be difficult to remove completely and haemorrhage can be difficult to control. Follow the standard care for haemorrhage: Rub up a contraction and give an oxytocic, followed by commencement of a Syntocinon® infusion.
- For suspected placenta accreta or placenta percreta urgent manual removal is indicated in theatre since both are responsible for adverse outcomes including maternal death (DoH, 2001). This high-risk situation should be managed by the consultant obstetrician, consultant anaesthetist and involve the haematologist to ensure the best outcome (DoH, 2001).

Home birth/birthing centre care

A woman who has given birth successfully at home or in a birthing centre, who then has a retained placenta, will naturally be very upset at the prospect of transferring to hospital. The midwife will need to closely monitor the woman's blood loss, pulse rate and general condition, and attempt to deliver the placenta described previously. If the placenta is retained then safe transfer to hospital is necessary for manual removal under anaesthetic. The woman will need to take in a bag to stay overnight with her baby. She will want to know what will happen when she reaches hospital and how soon she can return home afterwards.

Transfer of a woman with a retained placenta

- **Intravenous infusion (IVI)**. A woman with a retained placenta requires safe transfer to hospital by ambulance and an IV Syntocinon® infusion: 5–30 IU in 500 ml of normal saline run over 1–2 hours. (Run all IVIs through blood-giving sets, as a greater quantity of fluid can be administered quickly should haemorrhaging occur.)
- **Notes and bloods**. Remember to take the woman's maternity notes and emergency bloods to hospital.
- **Take a vomit bowl**. The woman may feel sick, or be sick, as a result of receiving oxytocics. Have plenty of incontinence pads (incos) to hand.
- **Accompany the woman**. Her baby should be tucked skin-to-skin down her top in the ambulance, providing her condition is stable. This direct contact has the potential to stimulate natural oxytocin and the midwife may discover the placenta delivers en route!

If active bleeding occurs at home/birthing centre or during transit

- Give oxytocic (for maximum dosage of ergometrine and synometrine see Table 23.5).
- Increase the speed of IV fluids and Syntocinon® infusion.
- Site a second cannula promptly and commence IV fluids.
- If bleeding is heavy and ongoing, and in the absence of medical aid, manual removal of the placenta should be undertaken by the midwife (UKCC, 1998). See also Box 11.1.

Summary

Haemorrhage

- Call for help.
- Site cannula(s).
- Take emergency bloods.
- Replace loss with IV fluids/blood products.
- Monitor vital signs.
- Beware that blood loss is often *underestimated*.
- Notes.
- De-brief everyone.

Placenta praevia

- Painless, fresh, vaginal blood loss.
- May experience some contractions.
- Monitor FHR, maternal pulse, BP and blood loss.
- Delivery is usually by caesarean section.
- Postpartum haemorrhage can be a problem.

Placental abruption

Is serious for the baby and the mother.

- Hard uterus/severe pain/possible FHR abnormalities.
- In severe cases the baby will have died.
- Monitor FHR, maternal pulse, BP and blood loss.
- Treat hypovolaemia, clotting can be a problem.
- In severe cases immediate delivery is required.

Postpartum haemorrhage

Uterine atony (tone)

- Relaxed, atonic uterus and heavy vaginal bleeding.
- Deliver the placenta if still *in situ*.
- Uterus well contracted/rub up a contraction/give oxytocics.
- Severe bleeding give carboprost and/or transfer to theatre for manual removal of placenta.

Trauma – tear/episiotomy

- 'Pumping' or trickle bleeding from the vaginal or external genitalia.
- Usually the uterus remains well contracted.
- Apply pressure over the bleeding point for several minutes.
- Clamp and tie off the bleeding vessel.
- Deep internal trauma may require suturing in theatre.

- Haematoma – not always visible but the woman describes acute pain and intolerable, internal pressure.
- Haematomas >3 cm or the woman is typically symptomatic – excision and drainage followed by packing or suturing, ideally in theatre.
- Blood loss is usually concealed and grossly *underestimated*.

Thrombophilias/clotting disorders

- A rare cause of haemorrhage.
- Bleeding from puncture sites.

Retained placenta

- Refer any woman with a prolonged third stage to an obstetrician.
- A retained placenta at a home birth or birthing centre requires safe transfer to hospital, with midwife escort. Use IV fluids and a Syntocinon® infusion.

References

AAFP (2000/2001) *Advanced Life Support in Obstetrics (ALSO). Course Syllabus Manual*, 4th edn. American Academy of Family Physicians, Leawood, Kansas.

Bobrowski, R. (1994) Trauma in pregnancy. In *High Risk Pregnancy: Management Options*, 2nd edn (James, D.K., Steer, P.J., Weiner, C.P. & Goink, B., eds), pp. 959–82. WB Saunders, London.

Campbell, S. & Lees, C. (2000) Obstetric emergencies. In *Obstetrics by Ten Teachers*, 17th edn (Campbell, S. & Lees, C., eds), pp. 303–17. Edward Arnold, London.

Carroli, G. & Bergel, E. (2002) Umbilical vein injection for management of retained placenta (Cochrane Review). *The Cochrane Library*, Issue 4. Update Software, Oxford.

Crafter, H. (2002) Intrapartum and primary postpartum haemorrhage. In *Emergencies Around Childbirth – A Handbook for Midwives* (Boyle, M., ed.), pp. 113–26. Radcliffe Medical Press, Oxford.

DoH (2001) *Why Mothers Die, 1997–1999. The fifth report of the Confidential Enquiries into Maternal Deaths in the United Kingdom*. Department of Health, RCOG Press, London.

Fraser, R. & Watson, R. (2000) Bleeding in the latter half of pregnancy. In *A Guide to Effective Care in Pregnancy and Childbirth*, 3rd edn (Enkin, M., Keirse, M.J.N.C., Neilson, J. *et al.*, eds), pp. 178–84. Oxford University Press, Oxford.

Hayashi, R. (2000) Obstetric collapse. In *Best Practice in Labor Ward Management* (Kean, L.H., Baker, P.N. & Edelstone, D.I., eds), pp. 415–33. WB Saunders, Edinburgh.

Johnson, C., Keirse, M.J.N.C., Enkin, M. & Chalmers, I. (2000) Hospital practices – nutrition and hydration in labor. In *A Guide to Effective Care in Pregnancy and Childbirth*, 3rd edn (Enkin, M., Keirse, M.J.N.C., Neilson, J., *et al.*, eds), pp. 255–66. Oxford University Press, Oxford.

Kean, L. (2000) Other problems of the third stage. In *Best Practice in Labour Ward Management* (Kean, L.H., Baker, P.N. & Edelstone, D.I., eds), pp. 435–50. WB Saunders, London.

Langdana, F., Geary, M., Haw, W. *et al.* (2001) Peripartum hysterectomy in the 1990s: any new lessons? *Journal of Obstetrics and Gynaecology* **21**, 121–3.

Lockwood, C. (1996) Third trimester bleeding. In *Protocols for High Risk Pregnancies*, 3rd edn (Queenan, J.T. & Hobbins, J.C., eds), pp. 568–72. Blackwell Science, Oxford.

McDonald, S. (1999) Physiology and management of the third stage of labour. In *Myles Textbook for Midwives*, 13th edn (Bennet, V.R. & Brown, L.K., eds), pp. 465–88. Churchill Livingstone, Edinburgh.

McGeown, P. (2001) Practice recommendations for obstetric emergencies. *British Journal of Midwifery* **9** (2), 71–3.

Mercer, J.C. (2001) Current best evidence: a review of the literature on umbilical cord clamping. *Journal of Midwifery and Women's Health* **46** (6), 402–14.

Prendiville, W. & Elbourne, D. (2000) The third stage of labor. In *A Guide to Effective Care in Pregnancy and Childbirth*, 3rd edn (Enkin, M., Keirse, M.J.N.C., Neilson, J., *et al.*, eds), pp. 300–309. Oxford University Press, Oxford.

Sleep, J., Roberts, J. & Chalmers, L. (2000) The second stage of labor. In *A Guide to Effective Care in Pregnancy and Childbirth*, 3rd edn (Enkin, M., Keirse, M.J.N.C., Neilson, J. *et al.*, eds) pp. 289–99. Oxford University Press, Oxford.

UKCC (1998) *Midwives Rules and Code of Practice*. United Kingdom Central Council for Nursing Midwifery and Health Visiting, London.

12 Childbirth emergencies

Introduction

'Even when serious emergencies occur, midwives can do much to create an environment which respects the woman as a person with feelings and emotions rather than an object to be rushed to theatre.' (Weston, 2001).

While 'choices' are sometimes taken from the woman in order to save time, midwives can do much to reassure her and her partner by briefly explaining what is happening. This can be achieved by simply touching her arm and saying calmly 'I know this is really frightening for you but we need to be quick now and do x, y and z to get the baby out'.

Increasingly protocols and emergency training drills are in place so that all clinicians can respond appropriately to serious emergencies in childbirth. At home, or in a birthing centre, midwives can be faced with serious emergencies and they need to have the skills, experience and confidence necessary to cope with problems safely. Prompt transfer of the woman or baby to hospital may also be indicated.

Cord prolapse

A *cord prolapse* is the prolapse of the umbilical cord alongside, or past, the presenting part where the membranes are absent. If the membranes are intact this is known as a *cord presentation*. It can be *occult*, alongside the presenting part, or *frank*, where the cord escapes through the cervical os and can even be visible outside the vagina.

Incidence and facts

- Cord prolapse occurs in 0.14–0.62% of births (Murphy & MacKenzie, 1995).
- Umbilical cord prolapse is associated with poor perinatal outcomes, even when the facilities exist to offer a rapid emergency delivery (Prabulos & Philipson, 1998).
- Squire (2002) suggests that mortality is predominantly associated with congenital abnormalies and prematurity rather than birth asphyxia per se.
- Occult cord prolapse is associated with less perinatal morbidity than frank prolapse (Prabulos & Philipson, 1998).
- In only 41% of cases, electronic fetal monitoring (EFM) aided the diagnosis of cord prolapse (Murphy & MacKenzie, 1995).

Associated risk factors

- Artificial rupture of the membranes (ARM) is a direct cause of cord prolapse in over 50% of cases (Prabulos & Philipson, 1998).
- Predisposing factors include a small or preterm baby, malpresentation (e.g. breech, twins), high parity, high head (McGeown, 2001), polyhydramnios.

Signs and symptoms

Signs and symptoms of cord prolapse are given in Box 12.1.

Box 12.1   Signs and symptoms of cord prolapse.

Vaginal examination
  - A vaginal examination will confirm a frank cord prolapse, in which the cord can be felt pulsating if touched.
  - Sometimes the cord can be visible hanging outside the vagina.

Artificial rupture of the membranes (ARM) or spontaneous prelabour rupture of the membranes (PROM)
  This can be complicated by the fact that the woman is in an unphysiological position such as lying flat or in lithotomy.
  - Sometimes the presenting part ballots away from the fingers following ARM.
  - In situations where ARM has been performed inappropriately (such as when the presenting part is high as for a second twin) then cord prolapse may occur.

Fetal heart rate (FHR)/palpation
  - On re-palpating the baby's body, the location of the fetal heart may have changed noticeably.
  - Following rupture of the membranes there may be a sudden deterioration in the baby's condition: abnormal FHR changes may occur or the baby may pass fresh meconium.

Practice recommendations/manoeuvres

- Call for help.
- The midwife should try to remain calm and briefly explain to the woman and her partner what is happening and what they may need to do.
- **Vaginal examination.** On performing a vaginal examination the midwife/clinician who discovers the cord prolapse should keep their fingers firmly pushing on the presenting part, particularly firmly during contractions, to relieve cord compression, until emergency delivery can take place.
- **Complete cord prolapse.** If the cord is 'hanging' out of the vagina gently place it back into the vagina. Davis (1997) suggests that if this it not possible cover it in warm, wet sterile gauze or a cloth then a polythene bag, as the cold air or touching it excessively can cause spasm and constriction and, therefore, hypoxia.
- **All-fours/knee-chest position.** Get the woman into the 'all-fours/knees-to-chest' position, to reduce the pressure caused by the presenting part, as seen in Fig. 12.1. This can be frightening for the woman as well as uncomfortable and undignified. Cover her lower half with the sheet for modesty.
- **Second stage.** In the second stage of labour, the woman can be encouraged to push and should be assisted to an upright position such as a squat, to facilitate effective pushing. Depending on the fetal heart rate (FHR), an instrumental delivery may be indicated.
- **Emergency delivery.** In hospital the midwife can let everyone else run around and get the woman to theatre. As the midwife keeps the pressure off the cord, this is the time to offer verbal reassurance and calmly talk to the woman and her partner. Due to the acute nature of this emergency the woman is wheeled directly to theatre on the bed, maintaining the knee-chest position. The midwife usually maintains the internal pressure on the presenting part while the caesarean is performed, until the actual delivery of the baby.

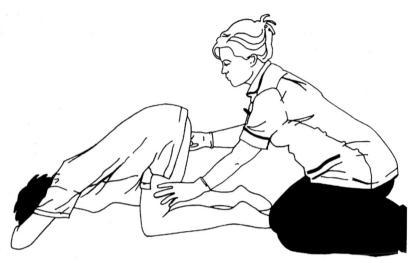

Fig. 12.1   Knee-chest position.

- **Paediatric resuscitation**. A baby with a frank cord prolapse is likely to require intensive resuscitation, so a paediatrician should be called for the birth. Help should still be summoned at a birthing centre or at home.

See also 'Alternative treatments' in the list below.

Birthing centre or home birth

A cord prolapse is less likely to happen at home/birthing centre since ARM is usually avoided in such settings and women considered 'high risk' are more likely to labour and birth in hospital. If a prolapse does occur:

- Try the 'Practice recommendations/manoeuvres' on page 187. Use internal pressure on the presenting part and place the mother in the knee-chest position.
- **Transfer to hospital** with the woman in the knee-chest position and the midwife's fingers pushing on the presenting part. This is unpleasant and frightening for the woman. Minutes may feel like hours. This scenario can also be very uncomfortable and stressful for the midwife.
- **Second stage**. There may not be time to transfer the mother but call a paramedic ambulance anyway. The midwife will need to encourage the woman to push effectively and assist her into an upright position. Alternatively, at a birthing centre, if available, a midwife ventouse practitioner could be contacted to perform a ventouse.
- **Alternative treatments**. McGeown (2001) discusses an additional possibility for treating this emergency. She discusses two studies reviewing 75 cases of cord prolapse (by Katz [1988] and Chetty [1980]). Both described filling the maternal bladder with 400–700 ml of saline. This apparently not only relieves cord compression but also inhibits uterine activity.

'Filling the bladder with saline may well prove useful if there is a delay in performing a caesarean section, such as when a cord prolapse occurs in a birthing centre or at home' (McGeown, 2001).

Amniotic fluid embolism

Amniotic fluid embolism (AFE) is a rare, usually fatal, cause of sudden maternal collapse in labour. Diagnosis is not always clear at the time of the woman's deterioration but it manifests itself with the woman gasping for breath, a drop in blood pressure and the sudden onset of shock which is usually followed by cardiac arrest.

In recent years, some clinicians have recommended that this condition should be reclassified, not as an embolic episode, but as an anaphylactic-type reaction to amniotic fluid which has entered the maternal circulation. Amniotic fluid embolism is now thought to be a combination of left ventricular failure (indicated by the woman's sudden breathlessness) and acute lung injury that is accompanied by the activation of clotting factors. An immunological basis for these effects, and the woman's sudden collapse, is thought to be the most likely cause (Fahy, 2001; Fletcher & Parr, 2001). This situation can be frightening for all those involved and the high maternal mortality makes it stressful and difficult emotionally, especially for the woman's birth partner(s) if present at her collapse.

Incidence and facts

- There were a dramatic 17 maternal deaths from AFE in the 1998 Report on Confidential Enquiries into Maternal Deaths in the United Kingdom (DoH, 1998). This had reduced by half in the subsequent 2001 report (DoH, 2001).
- There are no definitive diagnostic tests for this condition, even at post-mortem. Fahy (2001) suggests that AFE occurs in 1.52 per 10 000 child-bearing women. He suggests that the more knowledgeable clinicians become about AFE, the more frequently it is diagnosed.
- Little is known about how to improve maternal mortality. The interval between collapse and death is generally sudden, with an 85% maternal mortality rate, and with 25% of women dying within the first hour. Of those women who survive the initial collapse, most will then develop disseminated intravascular coagulation (DIC) (Davis, 1999; Fahy, 2001). The perinatal mortality rate is 40%.

Signs and symptoms

See Table 12.1 for signs and symptoms of AFE. Sometimes haemorrhage due to DIC may be the initial presentation (Davis, 1999).

Practice recommendations

- **Call for help/transfer to hospital**. Amniotic fluid embolism requires the co-ordinated care of anaesthetists, obstetricians, midwives and the haematology team.
- **Treat for sudden collapse/shock** (Fahy, 2001) (see also later in this chapter in Box 12.6).

Table 12.1 Signs and symptoms of amniotic fluid embolism (AFE) (Fahy, 2001).

Sign/symptom	% of women
Hypotension (shock)	100
Fetal distress (if undelivered)	100
Pulmonary oedema or adult respiratory distress syndrome	93
Cardiopulmonary arrest	86
Cyanosis	83
Coagulopathy	83
Dyspnoea (difficult or laboured breathing)	49
Seizure	48

- **Think ABC.** Airway, Breathing and Circulation. Maternal resuscitation is covered further in Chapter 21.
- In the event of maternal cardiac arrest *deliver the baby* within 5 minutes. Obstetricians do not need to prepare a sterile field and should go for the quickest incision possible (Bobrowski, 1994).

Aftercare

The mother will usually require intensive care.

Uterine rupture

Uterine rupture is the separation of the uterine wall. It can occur during the antenatal period, at induction, during labour/birth, and even during the third stage of labour. It has various degrees, a true rupture being the most serious as the baby can be expelled from the uterus into the peritoneal cavity (Kroll & Lyne, 2002).

For additional information see Chapter 6.

Incidence and facts

- This serious emergency occurs in less than 1% of women and is potentially life threatening for both the mother and the baby.
- Half of all cases occur in women with no uterine scar, mainly in multiparous women (Enkin, 2000).

Associated risk factors

- Uterine rupture is most commonly associated with previous uterine surgery including previous caesarean section(s). It can also be attributed to poor obstetric practice, such as the inappropriate use of oxytocics to induce/hasten labour and/or obstructed labour (Silverton, 1993).
- Other causes are varied and include trauma caused by high cavity forceps, manual manipulation for an unstable lie, manual removal of the placenta, a car accident or other blunt trauma including physical assault/domestic violence (Kroll & Lyne, 2002).

Box 12.2 Signs and symptoms of uterine scar rupture.

Pain
- Sudden uterine or scar pain.
- A feeling of 'giving way' (Silverton, 1993).
- Lower abdominal pain may come with a contraction, or be a constant unrelenting pain.
- The woman may find it too painful to have her uterus touched or palpated.

Uterus/contractions
- Solid, tonic uterus.
- Contractions may stop or dwindle.

Fetal heart rate (FHR)
Abnormal fetal heart changes may occur such as a prolonged or variable deceleration usually progressing to a serious bradycardia (Menihan, 1999).

Shock
- Changes may occur in the vital signs:
  - tachycardia
  - sometimes low blood pressure
  - breathlessness, respirations > 24 per minute
- The woman may:
  - look cool and clammy
  - appear restless, agitated or withdrawn
  - say she is frightened and that something is wrong
  - vomit

Bleeding
- Bleeding may sometimes be evident from the vagina, as blood-stained amniotic fluid or a fresh bleeding.
- Sometimes, such as after the baby is born, a ruptured uterus may start to rise as it fills with blood.
- Placenta accreta is undeliverable vaginally, as the placenta is imbedded into the myometrium. It is associated with a previous scar on the uterus. This serious complication can be life threatening for the woman and is associated with uncontrollable bleeding which may necessitate hysterectomy (Bakshi & Meyer, 2000; Langdana *et al.* 2001).

Signs and symptoms

Signs and symptoms of uterine scar rupture are given in Box 12.2.

Practice recommendations

- Call for help/transfer to hospital.
- Proceed to immediate delivery by caesarean section.
- If an instrumental delivery is possible to deliver the baby, the woman will need to go straight to theatre afterwards for uterine repair. Occasionally, if the bleeding is uncontrollable, the surgeon may need to proceed to a hysterectomy (Bakshi & Meyer, 2000).

Aftercare

- In severe cases the mother and baby may require intensive care. Unfortunately in such cases perinatal mortality remains high.

- Closely monitor the woman following surgery as she is at risk of postpartum haemorrhage (Silverton, 1993).
- An intravenous (IV) oxytocic infusion is advisable post delivery.

Shoulder dystocia

Shoulder dystocia is usually preceded by a slow delivery of the baby's head; the baby's chin then retracts against the perineum and 'turtlenecks'. By the next contraction, the baby will not deliver as the anterior shoulder of the baby has become impacted against the symphysis pubic bone.

Incidence and facts

- 0.1–1.4% of vaginal births (Gee & Glynn,1997).
- Normal-sized babies make up the majority of shoulder dystocias and 50% of cases of shoulder dystocia have *no* identifiable risk factors (AAFP, 2000/2001).
- Macrosomic babies (infants over 4 kg) are the single most important associated factor in shoulder dystocia (CESDI, 1997). Ultrasound scanning, fundal height measurements and fetal size estimation remain inaccurate and, therefore, the prediction of a macrosomic baby antenatally also remains inaccurate (Lewis *et al.*, 1998)
- Morbidity for the baby includes common injuries such as: brachial plexus palsies (20% of infants [AAFP, 2000/2001]), fractures of the clavicle/humerus, bruising and soft tissue damage. Unfortunately, in severe cases, fetal death can result.
- Morbidity for the woman includes trauma, blood loss, bruising to the perineum/ genital tract and surrounding tissues, episiotomy/serious tears, psychological trauma, as well as a possibly serious injury and, in severe cases, the death of her baby.
- At most births it rests with the midwife to manage this emergency promptly, following a pre-rehearsed sequence of manoeuvres.

Associated risk factors

- Macrosomia/prior delivery of a baby >4.0 kg (CESDI, 1997).
- Over half of all shoulder dystocia cases are in babies of normal weight (AAFP, 2000/2001).
- Birthing semi-recumbent on a bed can restrict the movement of the coccyx and sacrum contributing to 'bed-birth dystocia' (Mortimore & McNabb, 1998; McGeown, 2001).
- Maternal diabetes.
- Instrumental delivery (AAFP, 2000/2001).
- Previous shoulder dystocia.

Signs and symptoms

See Box 12.3 for signs and symptoms of shoulder dystocia.

Box 12.3 Signs and symptoms of shoulder dystocia in labour

- Suspected large baby (CESDI, 1997).
- Slow progress from 7 to 10 cm, despite good contractions.
- Slow progress in second stage.
- Instrumental delivery (AAFP, 2000/2001).
- Slow advancement and slow crowning and delivery of the head

Practice recommendations/manoeuvres

Because shoulder dystocia is unpredictable, it is not preventable. All midwives should be prepared to deal with this emergency. It is advisable to commit to memory a series of manoeuvres (see Figs 12.2, 12.3 and 12.4).

The HELPERR drill

HELPERR is an obstetric plan for dealing with a shoulder dystocia emergency and is taught by the American Association of Family Practitioners (AAFP, 2001)

H   Help! Call emergency number for direct access to switchboard.
E   Evaluate for episiotomy.
L   Legs hyperflexed (McRoberts manoeuvre) said to be effective 80% of the time.
P   Pressure suprapubic.
E   Enter the vagina. Internal manoeuvres.
R   Remove the posterior arm.
R   Roll on to all fours.

HELPERR has become a formalized and accepted approach to the management of shoulder dystocia. It has seven letters each representing an action and is a well-intentioned drill that many clinicians find very useful. Unfortunately, it appears from an obstetric perspective, and assumes that all women give birth lying flat or in lithotomy. The term is fairly long and some of the letters represent tenuous link words,

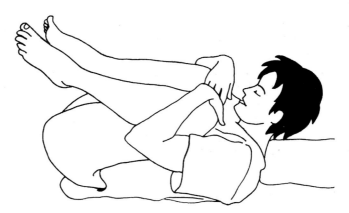

Fig. 12.2 McRoberts manoeuvre (side view).

(a) Semi-recumbent position

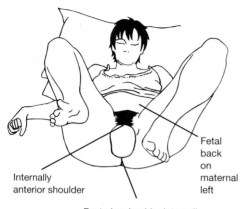

Internally
anterior shoulder

Fetal
back
on
maternal
left

Posterior shoulder internally

(b) McRoberts manoeuvre plus Rubins I and
Rubins II manoeuvres. The assistant stands
on the same side as the fetal back to apply
downward, lateral pressure or rocking to
the anterior shoulder

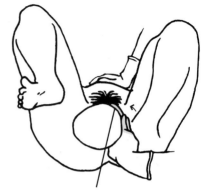

- Approach the anterior shoulder from behind
- Push it towards the fetal chest
  to reduce the shoulder girdle

(c) McRoberts manoeuvre, Rubins I and Rubins II
manoeuvres with the Woods screw manoeuvre

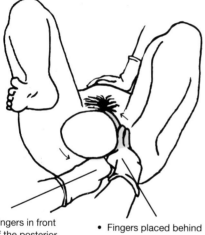

Fingers in front
of the posterior
shoulder

- Fingers placed behind
  the anterior shoulder
- Rotate/push towards
  the symphysis pubis

(d) Reverse Woods screw manoeuvre

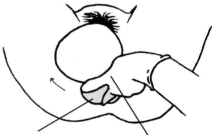

Posterior shoulder

- Fingers placed behind
  the posterior shoulder
- Push/rotate the baby
  towards the symphysis
  pubis

(e) Removal of the posterior shoulder

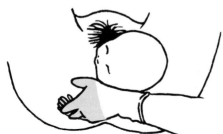

- Insert whole hand
- Flex arm at elbow
- Sweep arm out across
  fetal chest and face

Fig. 12.3 Manoeuvres for shoulder dystocia with the woman in the semi-recumbent position.

(a) Woman in all-fours position with midwife checking restitution of the shoulders

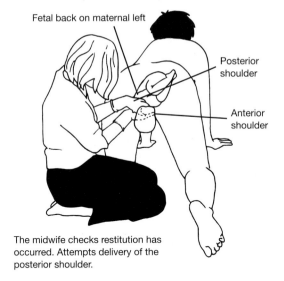

Fetal back on maternal left

Posterior shoulder

Anterior shoulder

The midwife checks restitution has occurred. Attempts delivery of the posterior shoulder.

(b) Rubins II manoeuvre

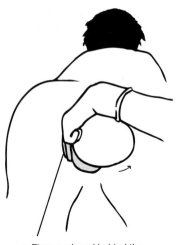

- Fingers placed behind the anterior shoulder
- Push towards the fetal chest to reduce the shoulder girdle

(c) Rubins II manoeuvre with the Woods screw manoeuvre

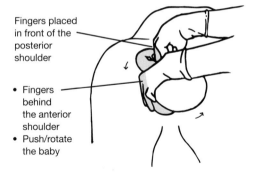

Fingers placed in front of the posterior shoulder

- Fingers behind the anterior shoulder
- Push/rotate the baby

(d) Reverse Woods screw manoeuvre

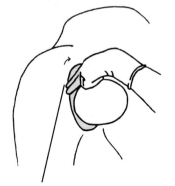

- Fingers push from behind the posterior shoulder
- Push/rotate the shoulders towards the symphysis pubis

(e) Removal of the posterior shoulder

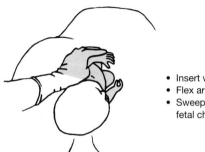

- Insert whole hand
- Flex arm at elbow
- Sweep arm out across fetal chest and face

Fig. 12.4 Manoeuvres for shoulder dystocia with the woman in the all-fours position.

which may leave the midwife struggling to recall exactly what some letters stand for. Therefore, below is a description of various manoeuvres, the ones the midwife tries will depend on what works for her, the woman's position at birth, as well as other factors detailed below. No protocol should serve as a substitute for clinical judgement because no one manoeuvre has been proven to be superior to another and none of the recommended, recognized manoeuvres for shoulder dystocia have been evaluated in trials (Nocon *et al.*, 1993; Nocon, 2000).

Bedbirth dystocia describes the iatrogenic effects caused by the semi-recumbent position, which restricts movement of the sacrum and coccyx (Mortimore & McNabb, 1998; McGeown, 2001). Some women naturally raise their buttocks off the bed at this point. Common sense suggests that any woman 'at risk' of shoulder dystocia should be discouraged from birthing in the semi-recumbent position.

Upright postures improve the alignment of the mobile pelvic bones, and improve the shape and capacity of the pelvis, optimizing the chances of a 'good fit' between baby and pelvis (Simpkin & Ancheta, 2000). Many midwives would suggest that a position change alone can be beneficial in shifting impacted shoulders from the symphysis pubis.

All-fours manoeuvre

- If appropriate, midwives should consider a change in position to all fours as a *first move*, before resorting to the more interventionalist and, subsequently, traumatic measures in order to deliver the baby's shoulders.
- Turning on to all fours often dislodges the impacted shoulder (AAFP, 2000/2001) as well as allowing the pelvis to move unrestricted.
- Many experienced midwives will be aware of the all-fours manoeuvre for shoulder dystocia (as described by Gaskin, 1990; Coates, 1995; Davis, 1997; AAFP, 2000/2001) where the coccyx can move freely while the baby's weight on the symphysis helps widen the anterior/posterior diameter a little. Gaskin (1990) notes that the posterior shoulder usually delivers first in this scenario.
- Anecdotally, in births managed on all fours, midwives report that there is enough room to insert the hand, up to the wrist, along the curve of the sacrum and to splint, then free the posterior shoulder if necessary (Gaskin, 1990).

Note: the all-fours position may be difficult for some women such as those with a dense epidural block. Also, consider where the anterior and posterior shoulders lie.

McRoberts manoeuvre

The McRoberts manoeuvre places the woman in the semi-recumbent position and abducts her thighs, pulling her knees to her chest and thus raising her coccyx off the bed and straightening her spine (see Fig. 12.2). When used, the McRoberts manoeuvre will deliver the baby in over 40% of cases, this increases to over 50% when used in conjunction with external pressure, see Rubins manoeuvre, p. 197 (AAFP, 2000/2001).

Rubins I and Rubins II manoeuvres

In addition to the McRoberts manoeuvre the application of external pressure, or a rocking side-to-side motion, can be provided by an assistant to dislodge the impacted anterior shoulder from the symphysis bone.

- Rubins I. This manoeuvre involves the application of downward, lateral pressure, or rocking with the palm of the hand, over the anterior shoulder. The clinician stands on the same side as the baby's back and directs pressure towards the midline (Coates, 1995; AAFP, 2001/2001) in order to help shift the impacted shoulder. If done incorrectly, this manoeuvre will simply impact the baby's shoulder further on to the pelvic bone. Try for 30–60 seconds (AAFP, 2000/2001).
- Rubins II (see Figs 12.3b and 12.4b). In addition to the external pressure, the delivering clinician inserts the fingers of one hand vaginally to approach the anterior shoulder *from behind*, thus pushing the anterior shoulder towards the fetal chest and collapsing the fetal shoulder girdle.

Internal manoeuvres

The following manoeuvres can be attempted, whatever the mother's position. Internal manoeuvres are painful and traumatic for the woman, while being difficult and uncomfortable for the midwife.

Episiotomy can aid accessibility in difficult internal manoeuvres but should remain at the judgement of the delivering clinician. Episiotomy will not aid delivery of the impacted anterior shoulder, does not improve the outcome in shoulder dystocia (Nocon *et al.*, 1993) and can cause extensive trauma to the woman's perineum. Some midwives therefore question its necessity (Gaskin, 1990).

The Woods screw manoeuvre

Woods applied the theory of physics to the problem of shoulder dystocia, developing the 'Woods screw manoeuvres'. The principle remains 'a direct pull is the most difficult way to release a screw' (Woods, 1943). AAFP (2000/2001) suggest that this manoeuvre is quite difficult to perform, they recommend, if necessary, pushing the shoulders up, back into the pelvis slightly, in order to accomplish the delivery.

- The Woods screw manoeuvre can be combined with the Rubins II (AAFP, 2000/2001). (The Rubins II manoeuvre involves placing fingers behind the anterior shoulder and pushing it towards the baby's chest.)
- The second hand is placed internally, with fingers in front of the posterior shoulder (see Figs 12.3c and 12.4c).
- The delivering clinician can internally push/rotate the baby towards the symphysis pubis.
- The idea is to shift the baby into the oblique so the anterior shoulder is freed from the pubic bone.
- **Reverse Woods screw**. Place fingers from behind, on to the posterior shoulder and attempt to rotate the baby towards the symphysis pubis (see Figs 12.3d and 12.4d).

Delivery of the posterior shoulder

- Insert the whole hand (lubricated) into the vagina to locate the baby's posterior arm and elbow.
- Flex the arm at the elbow and sweep across the fetal chest and out, delivery should follow.
- Do not pull on the baby's hand in order to try to deliver it as this may lead to fractures (AAFP, 2000/2001).

As a last resort

- **Deliberate clavicle fracture**. Although rarely required, it may be necessary to deliberately fracture the baby's clavicle. Davis (1997) describes a case where the midwife had to resort to fracturing the clavicle. She suggests it is simple to break, by placing two fingers on to the clavicle and pushing with the thumb between them to snap the bone.
- **Cephalic replacement/Zavanelli manoeuvre**. This is only possible in hospital and where the cord has not been clamped and cut. Squire (2002) suggests this should be a last resort until the applicability of this manoeuvre has been demonstrated more clearly. To perform, turn the baby's head to occipitoanterior (OA) or occipitoposterior (OP) (depending on the baby's position for delivery). Then flex the baby's head, push it back into the vagina, and proceed to immediate caesarean section.

Contraindicated manoeuvres

- **Incorrect application of supra-pubic pressure**. Pressure should not push the shoulders on to the symphysis pubis and further impact it.
- **Strong pulling/traction** on the baby's head will not release an impacted shoulder but will cause serious damage to the baby. Gentle traction should be attempted and if unsuccessful commence appropriate manoeuvres.
- **Fundal pressure** has been identified as being of no benefit and may even increase shoulder impaction and could cause serious injuries, including a ruptured uterus, haemorrhage and even maternal death.

Aftercare

- **Post-birth counselling**. The couple should be offered the opportunity to discuss what happened with the person who delivered their baby. They may wish to see the consultant obstetrician to discuss any long-term effects and the prospects for future pregnancies.
- **Litigation**. Solicitors can frequently find fault in the documented management of shoulder dystocia, questioning whether the care followed recognized manoeuvres. The documenting of all timings should be from the clock in the room and not people's individual watches (except in births at home). It is also sensible to work together in documenting how the case was managed after the event.

Uterine prolapse/inverted uterus

An inverted uterus is the inversion or prolapse of the uterus into the vagina, or at the vulva during the third stage of labour, resulting in the sudden and serious collapse of the woman (Magill-Cuerden, 2001).

Incidence and facts

- 1:2000 to 1:50 000 births (Kroll & Lyne, 2002).
- Kroll & Lyne (2002) suggest that the variation in statistics is dependent upon third stage management and the level of reporting.

Associated risk factors

- Oxytocic drug use.
- Suggested mismanagement of the third stage of labour, such as failing to effectively guard the uterus during controlled cord traction, or using fundal pressure while applying hard traction to the cord (Silverton, 1993).
- Can occasionally occur in cases of placenta accreta or a short umbilical cord (Kroll & Lyne, 2002).

Signs and symptoms

See Box 12.4 for signs and symptoms of a prolapsed uterus.

Box 12.4   Signs and symptoms of a prolapsed uterus.

Uterus visible
- The uterus may be visible as a shiny, mauve protrusion at the vagina.
- The placenta may be attached.

Haemorrhage
The most common sign of a prolapsed uterus is haemorrhage, but the woman's rapid collapse appears out of proportion to the amount of blood lost (Magill-Cuerden, 2001).

Profound shock
Immediate, often unexplained profound shock (Magill-Cuerden, 2001).

Pain
Great lower abdominal pain, caused by the traction on the ovaries and peritoneum and may be accompanied by a bearing-down sensation (Kroll & Lyne, 2002).

Practice recommendations/manoeuvres for replacing the uterus

Ideally, the uterus should be replaced manually when it has just 'inverted'. There are various medical descriptions of how to replace the uterus; most practitioners will consider any delay too long as it allows for the potential formation of a cervical constriction ring and the uterus can become oedematous and difficult to replace (Kroll & Lyne, 2002). Midwives who have been present when a woman has had an inverted uterus say that once they have registered what is actually happening, they then respond by simply pushing the uterus back into the vagina and up – promptly.

- Call for help/transfer to hospital.
- Replace the uterus promptly, see Box 12.5 for a description of how to replace the uterus.
- If unable to replace uterus:
  - ○ treat for shock (see Box 12.6)
  - ○ prepare for theatre
  - ○ withhold oxytocics until the uterus is replaced (Magill-Cuerden, 2001)
  - ○ provide support to the uterus, to minimize pulling on internal structures
  - ○ administer strong analgesia, such as morphine.

Box 12.5 Replacing a prolapsed uterus.

Prompt manual replacement
- It is usually possible to push the uterus all the way up, via the vagina, and back into place with the hand, even with the placenta attached. This is usually successful. This should be attempted at the immediate time of the prolapse (Campbell & Lees, 2000).
- Ensure the entire uterus is completely fed up through the cervix to avoid later complications. The uterus should be held in place for at least 5 minutes or until a firm contraction occurs (Kroll & Lyne, 2002).
- The woman will find the prolapse painful but replacement can be agonizing (Kroll & Lyne, 2002).

Uterine relaxant e.g. ritodrine
May be given prior to replacing the uterus.

Constriction ring
If a constriction ring is present (around the cervix) a general anaesthetic may be required to assist in replacing the uterus.

Placenta
Only after the uterus is replaced, can an oxytocic be administered and the placenta carefully delivered (Campbell & Lees, 2000; Magill-Cuerden 2001).

Aftercare

- Possible indwelling catheter for 24 hours, to avoid distention of the bladder (Silverton, 1993).
- Referral for physiotherapy to discuss pelvic floor muscle care and lifting/straining strategies.
- The mother may remember little of events but her partner will have seen her sudden collapse. The couple should be offered counselling as well as the opportunity to see an obstetrician to discuss what happened, and why. This is also the time to discuss any long-term effects of her collapse and the prospects for future pregnancies.

Box 12.6   Basic are for shock.

---

(1) Summon help.
(2) Ascertain the possible cause of the woman's shock
   • Commence appropriate treatment.
   • Deliver the baby.
   • If at home or birthing centre arrange urgent paramedic ambulance to hospital.
(3) Physical care
   • Site two large gauge cannula.
   • Take emergency bloods for:
      ○ group and cross-matching
      ○ full blood count (FBC)
      ○ clotting studies: fibrinogen levels, prothrombin time (international normalized ratio) (PT/INR)/activated partial thromboplastin time (APTT).
   • Commence intravenous (IV) fluids
   • Administer facial oxygen
   • Observations:
      ○ pulse
      ○ blood pressure (BP) } every few minutes
      ○ pulse oximetry
(4) Serious collapse (see 'Maternal resuscitation', Chapter 21)
   Stay calm, think ABC:
   A = Airway
   B = Breathing
   C = Circulation
(5) Ongoing resuscitation
   In hospital it is usually possible to assign a person to perform documentation of:
   • Vital signs.
   • Fluid chart in and out (including estimation of blood loss).
   • Drugs given, dosages and times.
(6) Transfer to intensive care unit
   'Intensive care is not simply a place – it is a service' (DoH, 2001)
   • Urinary catheter with urometer.
   • Central venous pressure (CVP) line.
   • Discussions with the family.

Maternal collapse/shock

Shock is a state where the woman deteriorates into a semi-conscious or unconscious state of collapse. It has many causes including massive blood loss, septicaemia, even an anaphylactic reaction. The woman's deterioration is usually preceded by a life-threatening event which causes the body to redirect blood to the vital organs. The woman will develop a tachycardia and her blood pressure can suddenly drop. The woman becomes peripherally shut down; she may vomit, look blue or pale, become frightened or agitated, and in severe cases even gasp for air.

If she becomes drowsy, even unconscious, collapse and cardiac arrest can rapidly follow. This serious emergency requires an emergency obstetric call. If at home/birthing centre, transfer to the nearest hospital under resuscitation.

In complete cardiac arrest, *deliver the baby within 5 minutes*. Obstetricians do not need to prepare a sterile field and should go for the quickest incision possible (Bobrowski, 1994).

Box 12.6 summarizes the basic care for shock including the taking of emergency bloods.

Summary

Cord prolapse

- Call for help.
- Vaginal examination to apply pressure to the presenting part until delivery.
- Woman to adopt the all-fours/knee-chest position.
- If at home/birthing centre transfer to a consultant unit.
- Explain to the woman calmly what is happening and why.
- Consider as a last resort filling the woman's bladder with 400–700 ml of saline.
- Emergency delivery – probable caesarean in the first stage, spontaneous vaginal or instrumental birth for the second stage.

Amniotic fluid embolism (AFE)

- Main symptoms of AFE are *breathlessness, shock* followed by *cardiac arrest* (Fahy, 2001).
- Treat for shock/collapse.

Uterine prolapse

- Call for help.
- Replace the uterus promptly (see Box 12.5 for a description of how to replace the uterus).
- Treat for shock (see Box 12.6).
- Offer analgesia.
- Withold oxytocics until delivery of placenta.
- If unable to replace uterus, prepare for theatre.

Useful contact

The Erb's Palsy Group   Telephone parent advisor: 024 764 3293. Website: www.erb-spalsygroup.co.uk.
Support for parents and professionals on brachial plexus injuries.

References

AAFP (2000/2001) *Advanced Life Support in Obstetrics (ALSO). Course Syllabus Manual*, 4th edn. American Academy of Family Physicians, Leawood, Kansas.

Bakshi, S., Meyer, B.A. (2000) Indications for and outcomes of emergency peripartum hysterectomy: a five year review. *Journal of Reproductive Medicine* **45** (9), 733–7.

Bobrowski, R. (1994) In *High Risk Pregnancy: Management Options*, 2nd edn (James, D.K., Steer, P.J., Weiner, C.P. & Goink, B., eds), pp. 959–82. WB Saunders, London.

Campbell, S. & Lees, C. (2000) Obstetric emergencies. In *Obstetrics by Ten Teachers*, 17th edn (Campbell, S. & Lees, C., eds), pp. 303–17. Edward Arnold, London.

CESDI (1997) *Confidential Enquiry into Stillbirths and Deaths in Infancy*, 4th Annual Report. Maternal and Child Health Research Consortium, London.

Chetty, R.M. (1980) Umbilical cord prolapse. *South African Medical Journal* **57** (4), 128–9.

Coates, T. (1995) Shoulder dystocia. In *Aspects of Midwifery Practice* (Alexander, J., Levy, V. & Roch, S., eds), Macmillan, Basingstoke.

Davis, E. (1997) *Hearts and Hands: A Midwife's Guide to Pregnancy and Birth*, 3rd edn. Celestial Arts, Berkeley, California.

Davis, S. (1999) Amniotic fluid embolism and isolated disseminated intravascular coagulation. *Canadian Journal of Anaesthesia* **46** (5), 456–9.

DoH (1998) *Why Mothers Die, 1994–1996. Report on Confidential Enquiries into Maternal Deaths in the United Kingdom.* Department of Health, The Stationery Office, London.

DoH (2001) *Why Mothers Die, 1997–1999. The fifth report of the Confidential Enquiries into Maternal Deaths in the United Kingdom.* Department of Health, RCOG Press, London.

Enkin, M. (2000) Labor and birth after a previous caesarean section. In *A Guide to Effective Care in Pregnancy and Childbirth*, 3rd edn (Enkin, M., Keirse, M.J.N.C., Neilson, J. *et al.*, ed), pp. 359–71. Oxford University Press, Oxford.

Fahy, K.M. (2001) Amniotic fluid embolism: a review of the research literature. *Australian Journal of Midwifery* **14** (1), 9–13.

Fletcher, J. & Parr, M.J. (2000) Amniotic fluid embolism: a case report and review. *Resuscitation* **43** (2), 141–6.

Gaskin, I. (1990) *Spiritual Midwifery*. The Book Publishing Co., Summertown, Tennessee.

Gee, H. & Glynn, M. (1997) The physiology and clinical management of labour. In *Essential Midwifery* (Henderson, C. & Jones, K., eds), pp. 171–202. Mosby, London.

Katz, Z. (1988) Management of labour with umbilical cord polapse: a 5 year study. *Obstetrics and Gynecology* **72**, 278–81.

Kroll, D. & Lyne, M. (2002) Uterine inversion and uterine rupture. In *Emergencies around Childbirth – A Handbook for Midwives* (Boyle, M., ed.), pp. 89–95. Radcliffe Medical Press, Oxford.

Langdana, F., Geary, M., Haw, W. *et al.* (2001) Peripartum hysterectomy in the 1990s: any new lessons? *Journal of Obstetrics and Gynaecology* **21**, 121–3.

Lewis, D.F., Edwards, M.S., Asrat, T. *et al.* (1998) Can shoulder dystocia be predicted? Preconceptive and prenatal factors. *Journal of Reproductive Medicine* **43** (8), 654–8.

McGeown, P. (2001) Practice recommendations for obstetric emergencies. *British Journal of Midwifery* **9** (2), 71–74.

Magill-Cuerden, J. (2001) Clinical file: case study. *The Practising Midwife* **4** (1), 29.

Menihan, C.A. (1999) The effect of uterine rupture on fetal heart rate patterns. *Journal of Nurse-Midwifery*, **44** (1), 40–46.

Mortimore, V. & McNabb, M. (1998) A six year retrospective analysis of shoulder dystocia and delivery of the shoulders. *Midwifery* **14**, 162–73.

Murphy, D.J. & MacKenzie, I.Z. (1995) The mortality and morbidity associated with umbilical cord prolapse. *British Journal of Obstetrics and Gynaecology* **102** (10), 826–30.

Nocon, J.J. (2000) Shoulder dystocia and macrosomia. In *Best Practice in Labour Ward Management* (Kean, L., ed.), pp. 167–86. WB Saunders, Edinburgh.

Nocon, J.J., McKenzie, D.K., Thomas, L.J. & Hansell, R.S. (1993) Shoulder dystocia: an analysis of risks and obstetric manoeuvres. *American Journal of Obstetrics and Gynecology* **168**, 1732–9.

Prabulos, A.M. & Philipson, E.H. (1998) Umbillical cord prolapse. Is time from diagnosis to delivery critical? *Journal of Reproductive Medicine* **43** (2), 129–32.

Silverton, L. (1993) *The Art and Science of Midwifery*. Prentice Hall International, London.

Simpkin, P. & Ancheta, R. (2000) *The Labor Progress Handbook*. Blackwell Science, Oxford.

Squire, C. (2002) Shoulder dystocia and umbilical cord prolapse. In *Emergencies around Childbirth – A Handbook for Midwives* (Boyle, M., ed.), Radcliffe Medical Press, Abingdon.

Weston, R. (2001) When birth goes wrong. *The Practising Midwife* **4** (8), 10–12.

Woods, C.E. (1943) A principle of physics applied to shoulder delivery. *American Journal of Obstetrics and Gynecology* **45**, 796–805.

13 Loss of a baby: stillbirth/ perinatal death

Barbara Kavanagh

Introduction

Perinatal loss has been described as a life crisis for both parents and professionals alike (Gardner, 1999). The death of a baby is not uncommon in maternity units. However, few staff feel comfortable when faced with this event. Healthcare professionals are expected to interact with the bereaved in a supportive manner whether or not they feel adequately prepared or disposed to do so (Gardner, 1999).

The bereaved parents not only have to face the loss of the person whom they have helped to create, there is also the loss of future aspirations, ambitions, hopes and dreams. So, when death occurs during pregnancy or childbirth, parents are stunned because death is not the expected outcome of pregnancy. These parents undergo intense grief reactions following the death of their baby; these feelings are very similar to any other form of bereavement (Golding, 1991). Although the experience of grieving is personal and intense, it is a normal healthy response to loss. Typical symptoms may include shock, numbness, disbelief, emptiness, a sense of failure, anger and guilt. There may also be a recurrence of feelings related to any previous loss(es). The midwife provides support in the very early stages of the grieving process, when denial, guilt and anger may be most in evidence (Butler, 2000). Kohner (1995) stresses that this is a difficult and demanding time for professionals. What they say and do may be critically important. Their words and actions are frequently remembered by parents for years to come, and may influence their memories and their grieving.

Definition

The perinatal mortality rate is defined as the number of stillbirths and early neonatal deaths (those occurring in the first week of life) per 1000 live and stillbirths.

Stillbirth is defined as 'a child, which has issued forth from its mother after the 24th week of pregnancy and did not at any time, after being completely expelled from its mother, breathe or show any other signs of life.' This is the legal definition in England and Wales.

Incidence and facts

- In the UK, in 1999, the stillbirth rate was 5.0 per 1000 total births (CESDI, 2001).
- Since 1992, the Confidential Enquiry into Stillbirths and Deaths in Infancy (CESDI) has been committed to improving outcomes in maternal and infant health. Since 1993–1999 there has been a significant downward trend in intrapartum related deaths (CESDI, 2001).
- Although the last 50 years have seen dramatic improvements in social welfare and maternity care, almost 1% of women entering the second half of pregnancy will suffer the loss of their baby (Fox *et al.*, 1997).
- It is vital that health professionals are aware of the fact that in many cases the loss of their baby will be many parents' first experience of death (Rajan, 1992).
- The immediate care a woman receives during a stillbirth can affect her emotional status 3 years after delivery (Radestad *et al.*, 1998).
- Formal burial or cremation is a legal requirement for all babies who are stillborn or die soon after birth.

Predisposing factors

While the cause of a baby's death may never be known, there can sometimes be certain predisposing factors (see Box 13.1).

Box 13.1 Predisposing factors.

Pregnancy related factors
- Placental abruption.
- Placenta praevia.
- Pre-eclampsia/eclampsia.
- Polyhydramnios.
- Blood group incompatibility.
- Prolonged pregnancy.
- Multiple pregnancy.
- Infections.
- Diabetes.
- Genitourinary.

Labour
- Placental abruption.
- Uterine rupture.
- Cord accident.
- Birth trauma.
- Hypoxia.

Conditions in the newborn
- Prematurity and associated complications.
- Confenital malformations.
- Infection.
- Hypoxia, pulmonary causes.

Diagnosing fetal death and decision making

The beginning of the grieving process

When a baby dies during labour or delivery, or immediately afterwards, parents should be told at once (Kohner, 1995). In the case of intrauterine death there should be minimum delay. Confirmation should be done with two doctors present and by ultrasound with a practitioner who is both skilled in real-time imaging and able to discuss the findings openly with the mother (Fox *et al.*, 1997). Delay in confirmation will inevitably cause greater stress. Confirmation should ideally take place with both parents present. The attitudes and empathy of midwives and doctors at the outset of this traumatic experience will influence from the beginning the grieving process, and the memories they take away with them.

Good communication and honesty are essential, full explanations should be given by midwives and doctors alike. Lovell (1983) cited in Moulder (1999), noted that some women were critical of the way staff handled the diagnosis of an intrauterine death or an abnormality; a succession of different staff were involved; staff were ill prepared and some unable to conceal their own distress at the diagnosis. When the mother first understands that death has occurred, there is a sense of shock and numbness temporarily preventing her from being overwhelmed by the full impact of the event (Jones, 1997). Some health professionals may find it difficult to know what to say at this point, if a partner is present it may be appropriate to give them a few moments alone before they are faced with painful decisions. Difficulties can arise if there is a language barrier; communication is vital, and a trained interpreter should always be made available to the family.

Decision making and choices

Midwives need to be conscious that decision making at this time, by the mother, can be hard. Due to the impact of this overwhelming shock and disbelief it may be that midwives and doctors find themselves having to re-iterate questions regarding major decisions. Repetition is often required, as difficult and emotional information is not always retained if given only once. This is a frightening and distressing situation, made worse if the woman is in pain.

Supporting parents whose baby has died and helping them to consider difficult and important decisions at a time of unbearable sorrow and anguish, is one of the most challenging roles undertaken by a midwife (Thomas, 1999). Bereaved parents will be looking for guidance about what to do next. To help parents make these difficult decisions the midwife caring for them should have established a good rapport through acknowledgment of the importance of the loss, effective communication and the use of basic counselling skills. She should employ a caring, sensitive and non-judgemental attitude, focusing on listening skills. Giving control and choices to parents and helping them to make their own decisions (which may be different to the decisions that professionals would make on their behalf) can be difficult and stressful (Kohner, 1995). Unless the cause of the fetal death threatens the mother's life, late fetal death seldom possesses a threat to maternal physical welfare (Howarth & Alfirevic, 2001).

Why vaginal birth?

It may be possible to discuss labour and delivery, the options available, and the support that will be offered throughout, in advance. Women whose baby has died *in utero* may be shocked to learn that they will have a vaginal delivery. It is a frightening thought to give birth to a dead baby. The mother's first reaction may be that she requests to have a caesarean section. Time should be taken to listen to her reasons for this, and dispel any worries that she may have regarding vaginal delivery. Gently pointing out that delivery by caesarean is thought to affect the woman's physical and mental recovery, in particular in relation to her ability to identify and accept the loss of her baby.

Induction or expectant management?

Awaiting spontaneous labour is usually safe, but research by Radestad *et al.* (1996) showed that it was advisable to induce the delivery as soon as feasible after the diagnosis of death *in utero*. They noted a strong association between waiting more than 24 hours before the start of delivery after the diagnosis of death *in utero* and anxiety related symptoms. Thus, postponing the delivery for a long time may induce an unnecessary psychological experience that is difficult to cope with. However, unless medically indicated, the decision of whether to induce or not rests with the parents themselves and that choice must be respected and supported.

Induction of labour following late intrauterine death differs from other inductions in two respects. There is no need to take account of fetal well-being, thus side effects and complications need only be considered from the maternal perspective. Second, most planned inductions with a live baby occur near term, while inductions for fetal death present over a wide range of gestational ages (Howarth & Alfirevic, 2001).

Home birth

The mother and father may consider a home delivery; they could make plans for what they would like to do with their baby. Thomas (1999) explains that in the presence of an experienced midwife, this sad event, occurring in the security of the home away from all the noise and intrusion of the hospital, can give parents positive memories of managing a difficult time. Parents would be able to feel in control and have a say in events rather than events controlling them.

Care in labour

Prior to induction for intrauterine death certain tests should be performed. Blood pressure (BP) should be measured, and urine tested for proteinuria to exclude pre-eclampsia. Temperature should be recorded, particularly in the case of ruptured membranes. If there is a suspicion that the baby died some weeks earlier then it is essential to take maternal blood for a platelet count and clotting studies as disseminated intravascular coagulation (DIC) could be a problem. These investigations are particularly important because they may influence the care options of the woman in labour and the puerperium (Fox *et al.*, 1997).

Observations

- Once labour has commenced BP, pulse and urine are observed.
- Monitoring the temperature is particularly important when using prostaglandins for induction as it can cause a pyrexia. Any significant rise in temperature may be a contraindication with epidural anaesthesia as a method of pain relief due to the possibility of maternal infection (Swanson & Madej, 1997). This information must be shared with the mother, otherwise if refused a promised epidural she may feel let down by the midwife.
- The use of cardiotocography (CTG) and pinard stethoscopes is obviously not required. The absence of the baby's heartbeat serves as a painful and constant reminder to the mother and midwife that there is to be a tragic outcome to this labour.

Pain relief

The emotional distress is worsened by the fact that the woman must undergo the labour experience, which is both psychologically and physically painful (Smith, 1999).

Radestad *et al.* (1998) studied 314 women whose babies were stillborn, they reported that they had pain relief more often during labour and delivery when compared with women who had delivered a live baby. They also remembered the labour and delivery as being physically 'insufferably hard'. Therefore, the woman must be reassured that support and adequate pain relief will be available to her at any time. However, as mentioned above, the use of an epidural may not be possible if a pyrexia is present.

Individualized care

The woman needs to be cared for in a sensitive manner by a midwife who is not afraid of her or her baby. She should be respectful and regard the baby as a precious, delicate little person. Moulder (1999), when reviewing findings from a large study of late pregnancy loss, found that the woman–midwife relationship should be based on *trust*, and was essential in providing *individualized care*. The diversity of these women's needs was understood and respected. The needs of one woman would not necessarily be right for another. Schott & Henley (1996) also explain that cultural differences and reaction to loss must be considered, it is important not to make assumptions based upon these. For example, the mother may be unwilling to see or hold her baby due to a specific religious or cultural prohibition against seeing a dead body.

The birth of the baby

- It would be ideal if the delivery could take place away from the main busy delivery suite area, in a quiet calm atmosphere.
- Giving comfort and support to the bereaved parents at this time of enormous sadness will help create a positive birth experience.
- A slow and gentle delivery of the baby would help to minimize any damage that may occur, as the skin will be very fragile.
- Small premature babies presenting by the breech can take longer to deliver the head. Reassurance needs to be conveyed to the parents at this crucial time.
- It may be appropriate to give the baby straight to the mother. If this is not acceptable, the baby could be wrapped in a small towel (not paper as it will be difficult to remove from the baby's skin later) and then offered to the parents to hold. Ideally discussion about this will have taken place, in the case of an intrauterine death, beforehand.

Third stage of labour

If the dead baby has been retained *in utero* for longer than 4 weeks or, if the woman has a suspected placental abruption (or other risk factors), she is at increased risk of postpartum haemorrhage. In such cases active management of the third stage is indicated. Any of these risk factors may have been determined at confirmation of the death and by blood tests for infection and clotting studies.

Following birth, the placenta should be transported according to local pathology guidelines. This varies greatly from hospital to hospital; some pathologists request the placenta is sent dry, others request it is transported in formaldehyde.

Precious moments with their baby

Following delivery of the placenta the mother should be made comfortable, and the midwife allow the parents some time alone with their baby if they so wish.

The research of Radested *et al.* (1996) suggested that the meeting and parting of the baby is important, and should be strengthened, to diminish the risk of long-term psychological problems. Therefore, the mother should be able to spend as much time as she wants with her newborn child. However, the study also found that staff should not force the mother to hold, caress, or kiss the dead child. Such actions were not beneficial in terms of a reduced risk for anxiety or depression. Thus, parents wanting to abstain should feel they could do so.

Following the birth

Attitudes to pregnancy loss and the care provided for women have undergone a revolution in the past 20 years. The prevailing view today is that parents should be encouraged to grieve and to be involved with their dead baby (Moulder, 1999). The added difficulty when grieving for a stillborn baby is that parents have not had the time to get to know their baby. There is no known person to talk about. Memories help to facilitate mourning. To assist parents to grieve normally, the most should be made of what is available to create special memories for them (Greaves, 1994). Many maternity units have recognized this need, and have devised a comprehensive checklist (see 'Checklists, tests and paperwork' on page 213).

Care following birth

Involving family members

If the parents and other members of the family wish to hold the baby, advising them beforehand how the baby will feel will go some way to allay any fears and anxieties they may have. For example, the baby will feel floppy, and large babies have some movement of the bones in their head (Dyer, 1992).

Parents can bathe and dress their baby in clothes they want him/her to wear; this process will take a long time and should not be hurried.

Parents need to be prepared for the honesty that children can show at these times. This may be a confusing time for them. They have often been looking forward to the birth of their baby brother or sister. They sometimes ask unexpected questions, and guiding the parents to be honest is the best course of action. Children are very accepting of death as long as they are able to participate and share the experience with their family (Dyer, 1992).

Creating mementoes

Parents are offered mementoes of their baby such as photographs, foot and hand-prints, a lock of hair. Polaroid photographs are usually taken with one remaining within the mother's notes. Parents need to know that if exposed to light they will eventually fade.

The practice in some units is to leave a camera and film with the bereaved family allowing them to take whatever pictures they want, enabling the parents to have the photographs developed in their own time. This also gives other members of the family, such as siblings and grandparents, time to become involved, create their own memories and say their own goodbyes to the baby.

Memory triggers and smells

The sensation of smell can be an emotional trigger. Dusting the clothes and shawl with baby powder and placing the keepsakes in a plastic bag will preserve the smell for many years, thus providing powerful memories.

Footprints and handprints can be taken, put on to card, and kept within a special memory booklet of the baby. This can also include locks of hair, name bands and the baby's personal details such as weight and measurements.

Spiritual beliefs and funeral arrangements

As previously mentioned, few parents have had little or no contact with death. They may never have had to think about making funeral arrangements, and when faced with such questions may have little idea of what is expected. Many women recall with great clarity events surrounding the death of their babies, and several were very hurt when asked how they would like the baby 'disposed of' (Rajan, 1992). This is such a sensitive issue and it should be handled with great respect.

The spiritual and religious outlook of individuals often takes on more importance at the time of bereavement (Jones, 1997). Asking the bereaved couple if they wish to see a hospital chaplain, or other religious person if appropriate, may help them to reach any decisions, and gain spiritual support. This may include having the baby baptised and named. However, this may not be suitable for every faith and culture.

There may be some parents, who do not wish to have any mementoes of their dead baby. This may be because of personal, cultural or religious reasons. Whilst these views would seem to be contrary to facilitating the grief process, they should not be viewed as abnormal or wrong (Schott & Henley, 1996).

Registering the baby's death

Box 13.2 describes the various certification steps required for registering a baby's death prior to burial or cremation.

Post-mortem

Many parents want to know the cause of their baby's death, though they may find the idea of a post-mortem distasteful. Parents often hope that a post-mortem will give them the reason for their baby's death, but they should be aware that this is not always the case.

Post-mortem must be discussed very gently but giving clear factual and unbiased information enabling them to be able to make the right decision for them. Explanation of the process, and how it is carefully done, may help to reassure the parents of the

Box 13.2   Registering a baby's death.

---

(1) **A Stillbirth Certificate** This is given to the parents which is completed by the midwife or doctor who attended the birth.

   If a post-mortem is to take place this may delay the proceedings and parents need to be conscious of this.

(2) The parents take the Stillbirth Certificate to the **Registrar for Births and Deaths**. This must be

   - within 21 days in Scotland
   - within 3 months in the rest of the UK.

   Typically parents often register the baby's death within a week or so of the birth. The Registrar will:

   - Issue a **Certificate for Burial or Cremation**, depending upon the parent's wishes.
   - Place the baby's name on the Stillbirth Register. This is an opportunity to give the baby a name if he or she does not yet have one.

   If the baby's father is not married to the mother both must attend the registration if they wish the father's name to be entered on the register.

(3) The parents take the Certificate for Burial or Cremation to the **hospital bereavement co-ordinator** or a **funeral director**. Either can arrange funerals for these parents and in many areas of the country this is free of charge, and may include a memorial service conducted by the couple's religious leader or hospital chaplain. Parents should be informed about the book of remembrance that most hospital chapels hold.

   Some parents request that their placenta is buried or cremated with their baby.

---

procedure itself. Some hospitals produce a written explanation of the post-mortem procedure for the parents. The Stillbirth and Neonatal Death Society (SANDS) also produce a leaflet suitable for parents.

Checklists, tests and paperwork

Checklists are used to avoid important tasks being overlooked and to prevent the parents being asked the same questions repeatedly. A checklist example is given in Appendix D. Schott & Henley (1996) argue that there is a danger that such a checklist can be used inflexibly and can become an end in itself, rather than a way of ensuring that the needs of the parents are met appropriately. They see that focusing on a checklist may also be a way of avoiding real contact, and believe that if midwives and other professionals are to offer appropriate care, they need to identify their own personal and cultural preferences and fears in relation to death and bereavement.

There are various maternal tests that can be undertaken to try to identify the cause of the fetal death (see Appendix D). Obstetricians and hospitals vary in the blood tests they offer. Common tests include full blood count (FBC), clotting studies and Kleihauer (regardless of the maternal blood group for evidence of a large feto-maternal haemorrhage). Other tests may include parvovirus serology, toxoplasmosis and glycosated Hb.

Care in the postnatal period

Staying in hospital

Simple measures can be taken to alleviate some of the parents' anxieties, for example in the ward environment, a private room with facilities and a double bed may be helpful. They should be able to spend as much time as they want with their baby. Ask the mother how she feels about her surroundings, and let her make the decision. Radestad *et al.* (1998) suggested that differences in the length of stay after fetal death, compared with live birth, may have depended on the mother's opinion of the maternity hospital environment. Naturally, many women disliked being confronted by newborn babies and their mothers, or pregnant women. The investigation showed that of the 314 women nearly half left the hospital within 24 hours after stillbirth, and almost one in ten women went home within 6 hours.

The option of taking baby home

It is important to offer parents choices. They may not realize that they can take their baby home before the funeral, allowing them to spend precious time together as a family before saying goodbye. Midwives may be uncomfortable with this idea and find it difficult to discuss this option with the parents. Nevertheless issues such as these should not be avoided, therefore help from colleagues or mentors may be needed.

Lactation

Suppression of lactation must be discussed. Mothers can become distressed at the knowledge that their breasts will produce milk yet there is no baby to feed. Drug therapy is available but there is little evidence to support the effectiveness of it. There are simple measures that can be suggested to the mother that will alleviate breast engorgement. For example cabbage leaves, gel packs and massage (Renfrew & Lang, 1997), hot towels and analgesia.

Mourning and planning for a future pregnancy

Mothers are very likely to ask midwives about the timing of a future pregnancy, the risks involved and the chances of a live healthy baby. It must be remembered that this is a very personal decision, and unless contraindicated, for example following a caesarean section, the timing of another baby will be up to the couple. However, difficulties can arise if the mother becomes pregnant while she is still mourning, or during a time when she has not been able to mourn for her stillborn baby. The new pregnancy can hinder the completion of the mourning process, as it deprives the mother of time and space to mourn (Greaves, 1994). These circumstances can be made worse if the baby is born near the anniversary of the lost baby.

Going home

- On discharge from hospital, appropriate information should be given to the parents. They must be reassured that they can return to see their baby whenever they wish before the funeral. Give them a contact number.
- Advise them that a community midwife will be visiting the next day who will have been informed of the baby's death. Also the mother's general practitioner and health visitor, who may be in touch.
- A consultant appointment will be arranged for about 6 weeks time, the parents need to know that this is a discussion about the baby's death, and does not include a physical examination of the mother.
- Information about support groups, up-to-date contact numbers, and any other relevant advice including contraception, should also be given to the parents.

Summary

- Good communication between health professionals and bereaved parents is vital.
- Midwives should have an honest, caring and non-judgemental approach, with an emphasis on listening skills.
- What professionals say and do following bereavement can have a lasting effect on the parents, and may affect the grieving process.
- Parents should be given individualized care to meet their particular needs. Cultural and religious backgrounds must be respected.
- Give parents information so they are able to make decisions and choices.
- Creating memories will help with mourning.
- Professionals need an awareness and understanding of the grieving process.
- Caregivers themselves need emotional support, and time for debriefing.

Useful contacts

Antenatal Results and Choices (ARC)   73 Charlotte Street, London W1T 4PN. Telephone: 020 7631 0285 Website: www.arc-uk.org

The Child Bereavement Trust   Aston House, West Wycombe, High Wycombe, Buckinghamshire HP14 3AG. Telephone: 01494 446648: Website: www.childbereavement.org.uk.

The Miscarriage Association   C/o Clayton Hospital, Northgate, Wakefield WF1 3JS. Telephone: 01924 200799. Website: www.miscarriageassociation.org.uk

Stillbirth and Neonatal Death Society (SANDS)   28 Portland Place, London E1N 4DE. Telephone: 020 7436 5881. Website: www.uk-sands.org

References

Butler, M. (2000) Facilitating the grief process: the role of the midwife. *The Practising Midwife* **3** (36), 37.

CESDI (2001) *Confidential Enquiry into Stillbirths and Deaths in Infancy*, 8th Anual Report. Maternal and Child Health Research Consortium, London.

Dyer, M. (1992) Stillborn – still precious. *MIDIRS Midwifery Digest* **2** (2), 341–4.

Fox, R., Pillai, M., Porter, H. & Gill, G. (1997) The management of late fetal death: a guide to comprehensive care. *Neonatal Intensive Care*, 56–64.

Gardner, J. (1999) Perinatal death: uncovering the needs of midwives and nurses and exploring helpful interventions in the United States, England, and Japan. *Journal of Transcultural Nursing* **10** (2), 120–30.

Golding, C. (1991) *Bereavement*. Redwood Press, Melksham, Wiltshire.

Greaves, J. (1994) Normal and abnormal grief reactions: midwifery care after stillbirth. *British Journal of Midwifery* **2** (2), 61–5.

Howarth, G.R. & Alfirevic, Z. (2001) Induction of labour following late fetal death (≥ 24 weeks) (protocol for a Cochrane Review). *The Cochrane Library*, Issue 4. Update Software, Oxford.

Jones, M. (1997) Mothers who need to grieve: the reality of mourning the loss of a baby. *British Journal of Midwifery* **5** (8), 478–81.

Kohner, N. (1995) *Pregnancy Loss and the Death of a Baby: Guidelines for Professionals*. Stillbirth and Neonatal Death Society (SANDS), London.

Lovell, A. (1983) Some question of identity. *Social Science and Medicine* **17** (11), 755–61.

Moulder, C. (1999) Late pregnancy loss: issues in hospital care. *British Journal of Midwifery* **1**, 244–7.

Radestad, I., Nordin, C., Steineck, G. & Sjogren, B. (1998) A comparison of women's memories of care during pregnancy, labour and delivery after stillbirth or live birth. *Midwifery* **14** 111–17.

Radestad, I., Steineck, G., Nordin, C. & Sjogren, B. (1996) Psychological complications after stillbirth – influence of memories and immediate management: population based study. *British Medical Journal* **312**, 1505–508.

Rajan, L. (1992) 'Not just me dreaming': parents mourning pregnancy loss. *Health Visitor* **65**, 354–7.

Renfrew, M.J. & Langs, S. (1997) Do cabbage leaves prevent breast engorgement? In Neilson, J.P., Crowther, C.A., Hodnett, E.D., Hofmeyr, G.J. & Keirse, M.J.N.C. (eds) *Pregnancy and Childbirth Module of the Cochrane Database of Systematic Reviews* (Updated 5.12.96), *The Cochrane Library*, Issue 1. Update Software, Oxford.

Schott, J. & Henley, A. (1996) Childbearing losses. *British Journal of Midwifery* **4** (10), 52.

Smith, S. (1999) The lost children. *Contemporary Nurse* **8** (1), 245–51.

Swanson, L. & Madey, T.H. (1997) The febrile obstetric patient. In *Clinical Problems in Obstetric Anaesthesia* (Russell, I.F. & Lyons, G., eds), pp. 123–31. Chapman & Hall, London.

Thomas, J. (1999) A baby's death – helping parents make difficult choices. *The Practising Midwife* **2** (7), 16–19.

Section 2
Support information

14   Record keeping and litigation

Introduction

This chapter focuses on the practical aspects of record keeping. Local protocols and the Nursing and Midwifery Council (NMC) guidelines on record keeping are commonly available in hospital libraries and on the labour ward/birthing suites.

Facts

- Medicolegal claims in obstetrics are increasing (Byrne, 1999).
- The NHS pays out £400 million per annum, 60% of costs are for obstetric and gynaecology cases (Andrews, 2002).
- Litigation experts advise that midwives' practice is likely to be judged as being only as good as their written notes (Mason & Edwards, 1993).
- Statute of limitations (legal time limit) for cases to be brought is usually when the child reaches adulthood, i.e. 18 years. However, a baby who is brain damaged is not considered legally to ever reach adulthood and so, technically, no time limit applies.

Record storage

Records, including all essential notes, test results, prescription charts and records of medicines administered, must be retained for 25 years (UKCC, 1998). Community and independent midwives will need to store their diaries and records, protected from damp, and kept secure for 25 years, even on retirement.

Consent

Informed consent is just that. The client is expected to decide, on the basis of information given to her, if she wishes to consent to the course of action proposed. The person giving consent must be:

- Of sufficient mental capacity to make the decision.
- In possession of all the important, relevant information (Griffith *et al.*, 1999).

Performing any invasive or intimate procedure requires maternal consent and the midwife should document if this has been given.

Example: Artificial rupture of the membranes (ARM)

The client should be informed of the indications and possible benefits for this procedure, and its possible risks and complications (common and rare). Only then can the woman make an informed decision and thus give or withhold consent.

- If the midwife performs artificial rupture of the membranes (ARM) without informed consent, this is could constitute assault or trespass on the person.
- If the ARM results in a cord prolapse with its subsequent consequences, and the midwife had not told the woman this was a possible complication of ARM, then although the woman consented, she did not do so in the light of the important, relevant information.

Keeping contemporaneous records

Basic standards

- Writen legibly in black, water-resistant ink. Print if others find your handwriting difficult to read.
- Date, time (use the 24-hour clock) and sign all entries. Since signatures can be difficult to read they should have the name printed alongside them on the first entry and subsequently on each new page.
- All referrals and consultations should be noted detailing the name and status of person. Avoid untraceable entries such as 'SR informed', is this sister informed, or senior registrar informed?
- Although frequently in use, try to avoid uncommon abbreviations or ambiguous terms. Many units have a formal, designated list of abbreviations.

Content and quality

Dr Thomas, an obstetrician with an interest in clinical risk management, suggests that the standard of record keeping is slipping, with clinicians writing too much yet missing important recordable aspects of care (Andrews, 2002).

Notes should contain accurate information about:

- Physical condition of the client.
- Psychological well-being.
- Care given.
- Brief points about the information given, if consent was given and any procedure carried out.
- Document the time and person to whom a referral has been made and the time that they responded or attended.
- Document decisions including the decision to 'wait and see'. 'A lack of documentation in "wait and see" decisions can make it appear as if no decision has been taken' (Symon, 1997).

> 'Narrative notes need to be written frequently enough to give a pictures of the woman's condition to anyone reading them ... women who have complications of pregnancy or women who are having contractions but are not yet in labour require frequent evaluation of their condition. The narrative notes should reflect the frequency with which these women are evaluated.' (Byrne, 1999).

Some content points often overlooked

- When describing liquor the midwife should mention its colour and the approximate quantity – minimal, moderate or large amount. This shows the midwife is observing for signs of polyhydramnios (excessive liquor) and oligohydramnios (minimal liquor) and making a note if all appears 'normal'.
- When describing any meconium staining of the liquor, be sure to clarify if it is thin or sparse, or, of greater concern, thick/fresh.
- Do not be afraid to comment when things are straightforward. For example, if the midwife thinks the cardiotocograph (CTG) is fine then she should document this.

Alterations

- Incorrect entries should be surrounded by brackets and one line drawn through the text, followed by writing 'incorrect entry' and signing it.
- Do not use correction fluid.
- Do not scribble out.

Times and late entries

'It should be clear what time events occurred and what time the entry was made.' (Bryne, 1999)

- All times should be entered in the margin using the 24-hour clock.
- All clinicians making entries in the notes should use the same clock. In hospital, this is usually the clock in the room, by which the CTG time should also be calibrated or at least noted on the trace with any time differences.
- At home, the midwife providing the care should clarify with any other clinicians, if in attendance, from which timepiece the time is being recorded and documented (usually their own watch).
- Note all late entries as such, giving the reason for the delay in documentation.

There are many situations, when providing one to one care in labour, during which it can be difficult to physically leave the woman in order to make notes about her labour, the fetal heart rate (FHR) and so on. Even when everything is 'normal', notes should be made with the evidence of this. At times, the attending midwife may well have no hands free with which to write the notes.

'Case records will be relied upon heavily in a legal investigation. Given the unexpected nature of legal claims, staff that fail to keep clear, contemporaneous records, particularly in the labour ward, may be putting their heads in a noose ... It may be difficult to maintain a good standard of record keeping when the unit is extremely busy or when emergencies occur but there is a clear duty to make adequate entries in the case notes as soon as is practicable.' (Symon, 1997)

Cardiotocographs (CTGs)

'Some of the most common problems relate to CTG traces that do not clearly state the woman's full name, the date and time or which contain unexplained gaps.' (Byrne, 1999)

For more information on correct documentation regarding CTGs See Chapter 17, pages 242–3.

References

Andrews, S. (2002) Clinical risk management study day review. *RCM Midwives Journal.* **5** (11), 366–7.

Byrne, U. (1999) Record keeping – a risk management perspective. *British Journal of Midwifery* **7** (7), 436–9.

Griffith, R., Tengnah, C. & Grey, R. (1999) Consent and women in labour: a review of the issues. *British Journal of Midwifery* **7** (2), 92–4.

Mason, D. & Edwards, P. (1993) *Litigation: A Risk Management Guide for Midwives.* Royal College of Midwives (RCM), London.

Symon, A. (1997) The standard of case records. *British Journal of Midwifery* **5** (8), 462–4.

UKCC (1998) *Midwives Rules and Code of Practice.* United Kingdom Central Council for Nursing, Midwifery and Health Visiting, London. (*Now the Nursing and Midwifery Council.*)

15   Midwifery skills to help women cope with labour

Virginia Howes

First meeting

Whilst some women do give birth in the secure surroundings of their own home, the vast majority of women still give birth in hospital and, therefore, it is vital to make the area of labour and birth as home like as possible. Society may have led women to believe that they will be safest in a hospital, but the primal part of their brain, which is used during labour (Odent, 1999; Ockenden, 2001) may be screaming 'danger' as they walk into the clinical environment and are faced with strangers. The adrenaline rush of this fear can have a detrimental effect on the oxytocin release needed for labour to continue.

First impressions have a huge impact on the physiology of labour and can alter its progression and so it is important to minimize this effect. The best way to do so is to welcome women to the ward with arms open (literally) and a smile. It may be just another day to the midwife but for the woman it is very special, it may be the best day ever or even her worst nightmare all rolled into one! Treat her like she is the only woman about to give birth in the world, make her feel special. This whole experience will be remembered by her for the rest of her life and will affect her relationship to her newborn, her self-esteem, as well as influence her attitude to childbearing, for herself and her children.

- Stop what you are doing.
- Give immediate welcome, even if you are busy.
- Make her feel special.
- Smile and give warmth.

The birth environment

Make sure the room is not full of equipment. All that is needed for normal labour is a listening device but not a cardiotocograph (CTG) monitor (NICE, 2001). Ensure there are lots of comfort things, such as pillows, drinks, a CD player, and hot and cold water. When the woman enters the room, encourage her away from the bed by sitting on it yourself and suggesting she takes a seat, or increase the height of the bed and suggest she leans forward on it. Remember that her partner is part of this scene and accommodating him/her too will help the woman to relax. Reinforce the fact the beds are not the place for labouring women and that baby will be born easier and quicker if she remains upright.

Keep the lights down low. Warm towels may be preferable to those in sterile packs and actually make drying the baby more effective and less uncomfortable. Keep all non-essential equipment out of the room or hidden and do not be afraid to change the layout of the room so the focus is not on the bed and the clock.

- Take all non-essential equipment out of the room.
- Move the bed so it is not the focus point.
- Have music playing softly.
- Turn off overhead lights.

Support

Kind words, the constant presence of the midwife and appropriate touch are proven powerful analgesia (Hodnett, 2002). A midwife continually present in the room, when wished by the woman, is the best labour support and pain management tactic a woman can have. Offer a bath or a shower. Provide food and drink. Use hot water bottles for pain comfort. Do not feel the need to look busy. Sit down and just be there. Maintain eye contact as appropriate and answer questions with total honesty. Support in labour was also covered in Chapter 1.

- Do not leave the woman alone.
- Remember that often the kindest and safest thing a midwife does is nothing.
- A midwife is not there to relieve pain but to help women through it.

Verbal support

Remember that all women are tired in strong labour. It is a normal physiological response so they relax between contractions. Those few minutes of sleep are like hours in the benefits obtained. Most women will close their eyes and relax between contractions but if not encourage them to do so.

Most women will get to a point where they think they cannot go on with this labour any longer. Midwives will recognize the words 'I can't do it', 'I'm too tired', 'get me ... drugs, caesarean, etc.', these words suggest that the woman is at the end of the first stage of labour (transition) and she can be reassured this usually heralds the approaching birth of her baby. A supportive midwife in constant attendance is best practice and what being a midwife is about. This is the time to offer words of encouragement, 'it's okay', 'you can do it', 'it will soon be gone', 'you are a strong woman', 'you are doing so well'.

- Use encouraging words and offer reassurance.
- Accept that things women say and do in labour are normal.
- Try changing the dynamics if the woman panics, suggest you go for a walk or a change of position.

Touch

Most women get a huge amount of comfort from massage, but some may feel hypersensitive and some women will dislike being touched. Find out what is right for her. Oil on your hands while rubbing her skin will have a warming, soothing effect that can bring huge relief. Touch can also be very invasive so judge the situation carefully. Her partner can help with massage and will serve to help them be together and gain comfort from each other. Hot water on a pad or in a bottle may help, so can immersing in a warm bath or shower.

- Find out what helps.
- Use massage and hot water to bring comfort.

Endorphin release

If labouring women are anxious, scared, facing a new environment or a new face, they release adrenalin. Adrenalin inhibits the release of the oxytocin that is needed for labour to progress, hence the midwife arrives at the house or the woman arrives at the hospital and it all stops! Once she is relaxed and calm, her brain will go into primitive mode (Odent, 1999) and the oxytocin will flow. She will soon be engulfed with pain-killing endorphins that give that 'on another planet' glaze in her eyes. Do not chatter and encourage others in the room to remain quiet as noise is distracting and may inhibit the progress of labour.

Turn off the lights. Tell her this is *her* room now and no one can enter without her permission and then ensure your word is kept. This woman now needs privacy, security, comfort and respect.

- Women *can* give birth unaided by intervention and drugs.
- The body has natural pain killers called endorphins.
- The labouring woman needs a caring midwife, relaxation, calm, quiet, dark and comforting surroundings for endorphins to be released.
- Women who do need pain relief should never be made to feel that they have failed. It is vital to reinforce how difficult her labour was and how well she has coped.

Useful contact

Doula UK   PO Box 26678, London N14 4WB. Website: www.doula.org.uk
  Trained birth supporters for women.

References

Hodnett, E.D. (2002) Caregiver support for women during childbirth, (Cochrane Review). *The Cochrane Library* Issue 4. Update Software, Oxford.
NICE (2001) *Clinical Guideline C – The Use of Electronic Fetal Monitoring.* National Institute for Clinical Excellence, London.
Ockenden, J. (2001) The hormonal dance of labour. *The Practising Midwife* **4** (6), 16–17.
Odent, M. (1999) *The Scientification of Love.* Free Association Books, London.

16 Vaginal examinations and artificial rupture of the membranes

Introduction

Vaginal examinations (VEs) are a common intervention performed during labour. While many question their necessity and routine frequency (Warren, 1999; Crowther, 2000; Walsh, 2000a), they do remain a skill that the midwife frequently undertakes. Many women are not aware that VEs are undertaken during the course of labour.

'Recent studies have reported that women find vaginal examinations traumatic, distressing, uncomfortable and embarrassing and that they can trigger issues of sexual intimacy, invasion of privacy and vulnerability especially for women who have been sexually abused'. (Nolan, 2001)

Explanations/information sharing

- Discuss the indication for the examination.
- Explain what it may feel like and typically how long it may last.
- In younger women, check if this is her first VE (this is surprisingly common).

In addition, the woman needs to know that if she wants the midwife to stop at any point, then the midwife will stop. If the examination 'hurts' or the woman has a contraction, or if she has been violated before, she needs to trust that her midwife will respond appropriately.

Consent or compliance?

Performing a VE or an artificial rupture of the membranes (ARM) without prior discussion and verbal consent is poor practice and may constitute assault. Many women conform or comply with suggestions which, when they later re-consider, they feel they were coerced into or their informed consent was not sought.

Document whether verbal consent was given or if consent was declined.

If consent is withheld:

- Remain sensitive, open and accept her decision.
- Seek alternative methods of assessing progress in labour as discussed in Chapter 1 under the heading 'Maternal and fetal well-being and progress in labour'.

Bear in mind that many women, including survivors of sexual abuse may not be able to cope with invasive, intimate procedures in labour (see later in this chapter).

Performing and documenting a vaginal examination

Modesty/comfort

- Never underestimate someone's potential for embarrassment or feelings of vulnerability (even if attending a birth at home). For the woman, a variety of factors from religious, cultural or personal issues, including having a partner present or others in the room, can all contribute to her embarrassment and how she perceives her situation.
- Cover up the woman's lower half with a sheet/towel/dressing gown.

- Ensure doors are shut/curtains drawn, etc.
- In hospital have a 'please knock and wait' sign on the door.

Procedure

Before the examination

- Ensure the woman's bladder is empty.
- Abdominal palpation first! This is a good habit to get into.
- Never perform a VE during a contraction as it is insensitive, painful and immobilizing for the woman.
- Sit next to the woman and chat to help her relax, before the examination.

During the examination

Some midwives are adept at performing VEs when the woman is in a different position or in the waterbirth tub. If the woman is in a forward leaning or upright position, the angle of the vagina is steep and more towards her bottom. It can sometimes be difficult to accurately assess the anterior section of cervix in such positions.

- The midwife should explain what she is doing and check the woman is fine.
- All midwives should be aware of their own body language, when performing a VE. Avoid looking worried, disappointed or disconnected from what is happening.
- Be aware of the woman's body language and ensure she is okay.

After the examination

- Help the woman into an upright position, ideally off the bed. (Lying is a suboptimum position and can cause a variety of complications.)
- Listen to the fetal heart rate (FHR) (again, ensure the woman isn't lying flat).
- Congratulate her on how well she coped with the examination and find something positive to say, even if there is little change (see 'Poor progress' on page 232).
- Discuss the findings with the woman. If approached with sensitivity and the findings are good news, then this can lift the woman's spirits and reassure her. However, the opposite is also true, if handled insensitively or the news is poor, an examination can be a distressing or negative experience.
- Document your findings (see Box 16.1).

Accuracy and timing of vaginal examinations

Warren (1999) suggests midwives ask themselves 'What decision has to be made at this time which requires information that can only be obtained from a vaginal examination?'.

- The timing of VEs should be relevant to each individual woman in order to permit adequate assessment of her progress and should not be performed too frequently or for the sake of 'routine' (Crowther, 2000).

Box 16.1   Documenting a vaginal examination (VE).

Vulva and vagina
  • Healthy – identify potential problems or conditions including female genital mutilation/circumcision, genital warts, offensive smelling discharge.

Cervix
  • Location (posterior, mid, central, anterior or lateral).
  • Consistency (soft, thick, firm, thin, stretchy).
  • Application (loosely, moderately or well applied).
  • Effacement (from uneffaced, to partially, to fully effaced).
  • Dilatation (os closed, 1 to 9 cm, anterior lip, 10 cm or fully dilated).

Presenting part (cephalic, breech, other)
  • Position (see Fig. 16.1 for examples of various vertex positions).
  • Station (ballotable, -3, -2, -1, at spines, +1, +2).
  • Caput/moulding (absent or present, approximate amount).

Membranes
  • Intact or absent/artificial rupture of the membranes (ARM).
  • Liquor (absent or present, colour and approximate quantity, +, ++, +++).

Document
  • VE findings.
  • Fetal heart rate (FHR).
  • Contractions.

  • These assessments (commonly 4 hourly) and definitions of progress (such as a cervical dilatation of 1 cm or 0.5 cm per hour) vary greatly between units and within the literature (Crowther, 2000).
  • Repeated VEs in labour are an invasive intervention of unproven benefit (Crowther, 2000).
  • VEs are not as accurate as clinicians would like to think. Results vary from one practitioner to another, and even from the same examiner on repeat examination (Crowther, 2000). At other times, the findings are superfluous to what is actually happening to the woman's body. For example, the multiparous woman who was 6 cm a few minutes ago and is now pushing, is not uncommon.
  • A VE is only part of the whole assessment of the progress of labour. Increasingly midwives are reclaiming traditional skills to utilize alternative ways of assessing progress in labour.

Some common problems

Poor progress

Poor progress can be hard to accept. It can be very demoralizing for the woman and creates self-doubt about her ability to labour and birth. Even if there is little or no change try to find something positive to say, such as 'the cervix is so much thinner and the baby's in a great position and moving down really well', or similar positive news! Chapter 4 also considers slow progress in labour.

Oedematous cervix

Oedematous cervix occurs when the anterior part of the cervix swells, feeling tense and enlarged, and occurs occasionally in the later stages of labour. Midwives have always thought that women who push prior to full dilatation have the greatest risk of swelling their cervix. However, Walsh (2000b) suggests that there is no evidence to show this happens in practice. Walmsley (2000) suggests that a premature urge to push, common in posterior position babies, may be physiologically desirable to rotate the baby into an optimum position prior to full dilatation and descent.

- If the cervix is oedematous, a common non-evidence based course of action is to get the pressure off by supporting the woman to resist the urge to push and adopting a position which reduces this sensation, such as side lying, all fours or knee-chest positions. The cervix usually becomes a tight lip, which can, if not too resistant, be slipped over the presenting part during a VE.
- If the oedematous cervix will not budge, more time and huge support are necessary for the woman to get her to cope with these distressing, expulsive contractions. In some cases an epidural may bring welcome relief.
- Anecdotally, midwives who discover a swollen cervix mid way through labour suggest it rarely resolves and a caesarean usually becomes necessary (ARM, 2000).

A 'shrinking' cervix

This issue has sparked debate among radical midwives. Presumably, the presenting part can subtly de-flex or flex, affecting the pressure, or lack of it, against the cervix (as can bulging membranes) which can cause changes between examinations. Anecdotal evidence suggests that a shrinking cervix is more common in occipitoposterior (OP) positions and can be a sign of dystocia (ARM, 2000).

Cervical dilatation and positions of the fetal head

The one question every woman, midwife or doctor usually wants to know following a VE is 'what is the dilatation?'. Assessing cervical dilatation has become the primary source of information gleaned from the examination. Figure 16.1a shows a template illustrating cervical dilatation and Figs 16.1b–e show some examples of positions of the fetal head.

Invasive examinations and sexual abuse

Providing intimate care for survivors of child sexual abuse and women who have been sexually assaulted or raped

Many women may not disclose if they have been sexually abused as a child or pre- viously sexually assaulted. Symptoms associated with survivors are often mis- interpreted and women can be labelled as 'difficult patients'. This lack of awareness by health professionals can result in inappropriate treatment, resulting in further damage (Aldcroft, 2001). Women experiencing any intervention, from having blood taken to a VE, are having to comply and let someone do something to their body, which is

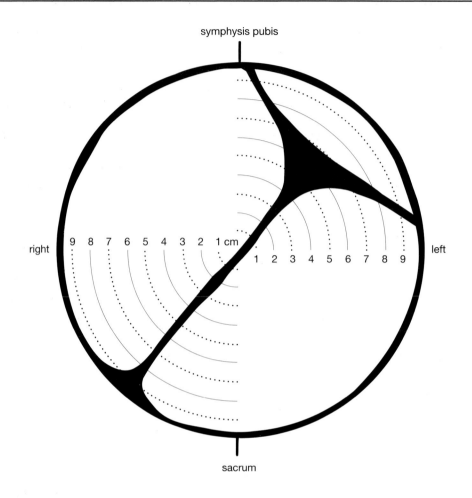

symphysis pubis

right   9 8 7 6 5 4 3 2 1 cm   left
                              1 2 3 4 5 6 7 8 9

sacrum

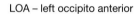

LOA – left occipito anterior

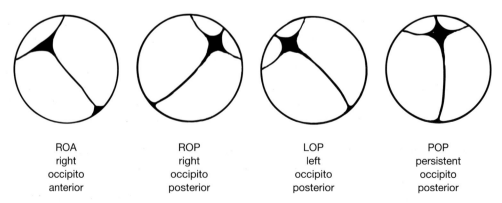

ROA	ROP	LOP	POP
right	right	left	persistent
occipito	occipito	occipito	occipito
anterior	posterior	posterior	posterior

Fig. 16.1   Cervical dilatation and positions of the fetal head.

invasive, unpleasant, and possibly painful. 'Submitting' to the midwife or doctor can be reminiscent of their past abuse. They may be left feeling vulnerable, powerless, violated and dirty (Kitzinger, 1992). Some points to bear in mind include:

- Women who have suffered previous sexual abuse are more likely to have a difficult birth experience which results in a higher level of obstetric interventions. (Gutteridge 2001).
- 20% of women have been subjected to some form of sexual physical contact in their childhood (Riley, 1995).
- Sociologists have observed how carers can act in a paternalistic manner, with the woman feeling powerless and childlike, regressing them back to their former role as a victim (Kitzinger, 1992).

Phobias and behaviours linked to past experiences of sexual abuse or rape

- Fear or obvious dislike of VEs, invasive procedures, needles or going to the dentist.
- History of depression, poor self-esteem and emotional problems (Riley, 1995).
- There is a correlation between women who have been sexually abused as children and psychiatric/emotional dysfunction and postnatal depression (Riley, 1995).
- Disclosure to the midwife of previous abuse.

Behaviour during intimate procedures may include:

- 'Shut off' during the procedure.
- May cry or become distressed by the procedure.
- Regressive or infantile behaviour (Gutteridge, 2001).
- May tense up or refuse to proceed with the examination.

What can the midwife do to help?

- **The midwife must try not to replicate abuse**. Ensure the woman is comfortable and, essentially, in control (Aldcroft, 2001).
- **Staying in control**. Squeezing the midwife's free hand during a VE, as a sign of when to stop, may be more helpful than expecting the woman to speak (Aldcroft, 2001).
- **Language**. Avoid patronizing or disempowering terms. Phrases offered to reassure or make suggestions can regress women back to themselves as former victims, with the midwife now as the perpetrator (Mayer, 1995), for example: 'That's a good girl', 'Open your legs a bit wider', 'Lie still, this won't hurt'; 'shhh' (Gutteridge, 2001).
- **Reality check**. Ground the woman in the 'here and now' explaining what is happening as it happens. Keep the situation focused on the cervix, the labour, and the baby … rather than letting her return to her former state as a victim (Aldcroft, 2001).
- **Eye contact**. During a VE the avoidance of eye contact is thought to further medicalize and depersonalize the situation (Aldcroft, 2001).
- The presence of others may appear voyeuristic, which can replicate abusive situations. So send others out of the room, particularly male midwives/doctors (Kitzinger, 1992).
- Ask yourself, is this examination really necessary? (Warren, 1999).

Artificial rupture of the membranes

For the vast majority of women experiencing a 'normal' labour, their membranes tend to remain intact during the first stage of labour, often rupturing spontaneously around the time of full dilatation, heralding the onset of the second stage. Artificial rupture of the membranes (ARM) is a widely practised intervention and is more common in units with high intervention rates and an active management approach to routine care (Rosser & Anderson, 1998).

Possible benefits of artificial rupture of the membranes

- Artificial rupture of the membranes results in shorter labour by 60–120 minutes and a decrease in the use of oxytocics, particularly in nulliparous women (Rosser & Anderson, 1998; Fraser *et al.*, 2002).
- Artificial rupture of the membranes allows for visualization of the colour and quantity of the liquor.

Consequences and contraindications to artificial rupture of the membranes

- Artificial rupture of the membranes is not advisable during the first stage of labour in any baby at increased susceptibility to cord compression or fetal compromise such as growth-restricted babies, oligohydramnios (Moore, 1996), babies presenting by the breech (Banks, 1998) or preterm infants.
- Artificial rupture of the membranes increases the risk of severe, variable FHR decelerations (Goffinet *et al.*, 1997), which possibly accounts for the small increase in caesarean sections (Walsh, 2000a; Fraser *et al.*, 2002).
- A high head or ballotable presenting part. In over 50% of cases of cord prolapse, ARM is a direct cause. Cord prolapse is associated with poor perinatal outcomes (Prabulos & Philipson, 1998).
- Artificial rupture of the membranes is contraindicated in women with a genital tract infection or in a woman suspected of carrying Group B Streptococcus (unless receiving appropriate antibiotic treatment).
- Women who are human immunodeficiency virus (HIV) positive increase the risk of transmission of HIV to their unborn baby if their membranes rupture, particularly if the rupture exceeds 4 hours (Enkin, 2000). Midwives should bear in mind that many women do not know they are HIV positive, and many will remain undiagnosed.

'Given the current state of knowledge, it would seem reasonable to reserve ARM for labours which are progressing slowly. It's use then would be as a treatment for dystocia rather than as a prevention.' (Rosser and Anderson, 1998)

Useful contact

FORWARD – Foundation for Women's Health, Research and Development 6th Floor, 50 Eastbourne Terrace, London W2 6LX. Telephone: 020 7725 2606. Website: www.forward.dircon.co.uk
Information, help and advice on the practice of female genital mutilation.

References

Aldcroft, D. (2001) A guide to providing care for survivors of child sex abuse. *British Journal of Midwifery* **9** (2), 81–5.

ARM (2000) *Association of Radical Midwives* Nettalk: Incredible shrinking cervices. *Midwifery Matters* Issue 87, 30.

Banks, M. (1998) *Breech Birth Woman Wise*. Birthspirit Books, Hamilton New Zealand.

Crowther, C., Enkin, M., Keirse, M.J.N.C. & Brown, I. (2000) Monitoring progress in labor. In *A Guide to Effective Care in Pregnancy and Childbirth*, 3rd edn (Enkin, M., Keirse, M.J.N.C., Neilson, J., eds), pp. 281–8. Oxford University Press, Oxford.

Enkin, M. (2000) Infection in pregnancy. In *Guide to Effective Care in Pregnancy and Childbirth*, 3rd edn (Enkin, M., Keirse, M.J.N.C., Neilson, J. *et al.*, eds), pp. 154–68. Oxford University Press, Oxford.

Fraser, W.D., Krauss, I., Brisson-Carrol, G. *et al.* (2002) Amniotomy for shortening spontaneous labour (Cochrane Review). *The Cochrane Library* Issue 4. Update Software, Oxford.

Goffinet, F., Fraser, W., Marcoux, S. *et al.* (1997) Early amniotomy increases the frequency of fetal heart rate abnormalities. *British Journal of Obstetrics and Gynaecology* **104**, 548–53.

Gutteridge, K. (2001) Failing women: the impact of sexual abuse on childbirth. *British Journal of Midwifery* **9** (5), 312–15.

Kitzinger, J.V. (1992) Counteracting, not re-enacting, the violation of women's bodies: the challenge for perinatal caregivers. *Birth* **19** (4), 219–22.

Mayer, L. (1995) The severely abused woman in obstetric and gynaecological care. Guidelines for recognition and management. *Journal of Reproductive Medicine* **40** (1), 13–18.

Moore, T.R. (1996) Oligohydramnios. In *Protocols for High Risk Pregnancies*, 3rd edn (Queenan, J.T. & Hobbins, J.C., eds), pp. 488–95. Blackwell Science, Oxford.

Nolan, M. (2001) Vaginal examinations in labour (Expert View). *The Practising Midwife* **4** (6), 22.

Prabulos, A.M. & Philipson, E.H. (1998) Umbilical cord prolapse. Is time from diagnosis to delivery critical? *Journal of Reproductive Medicine* **43** (2), 129–32.

Riley, D. (1995) *Perinatal Mental Health*. Radcliffe Medical Press, Oxford.

Rosser, J. & Anderson, T. (1998) Amniotomy to shorten spontaneous labour: a presentation of the main points from the Cochrane Database review on routine ARM. *MIDIRS Midwifery Digest* **8** (2), 201–202.

Walmsley, K. (2000) Managing the OP labour. *MIDIRS Midwifery Digest* **10** (1), 61–62.

Walsh, D. (2000a) Evidence-based care. Part 3: Assessing women's progress in labour. *British Journal of Midwifery* **8** (7), 449–57.

Walsh, D. (2000b) Evidence-based care. Part 6: Limits on pushing and time in the second stage. *British Journal of Midwifery* **8** (10), 604–608.

Warren, C. (1999) Why should I do vaginal examinations? *The Practising Midwife* **2** (6), 12–13.

17 Monitoring the fetal heart rate in labour

Introduction

'EFM was introduced with the aim of reducing perinatal mortality and cerebral palsy. This reduction has not been demonstrated in the systematic reviews of randomised controlled trials (RCTs). However an increase in maternal intervention rates has been shown.' (NICE, 2001)

Despite the lack of evidence to support electronic fetal monitoring (EFM), even for women deemed 'high-risk', NICE (2001) continue to recommend its routine use for any woman with a 'risk' factor. For a variety of complex reasons, EFM technology has become part of the hospital-birth culture (Walsh, 2001). As part of this culture, hospital doctors and midwives rely heavily on this form of monitoring as part of their skill base, even if evidence suggests their confidence may be misplaced. It may be difficult for many clinicians to re-skill themselves physically and psychologically and to, therefore, avoid coercing women into accepting EFM. The NICE (2001) recommendations for fetal heart rate (FHR) monitoring are summarized in Box 17.1.

Box 17.1 Recommendations for fetal heart rate (FHR) monitoring (NICE, 2001). (Reproduced with kind permission from the National Institute of Clinical Excellence [NICE].)

Guidelines for 'low-risk' women:

- The admission trace should be abandoned
- Low-risk women should be offered **intermittent auscultation**

Guideline for 'high-risk' women:

- EFM should be **offered** to 'high-risk' cases

EFM   Electronic fetal monitoring

Issues to consider in electronic fetal monitoring

Positive aspects of electronic fetal monitoring

- In studies reviewed by Grant (2000) parents said that EFM demonstrated that the baby was alive, giving them positive information. Some women and their partners felt reassured/'safe and secure' by hearing and seeing their baby's heartbeat (Sinclair, 2001). This was enhanced if they could see the monitor (Grant, 2000).
- Clinicians often feel reassured that they are actually doing something physical, measurable and observable when recording a trace of the fetal heart.
- Although not necessarily 'best practice', there are times when the midwife is unable to be with the woman in labour and she uses EFM to 'keep an eye' on the fetal heart when she is unavailable. This can happen when a unit is short staffed or busy and EFM is then used to monitor many women at the same time.

Informed decision making – consent or compliance?

NICE (2001) uses the term 'offered' as opposed to 'recommend' when discussing EFM with women. This is presumably because in the era of informed choice, EFM cannot be routinely recommended because of the lack of evidence to support any benefit even for 'high-risk' women.

The iatrogenic risks/complications of EFM are rarely discussed with women. 'Is this because clinicians are unaware of these complications?' questions Wagner (2000). Wagner provokes clinicians and asks 'Is ignorance misconduct?'

Interventions are at best unpleasant and stressful, and at worst physically painful and psychologically distressing. Interventions are particularly hard to justify when the delivery is brought forward (for example by an intervention such as an episiotomy or an instrumental delivery/caesarean section) and the baby is delivered without evidence of hypoxia. Wagner (2000), poignantly suggests doctors are rarely sued or criticised for unnecessary interventions.

Iatrogenic risks

Iatrogenesis is pathology that is caused by medical intervention which as Walsh (2001) states is abhorrent because it is entirely preventable.

Electronic fetal monitoring increases interventions (including performing fetal blood sampling, episiotomy, instrumental delivery, caesarean section) but does not improve fetal outcomes.

Beech Lawrence (2001) argues that not all risk is 'high risk' and that some conditions are notoriously misdiagnosed, such as oligohydramnois and growth-restricted babies, and that meconium-stained liquor has degrees of severity from irrelevant until birth to ominous. Preterm infants have different heart patterns to term infants due to the baby's immature autonomic nervous system and evidence that EFM offers any advantage over intermittent auscultation (IA) in preterm labours is not forthcoming (Atalla *et al.*, 2000).

Randomized controlled trials of women's experiences of electronic fetal monitoring compared to intermittent auscultation

In studies reviewed by Grant (2000), women in the electronic fetal monitoring (EFM) group experienced discomfort and restriction of movement. Evidence suggests that restricted maternal movement is more likely to prolong labour, to increase the need for analgesia and to increase the incidence of FHR abnormalities (Gupta & Nikodem, 2002). There was a tendency for the intermittent auscultation (IA) group to have a more positive experience of labour. Some women felt EFM interfered with their relationship with their partner and caregivers.

Walsh (2001) suggests that instead of the mother being the centre of the birth scenario, the monitor can become the stressful focus of many a labour and birth. Some women and their partners feel distracted or worried by hearing and seeing their baby's heartbeat during labour, and this can create 'accumulative anxiety' (Walsh, 2000). A trace that becomes worrying heightens anxieties, particularly if there is uncertainty about the significance of abnormalities (Grant, 2000).

Intermittent auscultation

Midwives have traditionally monitored according to the stage of labour and increased the frequency of auscultation when the woman is in established, advanced labour. Unfortunately, there have been no trials to compare the more flexible and individualized time intervals for monitoring the FHR, relative to the stage of labour and in the normality of the situation. Midwives have been given 'recommendations' (see Box 17.2) that are based only on 'medical expert committee reports/opinion'. This is because there were no randomized controlled trials (RCTs) on which NICE (2001) could base their recommendations for IA. As Beech Lawrence (2001) suggests, the medical bias here makes this recommendation as restrictive as continuous EFM. This view is also echoed by Spiby (2001) as being difficult to achieve in practice.

Box 17.2   Guidelines for intermittent auscultation (IA) (NICE, 2001). (Reproduced with kind permission from the National Institute of Clinical Excellence [NICE].)

> The FHR should be asucultated after a contraction for 1 minute:
>
> - every 15 minutes in the first stage of labour
> - every 5 minutes in the second stage of labour

FHR   fetal heart rate

Using a pinards/a sonicaid

Unlike other forms of monitoring, with a pinards what the midwife hears is the baby's, not the mother's heart rate. Using a pinards requires a degree of precision and is a fairly sure way of confirming the baby's position. Some midwives prefer to use the pinards throughout labour. However, as labour advances some midwives and women find this method of monitoring uncomfortable, as the midwife presses quite firmly for over a minute, and it requires the woman to be in an accessible position. A hand-held sonicaid can be substituted, as appropriate, which is portable and, if water resistant, it can be used in birthing pools or for women labouring in the bath.

To use a pinards, place the pinards bell end over the baby's torso, where the palpation suggested the baby's heart is located. Then the midwife can press her ear on to the flat end to secure it against the woman's bump. Then letting go of the pinards the midwife carefully listens for a muffled thudding, the same sound as putting an ear directly over someone's chest to hear their heart. If the midwife wears glasses, she may find it more comfortable to listen if she takes them off!

Midwives can purchase their own wooden pinards from the Association of Radical Midwives (ARM) (listed in the 'Useful contacts' section at the end of this chapter).

Continuous electronic fetal monitoring

Continuous EFM consists of applying two monitor heads, held in place by elastic belts, around the woman's uterus. The first monitor head, the toco, is sensitive to the contractions and is positioned around the top of the uterus. The second, the sonicaid is placed over the fetal heart, which should have ideally been located first using a pinards (this rules out mistakenly picking up the maternal heart rate).

- Taking the maternal pulse and documenting this at frequent intervals on the trace, differentiates the maternal from the fetal heart rate.
- The monitor belts can be uncomfortable and very restrictive to the mother's movements. It is important to undo them and encourage the woman to stretch her legs and mobilize to the toilet at frequent intervals if possible.

- The woman should be encouraged to move around, maintaining upright positions when on the monitor, to avoid common complications caused by restricted mobility (Gupta & Nikodem, 2002)
- Sinclair (2001) recommends that the midwife should always explain the basics of monitoring, such as which line represents the contractions and which represents the FHR, and should explain also that accelerations are fine and are a good sign that the baby is active. Also explain why it is common to have 'loss of contact' as this can be terrifying for parents when this happens, possibly fearing that their baby's heart may have stopped.

Procedures when using electronic fetal monitoring

According to the NICE (2001) recommendations the following points should be observed:

- **At risk women**. Only women considered 'high risk', should be 'offered' EFM in labour.
- **Fetal blood sampling (FBS)**. Units using EFM should have FBS available (for more information see 'Fetal blood tests' in Chapter 18).
- **Labelling**. Traces should be labelled with the mother's name, date and hospital number.
- **Labour events**. Any intrapartum events, such as a vaginal examination, siting an epidural, the woman vomiting, etc., can cause FHR changes that are usually isolated incidents and not of concern. These events, however, should be noted on the trace, signed and the time and date noted.
- **Consultations in labour**. Any member of staff who is asked to see the trace should note their findings on the trace and in more detail in the maternal notes, along with the date, time and signature.
- **After birth**. Following the birth, the caregiver should sign noting the date and time and type of birth on the EFM trace. Then the trace should be filed securely in the maternal notes.
- **Technical issues**. The date and time should be set correctly and the paper speed should be at 1 cm per minute.

Fetal scalp electrode

A fetal scalp electrode (FSE) is an accurate but invasive form of monitoring the FHR. On occasions, it can cause infection, scarring, abscess or injury to the baby. It is used far less today than years ago and is now only usually used in significant and serious fetal compromise, where external monitoring is found to be ineffectual.

Contraindications for applying a fetal scalp electrode

The FSE should *not* be applied if:

- The woman does not want one (most women do not like the idea of a clip piercing their baby's skin).
- The baby is very preterm.

- There is a non-cephalic, non-vertex presentation.
- The woman has an infection, human immunodeficiency virus (HIV), hepatitis, or any sexually transmitted disease, or the woman is in a high-risk group for these conditions (such as an intravenous [IV] drug user).

Applying a fetal scalp electrode

- The mother's consent must always be sought, and she should also be asked if she has any infections or knows of any reason why this should not be performed.
- The FSE is applied during a vaginal examination. The clinician passes the FSE splinted between their fingers and places the hook end flat against the baby's head. While one finger holds the FSE securely against the baby, the end visible at the vagina is rotated 180° to draw back the hook and released to close it. The skin is pierced and hooked by the electrode's closure, it is then very gently pulled to ensure it is securely attached to the baby. Simultaneously, a colleague should help ensure the FSE is receiving a signal and working. Then the clinician can carefully remove their fingers from the woman's vagina.
- The woman should be reassured that she has got through an uncomfortable moment. She should also be reassured that the monitor will now be making a different sound (which it should do) and that this represents her baby's heart beat.

Monitoring the fetal heart rate at home/birthing centre

Occasionally an abnormal FHR is detected during the course of a labour and birth in a birthing centre or home birth setting. While some are 'normal' and herald the approaching birth, such as second stage decelerations, less common are problems which occur earlier in the labour and can prompt a transfer to hospital. The midwife should always take into account any isolated intrapartum events which can affect the heart rate and resolve spontaneously, such as the woman's position, during a vaginal examination, if the woman is vomiting, etc.

Chapter 2 deals with care during a home birth and Box 17.2 gives guidelines for IA use.

Assessing baseline variability at home

If there are any factors of concern regarding the FHR, the assessment of variability becomes important. However, it is particularly difficult to assess by audibility alone. Unreactive baseline or 'metronome' FHR is a term used by Davis (1997) to describe a FHR that does not respond to the stresses and stimulus of labour. If viewed on a cardiotocograph it would present as a baseline with reduced variability. A 'metronome' FHR describes a heart rate that does not vary in sound and pace over a prolonged period in labour. A sonicaid that displays the FHR is useful, as it shows small but significant variations of the heart rate.

Simple stress test

If there is uncertainty regarding the fetal heart, a stress test can be done (Grant, 2000). This tests the baby's normal response to stimuli.

- One midwife should listen to the fetal heart which should accelerate if the baby is 'stimulated', for example during a vaginal examination by 'tickling' the fetal head with a gloved finger.
- Some stimulation tests have been performed by making a loud sound stimulus and again monitoring the fetal heart for an acceleration in response.
- Although this test is basic and has not been rigorously evaluated, the current evidence suggests a non-reactive test requires a fetal scalp acid–base estimation to be performed (Grant, 2000). At home/birthing centre this would require transfer to hospital.

Fetal compromise at home birth/birthing centre

The entire clinical situation must be taken into account before deciding if a mother requires transfer to hospital. Significant fetal heart changes at the onset of, or midway through, labour obviously require transfer to hospital, for observation and assessment, whereas approaching second stage decelerations become more common place, particularly in quick or multiparous labour.

Signs requiring closer fetal surveillance and transfer to hospital

- Fresh/thick meconium staining of the liqour.
- Any abnormal heart pattern or when the heart rate has two or more features that are non-reassuring (see Appendix E).
- A non-reactive stress-test.
- Clinical judgement should be used and consideration given to maternal risk factors, previous outcome and present stage of labour (especially if a multiparous woman) and discuss with colleagues if unsure.

Classification of fetal heart rate features

NICE (2001) have classified normal and abnormal features of the FHR to give clinicians guidance as to the level of monitoring and appropriate referral or intervention in a non-reassuring heart rate pattern (see Appendix E).

Useful contacts

Association of Radical Midwives (ARM)   6 Springfield Road, Kings Heath, Birmingham, B14 7DS. ARM Helpline: 01243 671673. Website: www.midwifery.org.uk
Suppliers of wooden pinards.

National Institute for Clinical Excellence (NICE)   Mid City Place, 71 High Holborn, London WC1V 6NA. Telephone: 020 7067 5800.
To order free copies of clinical guidelines telephone the NHS response line: 0870 1555 455. For *Guideline C The use of electronic fetal monitoring* quote ref 23807 or visit the Institute's website at www.nice.org.uk

References

Atalla, R., Kean, L. & McParland, P. (2000) Preterm labor and prelabor rupture of the membranes. In *Best Practice in Labor Ward Management* (Kean, L.H., Baker, P. & Edelstone, D.I., eds), pp. 111–39. WB Saunders, Edinburgh.

Beech Lawrence, B. (2001) Electronic fetal monitoring: do NICE's new guidelines owe too much to the medical model of childbirth? *The Practising Midwife* **4** (7), 31–3.

Davis, E. (1997) *Hearts and Hands: A Midwife's Guide to Pregnancy and Birth*, 3rd edn. Celestial Arts, Berkeley, California.

Grant, A. (2000) Care of the fetus during labor. In *A Guide to Effective Care in Pregnancy and Childbirth*, 3rd edn. (Enkin, M., Keirse, M.J.N.C., Neilson, J. *et al.*, eds), pp. 267–80. Oxford University Press, Oxford.

Gupta, J.K. & Nikodem, V.C. (2002) Woman's position during the second stage of labour (Cochrane Review). *The Cochrane Library* Issue 4. Update Software, Oxford.

NICE (2001) *Clinical Guideline C – The Use of Electronic Fetal Monitoring.* National Institute for Clinical Excellence, London.

Sinclair, M. (2001) Birth technology. *RCM Midwives Journal* **4** (6), 168.

Spiby, H. (2001) The NICE guidelines on electronic fetal monitoring. *British Journal of Midwifery* **9** (8), 489.

Wagner, M. (2000) Choosing caesarean section. *The Lancet* **356**, 1677–80.

Walsh, D. (2000) Evidence-based care. Part 4: Fetal monitoring should be controlled. *British Journal of Midwifery* **8** (8), 511–16.

Walsh, D. (2001) Midwives and birth technology: a debate that's overdue. *MIDIRS Midwifery Digest* **11** (Suppl. 2), S3–S6.

18 Intrapartum blood tests

Julie Davis

Maternal blood tests

Maternal blood may be taken for a variety of reasons, routinely or in an emergency during pregnancy or labour. Normal reference ranges for blood results may vary slightly between different hospitals or laboratories and are normally based on populous studies. The word 'normal' may need qualification. A measurement may have a value within the reference range, but the subject may be 'abnormal' in some way. A value may fall outside the range, yet the subject may be biologically normal but numerically non-standard (Brown, 1984). This needs consideration particularly when allowing for the changes in haemodynamics in pregnancy. The increase in circulating plasma volume is 50% above non-pregnant values by the 34th week of gestation, lowering haemoglobin, haematocrit and red cell counts as well as placing an increased demand on maternal organs. This evidence needs to be reflected upon when evaluating normal reference ranges in the pregnant women.

Venepuncture

Once consent has been gained to take blood, a site can be selected. The antecubital fossa is usually the site of choice, with the cephalic, median, cubital and basilic veins easily accessible and near the skin surface (Coates, 1998). The mother should know why her bloods are being taken and, subsequently, if her results fall within the normal ranges. The blood should be dispensed into the correct bottles (there is no national colour coding for blood bottles at present), stored appropriately with an accurately detailed laboratory card and sent to the laboratory as soon as possible. All details of the samples taken should be recorded in the mother's notes.

Biochemical tests

Electrolytes (Table 18.1)

Lithium heparin blood bottles

- Sodium (Na) is indirectly related to body water volume.
- Potassium (K) is important for normal cardiac electrical activity and very high or low concentrations are associated with cardiac electrical abnormality (such as ventricular fibrillation or asystole).

Table 18.1 Electrolytes – normal blood.

Constituent	Normal range
Na	135–145 mmol/l
K	3.4–5.2 mmol/l

Renal function tests (Table 18.2)

Lithium heparin blood bottles

- Creatinine is a nitrogenous end product of muscle metabolism. Creatinine is filtered by the glomeruli in the kidney, so that the renal clearance rate provides an approximate measurement of the glomerular filtration rate. As the concentration of creatinine can be readily measured in the plasma, it is a useful indicator of renal function, particularly when sequential observations are made (Walton *et al.*, 1994).

- Uric acid is the end product of protein metabolism. Elevated uric acid levels may reflect decreased renal blood flow caused by vasoconstriction.
- Urea is a waste product of metabolism which is excreted via the kidneys.

Table 18.2 Renal function tests – normal blood values for creatinine, uric acid and urea.

Constituent	Normal range
Creatinine	60–120 mmol/l
Uric acid	0.2–0.40 mmol/l
Urea	2.5–6.5 mmol/l

Liver function tests (Table 18.3)

Studies suggest that pregnancy liver enzymes are lower than the non-pregnant reference ranges often used and that, in the absence of altered hepatic blood flow, physiological haemodilution alone may result in lower values for alanine transaminase (ALT), aspartate transaminase (AST) and bilirubin levels (Girling *et al.*, 1997).

Table 18.3 Liver function tests – normal blood values for alanine transaminase (ALT), aspartate transaminase (AST), alkaline phosphatase, albumin and bilirubin.

Constituent	Normal range
ALT	6–40 U/L
AST	10–40 U/L
Alkaline phosphatase	40–120 IU/L (↑ to term)
Albumin	34 g/l (↓ to term)
Bilirubin	5–17 μmol/l

Alanine transaminase and aspartate transaminase

Lithium heparin blood bottles

The activities of these two aminotransferases are widely used as a sensitive, although non-specific, index of acute damage to liver cells, irrespective of its cause (Gaw *et al.*, 1999). Levels remain unchanged in normal pregnancy.

Alkaline phosphatase

Lithium heparin blood bottles

While other liver enzymes remain unchanged in normal pregnancy, alkaline phosphatase does not. It is produced by the placenta from the first trimester and increases into late pregnancy. Extremely abnormal increases in pre-eclampsia may indicate placental as well as liver damage.

Total albumin

Clotted blood sample

Plasma albumin is also synthesized in the liver and so indicates liver function. In normal pregnancy the decrease in albumin levels is caused by haemodilution and not as a result of liver insufficiency (McKay, 1999).

Total bilirubin

Lithium heparin blood bottles

This test is to screen the liver for damage and to investigate the causes of anaemia. Haemoglobin destruction results in the production of bilirubin, which is conjugated in the liver and excreted in the bile. Any overload or blockage of the system raises levels (Bratt-Wyton, 1998). During a normal pregnancy, levels do not usually rise. However, in HELLP syndrome levels can sometimes be affected and increase.

Haematological tests

Full blood count (Table 18.4)

Ethylenediamine-tetra-acetic acid (EDTA) blood bottles

- Haemoglobin (Hb) is the pigment contained in the red blood cells and enables them to transport oxygen around the body.
- Platelets are essential for normal haemostasis. Platelets may be reduced in pre-eclampsia and are low in HELLP syndrome. The function of platelets is related to the many factors that work within the body's coagulation system. A platelet count is an important test as thrombocytopaenia (deficiency of the platelets) frequency accompanies other disorders (Star & Peipert, 1996).
- White blood cells (WBC). This test calculates the number of all types of white cells together in one figure. It gives information about bone marrow health and indicates if the immune system is being stimulated for any reason (Frye, 1998).
- Haematocrit or packed cell volume (PCV). This is a measure of the concentration of red cells in the plasma. As with Hb, in normal pregnancy the haematocrit level will decrease during the second trimester.

Table 18.4 Full blood count (FBC) test – normal blood values for haemoglobin (Hb), platelets, white blood cells (WBC), packed cell volume (PCV) and mean corpuscular volume (MCV).

Constituent	Normal range
Hb	8–14 g/dl
Platelets	150–350 $\times$ 10^9/l
WBC	6–18 $\times$ 10^9/l
PCV	36–48%
MCV	80–95 fl

- Mean corpuscular volume (MCV) is the average volume of a single red cell. It has been regarded as the most sensitive red cell index for the identification of iron deficiency. Values below 70 fl occur only with iron deficiency anaemia or thalassaemia minor (Kirkpatrick & Alexander, 1996).

Clotting screening (Table 18.5)

Sodium citrate blood bottles

Samples must be tested as soon as possible on the day of collection.

- Activated partial thromboplastin time (APTT). This test measures the clotting time of plasma and indicates the overall efficiency of the intrinsic coagulation pathway.
- Prothrombin time (PT). This test measures the clotting time of plasma and indicates the efficiency of the extrinsic pathway.
- Fibrinogen is a protein formed in the liver. During tissue injury it is activated by thrombin to form fibrin, arresting haemorrhage (Tiran, 1997).

Table 18.5 Clotting tests – normal blood values for activated partial thromboplastin time (APTT), prothrombin time (PT) and fibrinogen.

Constituent	Normal range
Platelets	150–350 $\times$ 10^9/l
APTT	29–37 seconds
PT	11–15 seconds
Fibrinogen	20–40 g/l

Other tests

The Kleihauer test

Maternal blood 6 ml sample in EDTA bottle
Umbilical cord blood 1 ml sample in EDTA bottle

This test is offered to Rhesus negative women to detect if any fetal cells have crossed over into the maternal circulation. Blood is taken from the mother's vein and from the baby's umbilical cord following birth. If the baby is found to be Rhesus positive, an anti-immunoglobulin D injection can be offered to the mother. This directs any fetal cells away from stimulating the mother's immunological system.

Group and save

EDTA blood bottles

Blood is taken from the mother to determine her blood group, Rhesus status and then the serum is saved for between 5 and 7 days. Antibody screening is also carried out. This may be done prior to caesarean section, if a women presents with an antepartum haemorrhage, placenta praevia, has an intrauterine death or any other medical or obstetric problem that may necessitate the mother to require a blood transfusion.

Cross matching

EDTA Bottles

The donor's red blood cells and white cells are placed in the recipient's serum to confirm if the donated blood will be compatible with the potential recipient.

C-reactive protein

Clotted blood sample

The C-reactive protein (CRP) is present in low concentration in plasma, but its levels increase during an acute response phase, indicating a non-specific systemic response to inflammation or infection. Normal levels are no more than 10 mg/l.

The D-Dimer test

Sodium citrate bottles

This test is carried out to detect fibrin derivatives. The presence of a cross linked D-Dimer is diagnostic for the breaking down of a fibrin clot and is useful for detecting pulmonary, deep vein thrombosis and disseminated intravascular coagulation. Normal values are <500 ng/ml.

Blood tests for specific conditions and blood pictures

Pre-eclampsia (Table 18.6)

Bloods to take:
- Full blood count (FBC)
- Electrolytes
- Renal function tests (including uric acid)
- Liver function tests
- Clotting studies

Pre-eclampsia, is a syndrome that affects all maternal organ systems. Pathophysiological changes suggest reduced organ perfusion of the kidney, liver and brain (Roberts

Table 18.6 Blood picture for pregnancy induced hypertension (PIH). (The picture may appear normal.)

Sample	Level
Electrolytes	Unchanged
Haemoglobin (Hb)	May increase
Packed cell volume (PCV)	May increase
Platelets	May decrease
Clotting times	May be normal or prolonged in the severe stage of pre-eclampsia
Creatinine	May increase
Uric acid	Increased
Urea	May increase
Liver enzymes	Increased, with the exception of bilirubin which remains unchanged unless affected by HELLP syndrome

& Redman, 1993). The vascular system is subjected to a raised peripheral resistance, reduced plasma volume, reduced cardiac output and sometimes haemolysis. The renal system has a reduced uric acid clearance and reduced renal blood flow with reduced glomerular filtration rate. As the liver is put under stress, liver enzymes become raised and the clotting system has a tendency towards coagulation in severe cases.

HELLP syndrome (Table 18.7)

Bloods to take:
- FBC
- Electrolytes
- Clotting
- Liver function tests
- Renal functions tests

Table 18.7 Blood picture for HELLP syndrome. (Adapted from Poole, 1988.)

Sample	Level
Haemoglobin (Hb)	May decrease
Mean corpuscular volume (MCV)	Decreased
Platelets	Decreased
PT/APTT[a]	Unchanged
Fibrinogen	Increased
Creatinine	Increased
Urea	Increased
Uric acid	Increased
Liver enzymes	Increased

[a] Prothrombin time/activated partial thromboplastin time.

HELLP syndrome is characterized by haemolysis, elevated liver enzymes and low platelets. HELLP syndrome is a serious, potentially fatal complication of pregnancy most frequently found in conjunction with severe pre-eclampsia. It indicates that the pathophysiological changes in pre-eclampsia have resulted in injury to the vascular system with hypoxic changes in the liver (Nutt, 1997). Arterial vasospasms damage small blood vessels forming lesions. These allow platelet aggregation and formation of a fibrin network. As red cells are forced through the network under pressure, haemolysis results. As the haemolytic process continues, the haematocrit levels fall and bilirubin levels rise (Poole, 1988). Diagnosis is aided by laboratory findings and early diagnosis is essential to prevent further complications of disseminated intravascular coagulation (DIC), hepatic and renal failure.

Disseminated intravascular coagulation (Table 18.8)

Disseminated intravascular coagulation (DIC) is not a disease, it is more of an underlying disorder secondary to another syndrome. It is a contradictory process involving coagulation and anti-coagulation, and thrombosis can be overshadowed by

Table 18.8 Blood picture for disseminated intravascular coagulation (DIC).

Sample	Levels
Platelets	Decreased
PT[a]	Increased
APTT[b]	Increased
Fibrinogen	Decreased in acute DIC (may be normal in chronic DIC)
D-Dimer	Increased

[a] Prothrombin time.

[b] Activated partial thromboplastin time.

haemorrhage. Disseminated intravascular coagulation is characterized by widespread activation of blood coagulation, resulting in the intravascular formation of fibrin, which may lead to thrombotic occlusion of small and mid-sized vessels (Levi *et al.*, 2000). Acute DIC can occur after obstetric emergencies such as placental abruption, intrauterine death, amniotic fluid emboli, postpartum haemorrhage and infection, but is more commonly linked with eclampsia and HELLP syndrome.

Laboratory testing is indicated should the diagnosis of DIC require confirmation or if medication is planned. Tests should include a FBC with platelets, PT, APTT, fibrinogen, fibrin degradation products and the D-Dimer test. Research suggests that the D-Dimer test and fibrin degradation products are the best test panel for the diagnosis of DIC, and that the PT, APTT and platelet count, although sensitive are non-specific tests when examining DIC (Yu *et al.*, 2000).

Fetal blood tests

Fetal pH measurements

Fetal blood pH is an important diagnostic and prognostic test measured during pregnancy, labour or in the cord after birth. Severe fetal acidaemia is associated with increased perinatal mortality and increased risk for later impaired neurodevelopment (Huch *et al.*, 1994). Cord blood analysis is also useful to aid neonatal management, for medical audits and for litigation and legal purposes. There is no evidence to suggest that routine cord blood analysis should be the norm. Practices may vary from unit to unit. Selective reasons may be:

- Abnormal fetal heart rate (FHR) in labour.
- Following instrumental delivery or emergency caesarean section.
- Low Apgar score (see Table 19.1).
- Preterm birth.

Respiratory acidosis

Respiratory acidosis is due to the accumulation of carbon dioxide in the fetal blood. This is due to interference in the exchanges of gases between mother and baby. This can be caused by compression of the umbilical cord or hyperstimulation of the uterus. There will be a decrease in the PO_2 blood levels and an increase in the PCO_2 levels. The baby will suffer no serious effects as long as there is sufficient oxygen to maintain aerobic metabolism.

Metabolic acidosis

If oxygen levels continue to decrease, fetal metabolism changes from aerobic to anaerobic. During this time of reduced oxygen levels, the baby's body begins to metabolize glucose resulting in lactic acid as a waste product. In the absence of oxygen, lactic acid cannot be broken down and its accumulation causes a retention of hydrogen ions and therefore acidosis. The hydrogen ions are absorbed by a buffer base but as more lactic acid builds up further buffer bases have to be used. The base deficit will be higher in a metabolic acidosis where more buffering capacity has been needed. By measuring the base deficit it is possible to see if an acidaemia was respiratory or metabolic.

Vessels to sample

Umbilical arteries carry blood away from the baby. Arterial blood reflects fetal well-being and acid–base levels. The umbilical vein carries blood to the baby from the placenta. Venous blood reflects placental status and placental tissue acid–base levels (Wallman, 1997). When carrying out umbilical cord samples after delivery, both the artery and the vein should be sampled (Tables 18.9, 18.10). First, it will ensure that the umbilical artery value can be recognized (the artery has a lower O_2 tension and saturation, a lower pH, a greater base deficit and a higher CO_2 tension). Second, as the umbilical artery represents fetal circulation, and the umbilical vein blood shows the influence of the placenta, the balance between fetal acid production and placental oxygen can only be assessed by comparing both samples (Huch *et al.*, 1994).

The pH is a measure of the acid–base balance of the blood. The acid is the hydrogen ion donor, the base is the hydrogen ion receptor, and so by measuring pH values, hydrogen levels in the blood are determined. The base excess represents the deficit of bicarbonate in the blood.

Table 18.9 Umbilical arterial blood analysis. (Adapted from Westgate *et al.*, 1994.)

Arterial blood	Result	Median
pH	7.05 to 7.38	7.26
PCO_2	4.9 to 10.7 kPa	7.3
Base deficit	−2.5 mmol/l to 9.7 mmol/l	2.4 mmol/l

Table 18.10 Umbilical venous blood analysis. (Adapted from Westgate *et al.*, 1994.)

Venous blood	Result	Median
pH	7.17 to 7.48	7.35
PCO_2	3.5 to 7.9 kPa	5.3
Base deficit	−1.0 mmol/l to 8.9 mmol/l	3.0 mmol/l

Fetal blood sampling

Electronic fetal monitoring (EFM) of the heart during labour has been associated with increased caesarean section rates and instrumental deliveries for assumed fetal distress. The fetal blood sampling (FBS) technique developed by Saling in 1967 allows capillary blood to be taken from the baby during labour to assess pH values and to give a complete acid–base status, therefore giving a clearer picture of the baby's condition (Table 18.11). The mother needs to fully understand and consent to the procedure and she should be aware of the possible implications of an abnormal result. It is an uncomfortable procedure that can take 10 minutes or longer. The mother needs lots of support and can use entonox if required.

Table 18.11 Fetal blood pH as an indicator of action to be taken. (Adapted from NICE [2001] and reproduced with kind permission.)

Fetal blood pH	Subsequent action
7.25	FBS should be repeated if the fetal heart rate (FHR) abnormality persists
7.21–7.24	Repeat FBS within 30 minutes or consider delivery if there is a rapid fall since last sample
<7.20	Delivery is indicated

For the sampling to be performed:

- The cervix must be adequately dilated, to gain access to the presenting part, and membranes ruptured.
- The mother should be in the left lateral position to prevent compression of the vena cava.
- An amniscope can then be passed into the vagina and, once visualized, the presenting part can be cleaned and dried.
- Ethyl chloride may be sprayed on.
- A thin layer of liquid paraffin can then be applied to help give a good droplet of blood.
- A small incision is made and the blood collected in a dry heparin coated glass capillary tube to be analysed.

Contraindications for FBS are:

- When the mother is infected by HIV, hepatitis or herpes.
- Prematurity of less than 34 weeks.
- Fetal bleeding disorders.
- If during the second stage of labour, the cardiotocograph (CTG) trace is ominous and there is clear evidence suggestive of acute fetal compromise (NICE, 2001).

References

Brown, G.W. (1984) What makes a reference range? *Diagnostic Medicine* January, 61–9.
Bratt-Wyton, R. (1998) Interpretation of routine blood tests. *Nursing Standard* **13** (12), 42–6.

Coates, T. (1998) Venepuncture and intravenous cannulation. *The Practising Midwife* **1** (1), 28–31.

Frye, A. (1998) *Holistic Midwifery*, Vol. 1. Labrys Press, Portland, Oregon.

Gaw, A., Cowan, R.A., O'Reilly, D.S.J., Stewart, M.J. & Shephard, J. (1999) *Clinical Biochemistry*, 2nd edn. Churchill Livingstone, Edinburgh.

Girling, J.C., Dow, E. & Smith, J.H. (1997) Liver function tests in pre-eclampsia – importance of comparison with a reference range derived for normal pregnancy. *British Journal of Obstetrics and Gynaecology* **104**, 246–50.

Huch, A., Huch, R. & Rooth, G. (1994) Guidelines for blood sampling and measurement of pH and blood gas values in obstetrics. *European Journal of Obstetrics and Gynaecology and Reproductive Biology* **54**, 165–75.

Kirkpatrick, C. & Alexander, S. (1996) Antepartum and postpartum assessment of haemoglobin, haematocrit and serum ferritin. In *When to Screen in Obstetrics and Gynaecology* (Wildschut, H. Weiner, C.P. & Peters, T.J., eds), pp. 180–95. WB Saunders, London.

Levi, M., de Jong, E., Van der Poll, T. & Cate, H. (2000) Novel approaches to the management of DIC. *Critical Care Medicine* **28** (9), 520–24.

McKay, K. (1999) Biochemical and blood tests in midwifery practice. (1) Pre-eclampsia. *The Practising Midwife* **2** (8), 28–31.

NICE (2001) *Clinical Guideline C – The Use of Electronic Fetal Monitoring*. National Institute for Clinical Excellence, London.

Nutt, J. (1997) HELLP Syndrome. *British Journal of Midwifery* **5** (1), 8–11.

Poole, J.H. (1988) Getting a perspective on HELLP syndrome. *American Journal of Maternal and Child Health* **13**, 432–7.

Roberts, J.M. & Redman, C.W.G. (1993) Pre-eclampsia: more than pregnancy induced hypertension. *The Lancet* **341**, 1447–53.

Star, J. & Peipert, J.F. (1996) Intrapartum coagulation studies. In *When to Screen in Obstetrics and Gynaecology* (Wildschut, H., Weiner, C.P. & Peters, T.J., eds), pp. 219–27.

Tiran, D. (1997) *Baillière's Midwives Dictionary*, 9th edn. Baillière Tindall, London.

Wallman, C.M. (1997) Interpretation of fetal cord blood gases. *Neonatal Network* **16** (1), 72–4.

Walton, J., Barondess, J.A. & Lock, S. (1994) *The Oxford Medical Companion*. Oxford University Press, Oxford.

Westgate, J., Garibaldi, J.M. & Greene, K.R. (1994) Umbilical cord blood gas analysis at delivery. *British Journal of Obstetrics and Gynaecology* **101**, 1054–63.

Yu, M., Nardella, A. & Pechet, L. (2000) Screening tests of DIC. Guidelines for rapid and specific laboratory diagnosis. *Critical Care Medicine* **28** (6), 1777–80.

19 Examination of the newborn baby at birth

Introduction

The newborn check involves a thorough examination of the newborn baby and is usually carried out in the hours following birth. It is generally quite quick to perform once practised. With time the midwife becomes so familiar with the look and responses of the average newborn, that anything different, uncommon or abnormal tends to appear apparent.

It is important to involve the parents in the check of their baby, explaining all actions and reassuring them. If an abnormality is suspected a clear and simple explanation should be given. If the midwife is unable to answer the parents' questions, it is essential that a senior paediatrician is called immediately. The paediatrician can come and talk with the parents and examine the baby if necessary. If the breaking of bad news is handled poorly, rejection of the baby can occur (Kelnar & Harvey, 1987). For more information about breaking bad news see 'Giving upsetting news to parents' in Chapter 20.

The midwife's assessment of the baby at birth

Most babies are born responding well and these babies are given straight to their mother to get acquainted and for uninterrupted, essential skin-to skin contact. Occasionally, a baby may be born with an underlying problem or be hypoxic at birth. This may require a prompt response from the midwife (see pages 284–6). In addition, the Apgar score is used as a retrospective assessment of the condition of the baby following birth (Table 19.1).

Table 19.1   Apgar score assessment.

	Score		
Sign	0	1	2
Colour	Blue to pale	Body pink, limbs blue	Pink
Respiratory effort	Absent	Irregular gasps	Strong cry
Heart rate	Absent	<100 beats per minute	>100 beats per minute
Muscle tone	Limp	Some flexion of limbs	Strong active movements
Reflex irritability	Nil	Grimace or sneeze	Cry

Score 8–10: normal
Score 5–7: mild asphyxia
Score 4 or below: severe asphyxia

Colour

Caucasian babies should appear pink at birth, with the baby's extremities remaining blueish for several hours following delivery. Babies with darker skins tend to have a much paler version of their parents' skin tone with lighter extremities.

Possible problems are:

- **Cyanosis** is a blueness around the mouth and trunk and could indicate a respiratory or cardiac problem, darker skin babies can look greyish white when cyanosed. If a baby appears cyanosed, facial oxygen should be administered, respiratory effort and heart rate assessed, and a paediatrician contacted.

- A **very pale baby** may have a cardiac problem, anaemia or be shocked at birth and in need of resuscitation.
- Some babies have **facial congestion**. This can be caused by a rapid delivery or cord around the neck at birth. This facial congestion is a blue/mauve discoloration of the skin known as a petechiael rash, visible around the baby's face. The lips and mucous membranes should be pink. The midwife should bear in mind that facial congestion can be confused for a rash, which may be indicative of thrombocytopenia and may be found in congenital infections such as toxoplasmosis, meningitis or herpes (Baston & Durward, 2001).
- A **very red baby** may be plethoric (received a large placental transfusion) such as can occur in a baby who is a twin.
- Any degree of **jaundice** within 24 hours of birth is not normal and is likely to be due to haemolytic disease/Rhesus incompatibility or rarely from a congenital infection such as rubella, toxoplasmosis, herpes, cytomegalia virus or syphilis. In the latter case the baby will usually have other signs of infection (Hull & Johnston, 1999).

Respirations and cry

Not all newborns initiate respirations immediately at birth nor do all cry at delivery. This is especially true if the midwife has strived to maintain a relaxed atmosphere in the birthing room, with dim lights and hushed voices. However, some babies are seemingly inconsolable at birth! Once the baby is in the mother's arms and settled in skin-to-skin, the baby will usually relax and stop crying, often opening its eyes and with patience will eventually root towards the breast.

Possible problems are:

- If the baby is slow to initiate respiration and otherwise well (good heart rate and tone, colour) the midwife can stimulate the baby by rubbing the baby vigorously with a towel, or lifting it up into the cool air. If the baby fails to breath effectively, the midwife will need to consider more invasive resuscitation measures.
- A baby with tachypnoea (respirations >60 per minute in a term baby), grunting or sternal recession may have a serious infection, meconium aspiration, a respiratory or a cardiac problem.
- A very mucusy baby, who appears to be almost 'drowning' in its secretions, will require immediate suction. Such a baby may continue to produce excessive secretions and may have an oesophageal atresia.
- A healthy newborn cry is variable but some cries are distinctly high pitched or 'irritable', either of which could indicate cerebral irritation.

Heart rate

An instant assessment of the newborn's heart rate can easily be ascertained by placing two fingers on the chest directly over the heart, or by holding the base of the umbilical stump and counting the pulsating heart rate. With practice, this is an instant way of assessing any problems, such as a bradycardia.

Possible problems are:

- A bradycardia can recover quickly if all other signs are good. If not the midwife will need to consider more active resuscitation measures (dealt with in Chapter 21).
- A tachycardia can be present before birth and can indicate the baby has an infection, meconium aspiration, a respiratory or a cardiac problem.

Muscle tone

The newborn should have good muscle tone.
Possible problems are:

- A baby who is floppy at birth could be asphyxiated.
- Poor muscle tone can also be associated with certain abnormalities such as Down's syndrome.

Reflex/response

Not all newborns cry at birth but they should appear to have normal reflexes and responses, such as opening their eyes and responding to external stimuli and touch.
Possible problem is:

- Poor or no response can be a sign of asphyxia.

Routine measurements of the newborn baby

Weight

Place a warm towel directly in the scales and set to zero before placing the undressed baby into the scales. The weight is usually measured in kilograms (kg); however, most parents will want a conversion into pounds. A conversion chart is provided in Appendix F. Parents may also want the opportunity to take a photo of their newborn being weighed. At home, the midwife often uses traditional 'fish' scales, these provide a guide but ideally, for greater accuracy, the baby should be weighed on calibrated electric scales soon after birth.

A baby weighing under 2.500 kgs is usually considered to be of low birthweight; a very low birthweight is below 1.500 kg; a macrocosmic or large baby is one with its weight above the 90th centile for its gestational age.

Babies whose weights are either above the 90th, or below the 10th, centile for gestational age are at risk of becoming hypoglycaemic, so this information should be noted and blood glucose estimations considered (Newell *et al.*, 1997).

Length

Jokinen (2002) suggests, in the light of recommendations from the Joint Working Party on Child Health (Hall & Elliman, 2002), that a baseline length measurement remains important for assessment of a baby's future growth and well-being. She expresses concern that in the period following birth, the baby is still quite curled up and so this may not be the optimum time to obtain such a measurement. Jokinen (2002) also notes that this measurement can be inaccurate and suggests that the commonest method used, a tape measure held from the crown of the head to base of the foot on a gently extended leg, has been proven as being far from reliable (Wilshin *et al.*, 1999). Various studies have shown that midwives can get improved results if using the more accurate supine length measurement tools, such as a roll up mat (Jokinen, 2002).

Head circumference

This measurement is made by placing a tape measure around the occipitofrontal circumference. The measurement recorded should be the average of three readings. The normal range for a term baby is 32–37 cm (Baston & Durward, 2001).

Vitamin K prophylaxis

Vitamin K is essential for the formation of prothrombin, which enables blood to clot, and it is found in levels considered 'low' in the newborn. Haemorrhagic disease of the newborn (HDN) is a rare, potentially fatal, disorder that has been associated with vitamin K levels.

Wickham (2000) suggests that 'low' levels of vitamin K are for some reason normal and, therefore, physiologically desirable for the newborn baby. 'Low' levels are also found in breastmilk, leaving some to assume that this has occurred by design. In the early days and weeks following birth, babies build up a supply of vitamin K from feeding. Due to the low levels of vitamin K in breastmilk, totally breastfed babies are a group slightly more prone to late-onset haemorrhagic disease. However, it should be noted that in over half of the babies who develop late onset HDN, there was an underlying cause, such as malabsorption or liver disease, contributing to vitamin K deficiency (Puckett & Offringa, 2002).

Known factors in vitamin K prophylaxis

Haemorrhagic disease is an extremely *rare*, but potentially fatal, disease that affects:

- 1 in 17 000 babies without prophylaxis (without any vitamin K).
- 1 in 25 000 to 1 in 70 000 in babies who have had a single *oral* 1–2 mg dose at birth.
- 1 in 400 000 after a single intramuscular (IM) injection at birth (Puckett & Offringa, 2000).
- The incidence of haemorrhagic disease is significantly reduced in those babies receiving vitamin K at birth (Puckett & Offringa, 2002).
- Babies most at risk are those who have had traumatic deliveries, babies who are premature or babies who are 'unwell'.
- In the UK more than 97% of babies receive vitamin K after birth. This is similar to the 1993 figures, when the debates about its potential risks were at their peak (Ansell *et al.*, 2001).

Unknown factors in vitamin K prophylaxis

- Golding *et al.* (1992) suggested a tentative link with IM vitamin K and childhood leukaemia. Puckett & Offringa (2002) suggest that the debate about vitamin K and childhood cancer has not truly resolved, but that the weight of evidence favours no association.

- The DoH (1998) recommends that all babies should be offered an appropriate vitamin K regime as 'the available evidence does not support an increased risk of cancer caused by IM vitamin K – but that data limitations make it impossible to definitively exclude a small increased risk of leukaemia'.
- Wickham (2000) and other midwives fear that there may be (as yet undiscovered) complications associated with the administration of vitamin K. Anecdotal observation suggests vitamin K prophylaxis may increase prothombin levels and, subsequently, jaundice in the newborn (Wickham 2000).

In conclusion, the RCM (1999) and the DoH (1998) both advocate that newborns should receive an appropriate vitamin K regime but that the choice of administration (oral or IM) and whether to decline it altogether should rest with the parents.

Top-to-toe check of the newborn

Each midwife will have a system for checking the newborn baby (top to toe, front to back is one way). Ensure the baby is not exposed naked for too long as his/her body temperature will drop. The check can be performed in the cot, or on the bed or floor, wherever the baby's mother is resting, so the mother can observe what the midwife is doing.

Head

Newborn babies can have very misshapen heads at birth. Parents should be reassured that the shape does quickly return to normal and that moulding (overriding of the skull bones) and caput succedaneum (oedema of the scalp) are common at birth. A large, sometimes maroon, swelling known as a cephalohaematoma (an effusion of blood beneath the periosteum of the cranial bone) is not present at birth but can occur in the hours/days following delivery. It is quite slow to resolve and although a large unsightly swelling, it is not usually serious. The parents should be informed that a cephalohaematoma may take several weeks to resolve and may contribute to jaundice in a few days following birth.

Face

The appearance and symmetry of the face can be indicative of various syndromes such as Edward's, Down's or Turner's syndromes. Baston & Durward (2001) recommend seeing both parents before commenting on any unusual appearance as the baby may simply have inherited familial traits.

Eyes

The eyes should be clear from discharge or inflammation, which if present within 24 hours of birth should be investigated as it could be a result of a gonococcal infection which can lead to blindness. Other infections such as chlamydia and staphylococcal conjunctivitis usually occur a few days after birth. The eyes should be checked for the absence of cataracts (visible as a cloudy cornea), or a translucent iris which can be a sign of albinism. Subconjuctival haemorrhages (red, crescent-shaped lesions on the conjunctiva) are not uncommon, especially if the mother had been coerced into active pushing. These minor haemorrhages resolve in a matter of weeks.

Some babies are reluctant to open their eyes to be examined. Try darkening the room or, when checking the mouth with a clean, gloved finger, let the baby suck. Most babies then spontaneously open their eyes. Otherwise, observe the baby when it has a feed.

Ears

As with other areas of the body, the ears may have skin tags. These are usually small and are commonly tied with suture material by the paediatrician, until they drop off. Tags or dimpling are usually of no significance but can be indicative of renal problems and should be documented and mentioned to the paediatrician. Low set ears can be associated with various disorders such as Patau's syndrome/trisomy 13 (pages 276–7).

Mouth

To check the baby's mouth, the midwife should gently insert a clean, gloved finger, fleshy side up, to examine the roof of the baby's mouth to feel for a cleft palate. A visual inspection using a good light source is vital and may reveal a sub-mucous cleft, not easily felt. Unless small clefts are detected, babies can have difficultly with feeding and, later, with speech. Any baby with milk coming down their nose during a feed (not when vomiting) is very likely to have a cleft palate (Martin & Bannister, 2003). A cleft lip would be difficult not to miss and parents are often very shocked and distressed at how the baby with this problem looks. Cleft lips vary from almost unnoticeable to extensive – unilateral and bilateral. For more information on clefts see Chapter 21.

Finally, the midwife should check the whole of the mouth for problems such as congenital teeth (which may need removing) and for tongue-tie, here the tongue may appear short and square or heart shaped and have limited movement.

Neck, chest and abdomen

To check for fractures the midwife should trace her fingers along the clavicles feeling for irregularities. Breast enlargement is not uncommon in both boys and girls and the breasts may even secrete a small amount of milk ('witch's milk')(Hull & Johnston, 1999). There should be two nipples. If they are very widely located on a short chest, so that they look unusual, this could indicate a chromosomal abnormality such as Edward's syndrome (page 275).

It is wise to check that the umbilical clamp is secure and that there are no protrusions at the base of the umbilicus, which could indicate exomphalos (herniating bowel, page 274). The cord should have one vein and two arteries. The presence of only one artery in the cord can be associated with renal abnormalities.

Some babies will grunt or breathe loudly following birth. This is more common following a caesarean birth. If the breathing difficulties are accompanied by sternal recession and nasal flare the baby should be kept warm and be seen by a paediatrician.

Finally, the abdomen should feel soft and any obvious hernias should be reported.

Genitalia

The size and normal placement, and any skin pigmentation, should be noted. Parents who have darker skin may have babies with a darker discoloration of the scrotum or labia; however, this can also be a sign of congenital adrenal hyperplasia which can affect the sex of the baby. In cases where the sex is indeterminate and adrenal hyperplasia is suspected, staff should not try to 'guess' the sex of the baby as if this is later found to be incorrect it can prove even more distressing for the parents.

Baby boys

The size of the penis varies greatly. The midwife should ascertain the location of the urethral orifice. Hypospadias is where the urethral meatus opens on the under surface of the penis and occurs in 8.5 per 10 000 births (BDF, 2003). If the baby has a hypospadias, the midwife or mother should attempt to observe whether the baby passes a dribble of urine instead of a stream, as a dribble of urine could indicate a blockage of the urethra and surgery may be indicated to prevent renal damage. Babies with hypospadias should not be circumcized, as some of the skin may be needed for surgical repair later.

Some baby boys are born with large, swollen testes, known as a hydrocele. It is fairly common, and not serious in the newborn, and it resolves spontaneously over the following months. The scrotal sack is gently examined for the presence of testes, which if absent have usually descended by 6 weeks of age. A note should be made of their presence in case they later move out of the scrotal sac and are then, incorrectly, diagnosed as having not descended. It is advisable to also inform the parents of the presence or absence of the scrotum so they are aware for future baby checks.

Baby girls

The labia and clitoris can look large in preterm and small-for-dates newborns. A particularly large labia or clitoris could suggest the baby is of indeterminate sex, testes can sometimes even be felt beneath the 'labia'. The vaginal opening should be easy to see, but no vaginal orifice can sometimes be obvious by its absence. Withdrawal bleeding and mucus can be present at the vagina. Parents should be aware that withdrawal bleeding can continue for several days and that this can be normal.

Anus

Note and document any passage of meconium and always check that the baby has an anus and that it is correctly placed. A misaligned anus can be associated with malformation of the rectum (Baston & Durward, 2001).

Back and spine

The midwife should trace her finger down the spine to feel for any hidden swellings and observe for any degree of spina bifida/neural tube defect. Spina bifida can be found anywhere along the length of the spine, including the neck, and vary from small dimples to a large cyst or sac. A sinus, usually at the base of the spine, may require investigation using ultrasound to discover its end. Such a defect could be a meningocele but it is more likely to be a spina bifida occulta which is present in 10% of the population and rarely has any adverse effects. More information on spina bifida may be found in Chapter 20.

Limbs

The limbs should look symmetrical. Fingers and toes may have webbing or be overlapping, they may be deformed, fused, missing or have extra digits. All of these features can be hereditary or the features of various syndromes, so check the baby over thoroughly. Fused, malformed or missing digits can also be caused by the formation of amniotic bands *in utero*.

Talipes, a term describing congenital foot deformities, presents as the feet being either turned in with the toes pointing down, or out with the heel pointing down. If the foot can be pulled back into position, the condition is known as talipes equinovarus or 'positional talipes' and rights itself spontaneously. If the bones within the foot have developed abnormal positions this 'structural talipes' will need physiotherapy, splinting and occasionally requires surgery. These babies should all grow up normally and be able to walk and run (STEPS, 2003).

Skin

The baby born by caesarean has a 1.9% chance of being cut (lacerated) by the surgeon's knife, this rises to a 6% risk in non-vertex positions (Smith *et al.*, 1997). The midwife should explain to the parents what has happened and that it is not uncommon due to the proximity of the baby to the incised uterus. It may require a steri-strip and observing to ensure the wound does not become infected. Ensure also that the surgeon is aware and that this has been documented. Ideally, the surgeon should also see the parents to explain what happened and to answer any queries.

On examining the baby, commonly birthmarks can be found; some are more obvious than others. Parents can be naturally quite distressed at large or visible birthmarks, such as those on the baby's face, and will want to know if they are permanent or treatable. For more information on birth marks and skin discoloration see Box 19.1.

Summary

- **Assess:** Good colour, firm tone, responsive to handling, established respiration with a normal heart rate.
- **Measure:** weight, length and head circumference.
- **Head:** Feel for moulding, caput, haematomas and birth trauma.
- **Eyes:** Check for stickiness, cataracts, subconjunctival haemorrhages, albinism and their location.

Box 19.1   Birth marks and skin discoloration.

Mongolian blue spot
- Mongolian blue spot is a pigmentation of the skin and is occasionally found on the skin of babies who have dark skin tones.
- The areas of pigmentation are bluish and they tend to fade over the first year.
- Mongolian blue spots can also be found over the back, shoulders and limbs, but mainly over the sacrum.

Stork marks/naevus simplex
- These are fairly common, pink/purple areas which are superficial capillary haemangioma.
- They are present in one third of babies and almost always fade so that they are no longer visible after the first year.

Port-wine stains/capillary haemangioma
- Port-wine stains are present from birth and they grow with the baby.
- These are deeper, denser, large and bluish/purple in appearance and, unfortunately, are permanent.
- Laser therapy is often used to treat them, but careful cosmetic coverage is usually the recommended solution.

Pigmented naevi
- This is a large birthmark often involving a wide area of skin and may have a covering of hair.
- Excision and skin grafting in childhood is a possibility if the area is not too large.

Strawberry naevi
- These are pink or purple, raised areas of blood-filled capillaries above the surface of the skin. They are not obvious at birth but develop over the early days of life.
- Most are scarcely detectable by 8 years of age. Therefore, treatment is to leave them alone unless they are a real handicap, such as around the eye or nose area. Treatment would then involve laser therapy or surgery.

- **Ears:** Observe for skin tags, shape and position.
- **Mouth:** Examine for cleft lip, cleft palate, congenital teeth, protruding tongue.
- **Chest:** Check shape, recession, nipple location, respiration pattern, fractured clavicles.
- **Abdomen:** Examine for hernias, shape, umbilical clamp secure and three vessels in the cord.
- **Genitalia:** Check size, placement and for pigmentation.
- **Boys:** Check for hypospadias, hydrocele, descended testes.
- **Girls:** Check for a urethra and vagina, and in both sexes note any passage of urine and or meconium.
- **Back:** Check vertebrae and skin, spina bifida, sacrococcygeal dimple, Mongolian blue spot, anus, and note any passage of meconium.
- **Limbs:** Should be symmetrical, count fingers and toes; check for palmar creases, webbing, fused, malformed, overlapping digits; check for talipes.
- **Skin:** Check for lacerations, birthmarks, rashes, Mongolian blue spot, bruising and any birth trauma.
- Always **document** if the baby has passed meconium or urine and in boys the presence or absence of testes in the scrotum.
- **Refer** to a paediatrician anything of concern. Document any concerns carefully.

Useful contacts

For an extensive list see at the end of Chapter 20.

References

Ansell, P., Roman, E., Fear, N.T. *et al.* (2001) Vitamin K policies and midwives practice: questionnaire survey. *British Medical Journal* **322**, 150–52.

BDF (2003) The Birth Defects Foundation. Website www.birthdefects.co.uk (accessed May 2003).

Baston, H. & Durward, H. (2001) *Examination of the Newborn: A Practical Guide*. Routledge, London.

DoH (1998) *Vitamin K for Babies*. PLO/CNO/998/4 Department of Health, London.

Golding, J., Greenwood, R., Birmingham, K. & Mott, M. (1992) Childhood cancer, intramuscular vitamin K and pethidine given in labour. *British Medical Journal* **305**, 341–6.

Hall, D. & Elliman, D. (eds) (2002) *Health for all Children*, 4th edn. Joint Working Party On Child Health Surveillance. Oxford University Press, Oxford.

Hull, D. & Johnston, D. (1999) *Essential Paediatrics*, 4th edn. Churchill Livingstone, Edinburgh.

Jokinen, M. (2002) Measuring newborns: does size really matter? *Midwives Journal* **5** (5), 186–7.

Kelnar, C.J.H. & Harvey, D. (1987) *The Sick Newborn Baby*. Baillière Tindal, London.

Martin, V. & Bannister, P. (eds) (2003) *Cleft Care – A Practical Guide for Health Professionals on Cleft Lip and/or Palate*. Academic Publishing Services, Salisbury.

Newel, S.J., Miller, P., Morgan, I. & Salariya, E. (1997) Management of the newborn baby: midwifery and paediatric perspectives. In *Essential Midwifery* (Henderson, C. & Jones, K., eds), pp. 229–64. Mosby, London.

Puckett, R.M. & Offringa, M. (2002) Vitamin K for preventing haemorrhagic disease (Cochrane Review). *The Cochrane Library* Issue 4. Update Software, Oxford.

RCM (1999) Position Paper 13b: Vitamin K. *RCM Midwives Journal* **2** (8), 252–3.

Smith, J.F., Hernandez, C. & Wax, J.R. (1997) Fetal laceration injury at caesarean delivery. *Obstetrics and Gynaecology* **90**, 344–6.

STEPS (2003) National Association for Families of Children with Congential Abnormalities of the Lower Limbs. Information from: Website: www.steps-charity.org.uk. talipies- club foot (accessed MAY 2003).

Wickham, S. (2000) Vitamin K: a flaw in the Blueprint. *Midwifery Today* Issue 56, 39–41.

Wilshin, J., Geary, M., Persaud, M. & Hindmarsh, P. (1999) The reliability of newborn length measurement. *British Journal of Midwifery* **7** (4), 236–9.

20 Serious anomalies and disorders in the newborn

Introduction

The following serious anomalies and disorders at birth are given in order of frequency of occurrence.

Cardiac anomalies

Incidence: 17.9 per 10 000 births (ONS, 2001).

Antenatal ultrasound scanning will detect less than half the cases of congenital heart disease. So many defects go undiagnosed until after birth. Heart defects are sometimes associated with other anomalies or syndromes such as Down's syndrome and Edward's syndrome.

Depending on the severity of the defect, the baby's condition can deteriorate suddenly at birth, or in the hours/days following birth. Do not hesitate to emergency bleep the paediatric team if necessary. If attending a home birth the baby would require urgent transfer to hospital by paramedic ambulance.

Heart problems can lead to a dramatic deterioration in the baby's condition following birth, particularly if the circulation depends on their ductus arteriosus remaining open (Newel *et al.*, 1997).

The baby usually presents with:

- Signs of heart failure:
  - breathlessness
  - tachycardia
- Cyanosis, including when feeding or crying, failure to finish a feed.

These symptoms require urgent assessment by an experienced paediatrician.

There is a huge variety of heart disorders (as well as treatments) and some babies will not survive the newborn period. Parents can feel quite isolated when their baby is diagnosed with a rare heart condition (CHF, 2003). For many parents their baby's ongoing problems can be their significant difficulty with feeding. Such babies can be caught in a cycle of exhaustion when feeding, often crying, panting and going blue. Vomiting and wind also contribute to their exhaustion.

Down's syndrome (trisomy 21)

Incidence: 6.0 per 10 000 births (ONS, 2001).

Although each baby/child's abilities will vary, babies with Down's syndrome will develop their own personality and characteristics just like other children. They are usually capable of doing most things that other children do; many will read and write, go to mainstream school, pass GCSEs and look forward to a semi-independent life. Babies and children with Down's syndrome are usually a bit slower at reaching their milestones and they will have varying degrees of learning difficulty as well as some of the characteristic features of Down's syndrome (DSA, 2001).

One in three children born with Down's syndrome has a heart defect, around half of which usually require surgery (DSA, 2001). A minority of babies do not survive the newborn period due to major congenital heart disease, as well as the possibility of having gastrointestinal anomalies such as oesophageal atresia, duodenal atresia and/or an imperforate anus.

Diagnosis may be suspected at birth but blood can be taken for chromosomal studies, for which the results may take some time.

The baby usually presents with:

- Almond-shaped, slanted eyes with an extra fold of skin (epicanthic fold).
- A small mouth commonly with a protruding tongue.
- Flat occiput with a thin neck.
- Broad hands, short fingers, short incurving little finger and sometimes a singular palmar crease (simian).
- On handling the baby, he/she is usually noticeably floppy. This will improve as the baby gets older.

Some babies with Down's syndrome lack the strength and determination to feed in the early days. These problems, and co-ordinating feeding and breathing, are usually resolved during the first 2 weeks, although this can take longer when breastfeeding, and weight gain can be slow (DSA, 2001).

Sometimes parents feel they cannot cope with a baby who has Down's syndrome and will want to discuss adoption or fostering with the hospital social worker. Few parents go through with adoption once they have got to know their baby, although approximately 10–15% of couples do proceed (DSA, 2001).

Cleft lip and/or cleft palate

Incidence: Cleft lip – 2.2 per 10 000 births; cleft palate – 3.2 per 10 000 births; cleft lip and palate – 3.8 per 10 000 births (ONS, 2001).

A cleft lip can appear 'shocking' to parents who tend to focus on the baby's physical facial features. Baston & Durward (2001) suggest that parents often need a lot of support; they can feel betrayed and confused if this condition has not been picked up by antenatal ultrasound scanning. A member of the cleft team should speak to parents within 24 hours of the birth (HSC, 1998). These experts can bring parents huge reassurance and information. They can discuss feeding, surgery and usually show parents before and after photos of other babies who have had successful surgical repair.

Surgery is dependent on the type of cleft and the individual surgeon. A cleft lip is repaired within the first 6 months, some within a month of birth. A cleft palate is usually repaired by the time the baby is a 1 year old (CLAPA, 2003).

Babies with cleft palates can choke easily and run the risk of aspiration if they are 'force-fed' milk. In order to prevent choking/aspiration, parents and staff should be reminded not to position the baby on its back (Martin & Bannister, 2003).

Babies with cleft palates have incorrect positioning of the levator and tensor palati muscles which results in ineffectual soft palate movement needed to form oral negative pressure and can cause difficulty with efficient breastfeeding, despite the fact that the baby will look and sound as if it is feeding well. The latch must be exaggerated to ensure that the baby is able to keep hold of the breast and not 'fall off', and to enable the baby to actually 'milk' the breast successfully (Martin & Bannister, 2003). Cleft experts advise that the mother should express breast milk from day one in order to 'top-up' her baby.

Local support groups. While there is no substitute for support and sensitive explanations, parents may benefit from contacting the Cleft Lip and Palate Association (CLAPA) (see 'Useful contacts and organizations' at the end of Chapter 21).

Exomphalos/gastroschisis

Incidence: Exomphalos 1.0 per 10 000 births; gastroschisis 1.8 per 10 000 births (ONS, 2001).

This is a herniation of the abdominal contents at the umbilicus.

Exomphalos is the herniation of the bowel into the extra-embryonic part of the umbilical cord and so is covered in a membranous sac. Exomphalos is sometimes associated with other chromosomal defects such as Edward's syndrome (Hull & Johnston, 1999).

Gastroschisis is the protrusion of the gut through a defect in the abdominal wall (usually to the right of an otherwise normal umbilical cord). The gut is uncovered and therefore at risk of infection and trauma. Gatroschisis is not usually associated with chromosomal abnormalities (Hull & Johnston, 1999).

The success of surgery depends upon the size and degree of herniation that has occurred, as occasionally necrosis of the gut occurs. At birth the area is covered with non-adhesive film, to avoid trauma and sepsis until prompt surgery is carried out. Intravenous (IV) fluids are commenced to compensate for heat and fluid loss (Baston & Durward, 2001).

Diaphragmatic hernia

Incidence: 1.4 per 10 000 births (Office for National Statistics, personal communication, 2003).

A diaphragmatic hernia is a herniation of the stomach and surrounding organs, such as the liver, spleen and intestines, through the diaphragm and into the chest cavity. The baby may be pre-diagnosed by an ultrasound scan or diagnosis may be made at birth. If it occurs to a severe degree *in utero*, the lungs cannot develop properly and so the prognosis is poor.

Some herniations occur at birth or later, and all require emergency treatment as the lungs cannot expand fully and the heart is displaced. If the condition is identified antenatally it is important that the baby is delivered in a specialist unit and resuscitated by endotracheal intubation at birth. Positive pressure by mask is avoided. Bag and mask resuscitation can prove fatal as it increases air in the stomach, which increases the pressure of the hernia on the lungs and heart, and will further compromise respiration (Baston & Durward, 2001).

The baby usually presents with:

- Polyhydramnios during pregnancy.
- A visibly hollowed abdomen.
- Severe respiratory distress and cyanosis at birth.

Emergency surgery may be life saving, as the hypoxia results in a high mortality, especially in preterm infants:

- Intubate and ventilate.
- Pass a stiff naso-gastric tube into the stomach on free drainage, to avoid the accumulation of air in the herniated bowel (Baston & Durward, 2001).
- The paediatrician may detect heart sounds on the right side of the chest and may request an X-ray.

Edward's syndrome (trisomy 18)

Incidence: 1.0 per 10 000 births (Office for National Statistics, personal communication, 2003).

This condition affects mainly girls (SOFT, 2003) and is usually fatal during the early weeks of life as congenital heart disease is almost universal and usually the immediate cause of death. Most babies (90%) will have died within the first year of life (Baston & Durward, 2001).

The baby usually presents with:

- A long narrow skull with malformed low set ears.
- A short chest with broad-spaced nipples.
- Prominent heels, 'rocker bottom' feet.
- Cardiac abnormalities and mental deficiency are common.

Neural tube defects/spina bifida

Incidence: 1.0 per 10 000 births (ONS, 2001).

Spina bifida has varying degrees of severity, and children affected by this condition are usually quite capable of entering mainstream education, many go on to have families of their own (ASBAH, 2003). Lesions can range anywhere along the spinal cord, in differing degrees from the less serious and commonly asymptomatic spina bifida occulta (often just visible as a dimple) to an exposed spinal cord – spina bifida cystica. When there is a sac over the cord it is called a meningocele or if nerves are involved/exposed in a sac it is known as a myelomeningocele and this is the most serious defect. Neurological damage usually occurs below the level of the lesion, which can result in physical paralysis, difficulty in walking, and bladder and bowel control problems (ASBAH, 2003).

Children affected by spina bifida tend to be slower sitting and getting up but most will manage to walk with aids, others will find it easier with wheelchairs. Parents can be reassured that bladder and bowel problems can be well managed, in fact quite early on by the child themselves. This can involve regular catheterization and a routine for toileting (ASBAH, 2003).

Some babies also have the added complication of hydrocephalus where there are high levels of cerebral spinal fluid which distends the ventricles of the brain. Hydrocephalus is usually well controlled upon the insertion of a shunt, an internal tube to drain fluid from around the brain into the peritoneal cavity. However, severe cases can be incompatible with life. In most cases, the baby is likely to grow up with some degree of learning disorder. The degree of each child's ability will vary considerably, and co-ordination and concentration can also be affected.

Tracheo-oesophageal fistula/atresia

Incidence: Oesophageal atresia 0.4 per 10 000 births; oesophageal fistula 0.7 per 10 000 births (ONS, 2001).

Oesophageal atresia is an absence of the opening of the oesophagus. It is commonly associated with polyhydramnios in the mother. Tracheo-oesophageal fistula is a congenital defect between the opening of the trachea and the lower oesophagus.

The baby usually presents with:

- Polyhydramnios.
- Excessive, frothy saliva requiring suction to assist the baby in clearing it.
- Choking, even cyanosis, caused by build-up of mucus.

Treatment involves:

- A stiff naso-gastric tube is attempted to be passed but will not usually pass down the oesophagus. In the case of a fistula the tube should be X-rayed to identify its position.
- The baby should not be fed and will require frequent suction.
- Do not lie the baby on its back as it may aspirate.
- Corrective surgery is required fairly urgently.

Pierre Robin syndrome

Incidence: Estimated 0.6 per 10 000 births (Office for National Statistics, personal communication, 2003).

Pierre Robin syndrome is an abnormality of the mandible area in otherwise normal babies. The jawbone grows and usually corrects itself by adult life. In the early days (and in severe cases months) babies can have difficulty learning to co-ordinate feeding and breathing as the tongue tends to ball up and fall back, obstructing the airway (Patton, 2003). Babies should not be laid on their backs to sleep as aspiration can be a complication in severe cases. Most babies learn how to lay and avoid getting their tongue stuck in their cleft. While most babies cope well a minority require assistance with breathing which might include the use of a nasal prong or a tracheotomy (see also earlier in this chapter for information on cleft palates).

The baby will present with:

- A small lower jaw.
- A midline cleft palate without cleft lip or high arched palate.
- Glossoptosis – protruding tongue.

Patau's syndrome (trisomy 13)

Incidence: 0.3 per 10 000 births (Office for National Statistics, personal communication, 2003).

Patau's syndrome is quite rare and the baby will have severe mental retardation and cardiac problems. The majority (82%) will not live beyond the first month of life.

The baby usually presents with:

- An abnormal-shaped head, a depressed saddle nose with low-set malformed ears, cleft lip and/or cleft palate.
- Overlapping of the fingers and extra digits.

Potter's syndrome (renal agenesis)

Incidence: 0.1 per 10 000 births (Office for National Statistics, personal communications, 2003).

Unfortunately renal agenesis is incompatible with life and the baby will either be stillborn or die at birth due to pulmonary hypoplasia (the lungs have not developed normally). The mother will have had oligohydramnios, with its compression effects evident on the baby – talipes equinovarus, dislocated hips, squashed face, flattened nose. One obvious characteristic is the large, low-set, poorly cartilaginized ears.

Giving upsetting news to parents

Many parents assume that antenatal screening and scans will have picked up any problems with their baby. Therefore, the birth of a baby with an anomaly can come as a profound shock to parents who were expecting a 'normal' baby. Some parents' initial reaction at the time of their baby's birth can be one of rejection or extreme grief.

'I had no knowledge of reactions to birth, and it seemed as in some way I had rejected her because of her handicap.' (STEPS, 2003)

Grief is commonly felt and many tears may be cried. Feelings are often contradictory, of rejection and guilt towards their newborn baby. Many people ask 'Why us?', unable to understand why their baby is physically imperfect when the rest of the world seems full of perfect, healthy children. Parents need to be reassured and told, 'This is not your fault'.

For the midwife who delivers a baby with a problem, it can also be an unexpected shock. The midwife may herself feel useless and lost for words or ways to 'make things better'. Parents will take their cue from the midwife, if she can sound positive (not unrealistic) then they will be less likely to 'reject' their baby. Kelnar & Harvey (1987) suggest

'Try to talk to both parents together; it often helps for them to hold the baby while you explain the problem simply and clearly. You will need to repeat the explanation several times because parents in their panic often do not take in what you say ... it is a mistake to remove the baby from the mother or tell her that he is abnormal as he will then usually be rejected.'

Robb (1999) suggests that there is no perfect way of giving someone upsetting news. However, a few simple guidelines, sensitively followed, can mitigate some of the distress. Robb also advocates providing parents with privacy and explaining clearly in simple language what the problem may be. It is also useful to hold the baby's problem in a positive light and to personalize information to the baby and his/her family.

'As I began to know my child her condition became less predominant in my thoughts; although the shock, at the time of her birth, had been great.' (STEPS, 2003)

Who should tell the parents? In some situations, the midwife needs to respond immediately to a visible or obvious problem with a baby at birth. In other situations, there will be time to involve the paediatrician, who can check the baby and they may be the appropriate person to inform the parents of a problem.

Practise makes perfect. Robb (1999) recommends that midwives should practise the breaking of bad news amongst colleagues. It is not something that most midwives feel confident doing or do regularly enough to feel that they are proficient at it. Parents are usually shocked and only remember pieces of what they are told. However, they do remember who told them and if it was handled positively or not (Robb, 1999).

In summary then:

- Keep it simple.
- Remember to say something positive about their baby 'you have a gorgeous baby … beautiful eyes … he's so strong' or other such comments.
- Repeat clear and simple explanations as many times as seems necessary.
- Personalize the information to that family and baby. Use the baby's name (if the baby has been given one).
- If the midwife does not know the answers to the parents' questions, it is vital to get a senior paediatrician to come quickly, to avoid the midwife giving possibly inaccurate, even personal information, which may not be correct.
- Provide privacy.
- Do not forget other colleagues, referrals and early follow-up.
- Written information, support groups and contact numbers are important but they are no substitute for giving time and explanations.

Useful contacts

Association for Spina Bifida and Hydrocephalus (ASBAH)   42 Park Road, Peterborough, Cambridgeshire PE1 2UQ. Telephone: 01733 555988. Website: www.asbah.org
Support, advice, practical and financial help for carers of children with spina bifida and/or hydrocephalus.

The Birth Defects Foundation (BDF)   BDF Centre, Hemlock Business Park, Hemlock Way, Cannock, Staffordshire WS11 2GF. Telephone: 01543 468888.
Website: www.birthdefects.co.uk
BDF is a UK-based registered charity, founded by parents, doctors and business people to improve child health, aid families and create awareness of birth defects.

Birthmark Support Group   PO Box 3932, Weymouth, Dorset DT4 9YG. Fax: 01202 257703.
Website: www.btinternet.com/~birthmarksupportgroup
Support and information for parents of children with birthmarks.

The Child Bereavement Trust   Aston House, West Wycombe, High Wycombe, Buckinghamshire HP14 3AG. Telephone: 01494 446648.
Website: www.childbereavement.org.uk

Children's Heart Federation   52–54 Kennington Oval, London SE11 5SW. Telephone helpline: 0808 808 5000. Website: www.childrens-heart-fed.org.uk
Information, support and advice for parents/carers of children with heart disorders.

Cleft Lip and Palate Association (CLAPA)   235–237 Finchley Road, London NW3 6LS. Telephone: 020 7431 0033. Website: www.clapa.com

Cystic Hygroma and Haemangioma Support Group (CHHSG)   Villa Fontana, Church Road, Worth, Crawley, West Sussex RH10 7RS. Telephone: 01293 885901.

Down's Syndrome Association (DSA)   155 Mitcham Road, London SW17 9PG. Telephone helpline: 020 8682 4001. Website: www.downs-syndrome.org.uk

Pierre Robin Support Group UK   PO Box 27913, London SE7 7WL. Telephone/fax: 020 8858 6274. Website: www.pierrerobinuk.org

REACH (The Association for Children with Hand or Arm Deficiency)   REACH Head Office, PO Box 54, Helston, Cornwall, TR13 8WD. Telephone: 0845 1306225. Website: www.reach.org.uk
Regional support and information for carers of children with hand or arm problems.

STEPS (National Association for Children with Lower Limb Abnormalities)   Lymm Court, 11 Eagle Brow, Lymm, Cheshire WA13 0LP. Telephone: 0871 717 0044. Website: www.steps-charity.org.uk

SCOPE   Library and Information Unit, 6 Market Road, London N7 9PW. Cerebral Palsy Helpline: 0808 800 3333. Website: www.scope.org.uk
Advice and support for carers of children with cerebral palsy.

SOFT (Support Organisation for Trisomy 13/18 and Related Disorders)   Telephone helpline: 0121 351 3122. Website: www.soft.org.uk

References

ASBAH (2003) Association For Spina Bifida and Hydrocephalus website: www.asbah.org.uk (accessed May 2003).

Baston, H. & Durward, H. (2001) *Examination of the Newborn: A Practical Guide*. Routledge, London.

CHF (2003) Children's Heart Federation Website: www.childrens-heart-fed.org.uk (accessed May 2003).

CLAPA (2003) Cleft Lip and Palate Association Website: www.clapa.com (accessed May 2003).

DSA (2001) *Your Baby has Down's Syndrome – A Guide for Parents*. Down's Syndrome Association, London.

Hull, D. & Johnston, D. (1999) *Essential Paediatrics*, 4th edn. Churchill Livingstone, Edinburgh.

HSC (1998) Cleft Lip and Palate Services commissioning specialist services. Health Service Circular 1998/238. Department of Health, London.

Kelnar, C.J.H. & Harvey, D. (1987) *The Sick Newborn Baby*. Baillière Tindal, London.

Martin, V. & Bannister, P. (2003) *Cleft Care: A Practical Guide for Health Professionals on Cleft Lip and/or Palate*. Academic Publishing Services, Salisbury.

Newel, S.J., Miller, P., Morgan, I. & Salariya, E. (1997) Management of the newborn baby: midwifery and paediatric perspectives. In *Essential Midwifery* (Henderson, C. & Jones, K., eds), pp. 229–64. Mosby, London.

ONS (2001) *Congenital Anomaly Statistics Notifications*. A statistical review of notifications of congenital anomalies received as part of the England and Wales National Congenital Anomaly System. Series MB3 No. 16, section 5b. www.statistics.gov.uk

Patton, M. (2003) Professor of Clinical Genetics, St. George's Hospital Medical School, London. *Pierre Robin Website*. www.pierrerobinuk.org/ (accessed May 2003).

Robb, F. (1999) Congenital malformations: breaking bad news. *British Journal of Midwifery* **7** (1), 26–31.

SOFT (2003) Support Organization for Trisomy 13 and 18. Website: www.soft.org.uk (accessed May 2003).

STEPS (2001) National Association for Families of Children with Congenital Abnormalities of the Lower Limbs. Information from: Website: www.steps-charity.org.uk. talipies- club foot (accessed May 2003).

21 Neonatal and maternal resuscitation

Nick Castle

Introduction

A midwife must be able to instigate resuscitation on the newborn baby and mother. It is therefore vital that a midwife receive annual resuscitation training in neonatal and maternal resuscitation, and that during this training there is an opportunity to practise standard adult resuscitation.

Incidence and facts

- In the western world an estimated 5–10% of newborn babies require some form of resuscitation at birth (typically active stimulation), this number is higher in the developing world (American Heart Association *et al.*, 2000; Ergenekon *et al.*, 2000).
- Only 1% of babies weighing >2.5 kg require assisted ventilation and only 20% of these babies will require intubation. When low-risk births were reviewed, only 0.2% of babies required assisted ventilation and only 10% of these babies required intubation (Palme-Kilander, 1992).
- It has been estimated that up to 800 000 newborn babies who currently die, could be saved by the prompt instigation of basic resuscitation techniques (Zideman *et al.*, 1998).
- Anticipation remains the most important aspect of resuscitation of the newborn so that an appropriate team can be assembled prior to the birth (American Heart Association *et al.*, 2000). Some babies are born unexpectantly 'flat', this is an uncommon occurrence that can be effectively managed by basic resuscitation techniques (Palme-Kilander, 1992).

Risk management – anticipation

There are numerous, potential causes that will result in a newborn baby requiring some degree of active resuscitation as listed in Box 21.1. These causes can be subdivided into antepartum, intrapartum and neonatal conditions. In addition, any unexpected birth in the community or the Accident & Emergency (A&E) department should be considered as 'high-risk', although typically they are problem free.

Once a possible 'high-risk' birth is identified, paediatricians should be summoned prior to delivery (Royal College of Paediatrics and Child Health and Royal College of Obstetricians and Gynaecologists, 1997). Midwives caring for women at home or in a birthing centre environment should be aware of factors that can influence the baby's condition at birth and that may necessitate transfer. For a list of resuscitation equipment the community midwive should carry see Box 21.2.

Basic neonatal resuscitation

There have been numerous guidelines regarding resuscitation of the newborn, however, these guidelines have been superseded by the consensus document on resuscitation (American Heart Association *et al.*, 2000).

Successful resuscitation of the newborn is based around anticipation, environmental control, assessment, stimulation, effective ventilation and, rarely, cardiac com-

Box 21.1   Anticipation (American Heart Association *et al.*, 2000; Royal College of Paediatrics and Child Health and Royal College of Obstetricians and Gynaecologists, 1997).

Antepartum risk factors
- Maternal diabetes.
- Pregnancy-induced hypertension/pre-eclampsia/chronic hypertension.
- Chronic maternal illness:
  - Cardiovascular
  - Thyroid
  - Neurological
  - Pulmonary
  - Renal
- Previous fetal or neonatal death.
- Haemorrhage.
- Polyhydramnios/oligohydramnois.
- Size versus dates discrepancy/diminished fetal activity.
- Alcohol or drug misuse/abuse.
- Drug use:
  - Lithium carbonate
  - Magnesium
  - Adrenergic-blocking drugs
- No prenatal care.

Intrapartum risk factors
- Preterm birth.
- Infection/Chorioamnionitis/prolonged rupture of membranes.
- Abnormal fetal heart rate including bradycardia, tachycardia, declerations.
- Meconium-stained amniotic fluid.
- Breech or abnormal presentation.
- Maternal opioid analgesia prior (<4 hours).
- Prolapsed cord.
- Abruptio placentae/placenta praevia.
- Fetal abnormality.
- Instrumental delivery.
- Emergency caesarean section.
- General anaesthetic.

pressions, intubation and drug administration. Resuscitation involves a number of processes that occur simultaneously. Each step will be considered separately although the initial assessment, stimulation and the administration of facial oxygen should occur as one swift action, see Fig. 21.1.

Environment

It is essential to ensure that the newborn baby does not become cold, as acidosis is worsened by hypothermia (Stephenson *et al.*, 1970; Tyson, 2000). Within a hospital or birthing centre an over-head heater, typically incorporated into a resuscitaire, will be available for all births. Such equipment is not routinely available in the community or A&E departments, so the attending midwife should minimize all draughts, ensure that the area is warm and that warm, dry towels are available to wrap-up the newborn baby. Although this seems to be common sense, it is typically simple procedures that are forgotten during the initial phase of any resuscitation attempt.

Box 21.2 Resuscitation equipment for birth at home.

Baby resuscitation equipment
- Suction device.
- O_2 funnel.
- Self-inflating 500 ml bag-valve-mask (BVM) device (sizes 0, 00 and 000).
  The use of the 500 ml bag-valve-mask device, in association with a slow, steady and controlled breath, will reduce the risk of under-ventilation and/or barotrauma. The traditional 240 ml BVM device is now no longer recommended as with it, it is difficult/impossible to provide a slow, constant inflation pressure (Zideman *et al.*, 1998).
- Oxygen cylinder regulated flow rate at a minimum flow rate of 8 lpm.

Maternal resuscitation equipment
- Suction device.
- Medium concentration oxygen mask.
- Pocket mask with one-way valve and various oral airways.
- Bag-value-mask (BVM) device (optional as a pocket mask with oxygen is an effective basic life support (BLS) airway device).
- Oxygen cylinder (minimum of 8 lpm).

Miscellaneous: towels, gloves, syringes, needles and disposable sharps box, torch, scissors, watch/stop watch, stethoscope.

Access to phone to call for assistance.

Note: An oxygen flow rate of 8 lpm will provide a minimum of 40% inspired oxygen via a medium concentration mask, and via a pocket mask, as well as a minimum of 60% inspired oxygen via a BVM with a reservoir bag. The main benefit is that the oxygen cylinder will last longer.

D size cylinder (approximately 200 litres) is the typical size cylinder available to a community midwife providing

Rate	*Oxygen therapy*
8 litres per min	42 minutes
10 litres per min	34 minutes
15 litres per min	22 minutes

Assessment

Although the Apgar score is well established, such a formal assessment is not required prior to the commencement of resuscitation. A rapid assessment of tone, colour, respiratory rate, heart rate, and the gut instinct that things are not right, will indicate the need to instigate resuscitation procedures.

A step-wise approach is recommended in the assessment of the newborn, who may require resuscitation and this includes active stimulation, opening the airway and the administration of free-flow oxygen therapy.

Follow the ABC of resuscitation:

- **(A) Airway**. Place the newborn on a firm surface with the head in a neutral position. The newborn has a large head and a small neck and this can lead to airway obstruction.
- **(B) Breathing**. Assess rate, rhythm and depth of ventilation. During this period, administer facial oxygen directly to the baby.
- **(C) Circulation**. Observe the baby's colour (if floppy and pale, circulation is

---

Dry the baby, remove any wet cloth and cover

↓

Initial assessment at birth Start the clock or note the time Assess: COLOUR, TONE, BREATHING, HEART RATE

↓

If not breathing . . .

↓

Control the airway Head in the neutral position

↓

Support the breathing If not breathing give FIVE INFLATION BREATHS (each 2–3 seconds duration) Confirm a response: increase in HEART RATE or visible CHEST MOVEMENT

↓

If there is no response Double check head position and apply JAW THRUST 5 inflation breaths Confirm a response: increase in HEART RATE or visible CHEST MOVEMENT

↓

If there is *still* no response (a) Use a second person (if available) to help with airway control and repeat inflation breaths (b) Inspect the oropharynx under direct vision (is suction needed?) and repeat inflation breaths (c) Insert an oropharyngeal (Guede) airway and repeat inflation breaths **Consider intubation** Confirm a response: increase in HEART RATE or visible CHEST MOVEMENT

↓

When the chest is moving Continue the ventilation breaths if no spontaneous breathing

↓

Check the heart rate If the heart rate is not detectable *or* slow (less than around 60 bpm) and NOT increasing

↓

Start chest compressions First confirm chest movement. If chest not moving *return to airway* 3 chest compressions to 1 breath for 30 seconds

↓

Reassess heart rate If improving stop chest compressions, continue ventilation if not breathing If heart rate still slow continue ventilation and chest compressions Consider venous access and drugs at this stage

AT **ALL** STAGES ASK . . . DO YOU NEED HELP?
In the presence of meconium, remember:
- Screaming babies have an open airway
- Floppy babies – have a look

Fig. 21.1 Neonatal life support resuscitation algorithm. Reproduced with kind permission from the Resuscitation Council (UK).

inadequate) and record the baby's heart rate. This may be with a stethoscope (arguably the best method) or by palpating the umbilical cord or the apex beat.

Stimulation

- Dry and warm the baby as this will provide sufficient stimulus and will prevent heat loss.
- Aggressive forms of stimulus should be avoided although flicking/rubbing feet or rubbing the back of a baby may be considered if drying fails to provide adequate stimulus (American Heart Association *et al.*, 2000).

Supplementary oxygen

Oxygen should be administered during the initial phases of assessment, at a minimum of 5 litres per min (American Heart Association *et al.*, 2000), as a number of newborn babies with gasping respiratory patterns but who maintain a heart rate >100 bpm will respond rapidly with drying/stimulation and oxygen therapy (Zideman *et al.*, 1998).

- Supplementary oxygen can be administered via a funnel, a facemask or via a cupped hand over the baby's face.
- It is important not to waft oxygen over the baby as this will actively cool the newborn and a bag-valve-mask (BVM) device should never be used to deliver oxygen to a spontaneously breathing or gasping baby as it increases respiratory workload (American Heart Association *et al.*, 2000).

Suction (non-meconium)

- The baby's face should be wiped clean and in the absence of meconium or blood only a brief period of gentle suction is required to remove residual amniotic fluid from the upper airway.
- There is a tendency to over suction the airway of a baby requiring resuscitation and this can lead to localized trauma, delay in commencing ventilation and may lead to vagal-induced bradycardia (Codero & How, 1971).

The first five breaths

The initial breaths are of paramount importance and, if delivered effectively, can rapidly restore spontaneous breathing. There has been a tendency to deliver the initial breaths as a series of short, sharp and fast ventilations, but this approach is doomed to failure.

- The initial breaths need to be delivered slowly (2 seconds per breath) with a slow constant pressure to achieve an inspiratory pressure of 30 cm of water. These initial breaths have been described as 'inflationary breaths' and are designed to inflate the lungs and remove amniotic fluid (American Heart Association *et al.*, 2000).
- Following the initial breaths, the baby should be reassessed. At this point the baby will have either improved and be spontaneously breathing/crying, continue to be apnoeic but with a heart rate 60–100 bpm or be apnoeic with a heart rate less than 60 bpm.

- Ventilation should continue at a faster rate of 30–40 breaths per minute (1 complete breath every 1.5–2 seconds) and cardiac compressions should be commenced in all babies with a heart rate <60 bpm.

Refer also to Fig. 21.1 for a neonatal life support resuscitation algorithm and Table 21.1 for technique trouble shooting when a baby does not respond to assisted ventilation.

Table 21.1 Baby not responding to assisted ventilation.

Problem	Possible cause	Action
Poor technique	• Ventilating too fast	• Slow down. Administer the first 5 breaths over 2–3 seconds • Subsequent breaths at a rate of 30–40 breaths per minute
Chest not raising	• Poor seal • Wrong size bag-valve-mask (BVM) device • Airway obstruction • Neonatal airway problem	• Readjust mask position • Use a 500 ml BVM • Reposition baby's airway • Consider using an oral airway
Pressure release valve activated (Pressure relief valve is in place to reduce the risk of pulmonary barotrauma)	• Airway obstructed • Operator ventilating too fast	• Reposition baby • Slow down (see 'Poor technique' described above) *Note:* It is feasible that the pressure relief valve *may* need to be over-ridden. This can be achieved by pressing on the valve (some BVMs include a clip for this purpose). This is rarely required, especially if a 500 ml BVM is used

Ongoing resuscitation/complications

Compressions

The point at which to start cardiac compressions is arbitrary and is not evidence-based, although the general consensus is that cardiac compressions should be commenced once effective ventilation has been instigated and if the heart rate remains below 60 bpm.

The ratio of breaths to compression is set at 3:1 and this emphasizes the importance of effective ventilation in the management of the newborn baby.

Once compressions have been started it is impossible for a lone rescuer and difficult for a two-person team to provide a respiratory rate of 30 breaths per minute and a compression rate of 90 bpm as recommended by neonatal resuscitation guidelines (Whyte *et al.*, 1999; American Heart Association *et al.*, 2000). Therefore, the requirement to perform compressions is one indication for endotracheal intubation.

Cardiac compression technique

Two-finger method

- Place the tips of two fingers just below the nipple line in the centre of the baby's chest.
- This is the preferred method for the lay-public and for the lone healthcare resuscitator.

Two-thumb method

- The clinician encircles the baby's chest with her hands placing two thumbs just below the baby's nipple line in the centre of the chest.
- This is now the preferred technique for healthcare professionals but it can only be performed when two rescuers are available.

The international guidelines now recommend the two-thumb method for resuscitation of all babies less than 1 year old (American Heart Association *et al.*, 2000). These recommendations are based on evidence in both infant and animal models. Despite this, all midwives should be able to perform both resuscitation techniques, as the two-thumb method is not suitable for single-person resuscitation.

Meconium aspiration

The principle aim during the management of the newborn baby with meconium is to prevent inhalation of meconium. Suction of the mouth, nose and pharynx prior to delivery of the baby's chest may help to prevent meconium aspiration (Tyson, 2000). Figure 21.2 shows the procedure for managing a baby with meconium-stained amniotic liquor.

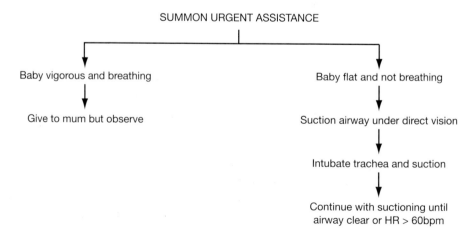

Suction mouth and nose before the shoulders are delivered (if possible)

SUMMON URGENT ASSISTANCE

Baby vigorous and breathing	Baby flat and not breathing
Give to mum but observe	Suction airway under direct vision
	Intubate trachea and suction
	Continue with suctioning until airway clear or HR > 60bpm

Fig. 21.2 Meconium aspiration algorithm.

The community midwife should concentrate on clearing the baby's upper airway of meconium with the use of suction. However, in the absence of a skilled intubator, ventilations will have to be commenced in the apnoeic newborn baby with a heart rate of less than 60 bpm (American Heart Association *et al.*, 2000).

Intubation

Palme-Kilander (1992) demonstrated that intubation is rarely required. The work by Palme-Kilander has resulted in fewer people being trained to intubate and a greater emphasis being placed on effective ventilation with a BVM device. Despite this, there are still a number of situations where intubation remains crucial:

• Prolonged/ineffective BVM ventilation.
• When chest compressions are required.
• Drug administration.
• Special circumstances, e.g. diaphragmatic hernia.

Drugs

With the exception of oxygen, few drugs are regularly used during routine resuscitation of the newborn baby. Table 21.2 gives details about the dose and administration of these drugs.

Table 21.2   Resuscitation drugs for neonates (American Heart Association *et al.*, 2000).

Drug	Dose/concentration	Route	Average dose
Epinephrine (formerly known as adrenaline)	10–30 µg/kg 0.1–0.3 ml/kg of 1:10 000 (1 mg in 10 ml)	Intravenous (IV) or via endotracheal (ET) tube	0.3–0.9 ml of 1:10 000
Sodium bicarbonate	1–2 ml/kg of 4.2% solution	Intravenous *only*	3–6 ml of 4.2% solution
Fluid bolus	0.9% saline 10 ml/kg Same amount is used for blood	Intravenous *only*	30 ml 0.9% saline
Naloxone	100 µg/kg	Usually intramuscular although the intravenous or endotracheal tube route may also be used	200 µg intramuscularly
10% dextrose	5 ml/kg	Intravenous *only*	10–15 ml

• **Epinephrine** (formerly known as **adrenaline**) is the principal resuscitation drug and is typically given to the newborn baby who, despite effective ventilation via an endotracheal (ET) tube and cardiac compressions, has a heart rate <60 bpm (American Heart Association *et al.*, 2000). Ideally, epinephrine should be administered via the umbilical vein, although it can be administered via a peripheral vein or via the ET tube.

- **Sodium bicarbonate**. There is little evidence to support its routine use and it is therefore reserved for the newborn baby who has not responded to effective ventilation, cardiac compressions and an epinephrine bolus (American Heart Association *et al.*, 2000).
- **'Normal' saline** is the first choice fluid for use in the resuscitation of the newborn, taking over from human albumin (American Heart Association *et al.*, 2000). A fluid challenge should be administered over at least 5 minutes in all babies where hypovolaemia is suspected, or where initial attempts at resuscitation have failed.
- **Dextrose** should be administered to all 'flat newborn babies' who have a capillary blood sugar <2 mmols.
- **Naloxone** has traditionally been given early in the management of the newborn with suspected respiratory depression secondary to maternal opioid analgesia. This approach should be discouraged. Naloxone is indicated where stimulation and ventilation fails to stimulate effective breathing despite the presence of effective cardiac output (American Heart Association *et al.*, 2000). In addition naloxone should not be used to treat newborn babies where there is a history of maternal opioid abuse as this represents a significant risk to the baby (American Heart Association *et al.*, 2000).

Extremely preterm babies

This is a highly emotive subject especially as neonatal intensive care has improved the outcome for even the smallest newborn (Van Reempts & Van Acker, 2001). It is recommended that each midwife refer to their individual unit's policies on very low birthweight babies and those babies born around the 24th week. However, if there is any doubt resuscitation should be implemented as estimated gestational dates can be inaccurate.

Maternal resuscitation

Incidence and facts

Cardiac arrest in pregnancy has been estimated to be 1:30000 pregnancies and one review estimated that in the UK there would be one peri-mortem or one post-mortem caesarean section for every 170000 deliveries (Whitten & Montgomery, 2000).

Maternal cardiac arrest

- The risk of accidental death remains regardless of whether somebody is pregnant or not.
- Road traffic accidents remain a common cause of maternal death as well as being the most common reason for peri-/post-mortem caesarean sections (Whitten & Montgomery, 2000).
- Maternal deaths from other causes, including sepsis and anaesthesia, have significantly reduced.
- The treatment of maternal cardiac arrest is dictated by the needs to treat the underlying cause, the provision of effective basic life support (BLS) supported by

supplementary oxygen and epinephrine, as well as the prompt performance of an emergency caesarean section (where appropriate).

Resuscitation procedures

The anatomical and physiological changes associated with pregnancy make resuscitation more difficult, see Box 21.3, and therefore require some changes to established resuscitation procedures (American Heart Association *et al.*, 2000).

Box 21.3 Factors affecting maternal resuscitation.

Difficult intubation
- Full dentation.
- Large breasts.
- Raised thoracic cage/flared rib cage.
- Oedema/obesity of the neck.
- Supraglottic oedema.

Difficult chest compressions
- Left lateral tilt position (to avoid inferior vena caval compression).
- Flared rib cage.
- Raised diaphragm.

Respiratory
- Increased tidal volume requirements.
- Increased O_2 demand.
- Reduced chest compliance.
- Reduced functional residual capacity.

Cardiovascular
- Incompetent gastro-oesophageal sphincter.
- Increased intragastric pressure.
- Increased risk of regurgitation.

Basic life support

The principle of BLS remains unchanged in the pregnant and non-pregnant patient, with equal emphasis being placed on airway management, assisted ventilations and cardiac compressions. The main difficulties are due to an increased risk of aspiration/regurgitation, higher than normal oxygen demand and the patient needing to be in the tilted left lateral position.

The ABC of resuscitation should be followed:

- **(A) Airway**. The patient's airway should be opened with a 'head tilt–jaw lift' manoeuvre once it has been checked visually for foreign bodies. The jaw thrust manoeuvre can then be used once in conjuction with airway adjuncts to facilitate effective ventilation.
- **(B) Breathing**. Regardless of what device is chosen to provide supplementary ventilation, it is of paramount importance that all breaths are given slowly to reduce the risk of gastric distension (American Heart Association *et al.*, 2000). Table 21.3 provides a comparison of the various devices available.

Table 21.3 Ventilation.

Device	Advantages	Disadvantages	Comments
Mouth-to-mouth	• Easy to learn • Provides a good seal	• Socially unpleasant • Difficult to provide additional oxygen	Remains a priority skill to learn but within a hospital basic airway devices should be available
Pocket mask	• Easy to learn • Provides a good seal • Can be used by one person • Some types provide O_2 ports	• Still require training to use effectively • Maximum O_2 is 50% (at 10–15 litres per min)	This remains the ideal first response device as it is easy and effective to use Ideal for community midwifery use
Bag-valve-mask (BVM) device	• Can provide high flow O_2 • Less tiring on the rescuer	• Difficult to use and often results in under ventilation • Typically less available at the bedside	This remains a device for anaesthetic staff to use or for midwives to use as a two-person technique with one midwife securing the mask to the face with two hands and a second midwife slowly squeezing the bag

- **(C) Circulation**. Cardiac compressions are performed at a ratio of 15 compressions to 2 breaths in all non-intubated adults (American Heart Association *et al.*, 2000). Once the patient is intubated, ventilation and cardiac compression are performed continuously with a minimum of 12 breaths per minute (American Heart Association *et al.*, 2000).

The left lateral tilt position/wedges

To minimize the affects of aortocaval compression, a wedge or the left lateral tilt position should be used in all critically ill visibly pregnant women. This can be achieved using a specially design wedge, by using upturned chairs (if patient is on the floor) or by using a human wedge approach. The general principles are to first ensure the patient achieves a 30° left lateral tilt; second, make sure that the wedge is non-compressible during chest compressions; and third the technique requires minimal training and patient movement to use.

Advanced life support

The resuscitation team will usually co-ordinate advanced life support. The principles of advanced life support remain the same regardless of the patient being pregnant (see Fig. 21.3), with one significant change, emergency peri-/post-mortem caesarean section.

Advanced airway management

Airway protection during cardiac arrest of the mother is of paramount importance to reduce the risk of pulmonary aspiration. The difficulties associated with intubating a

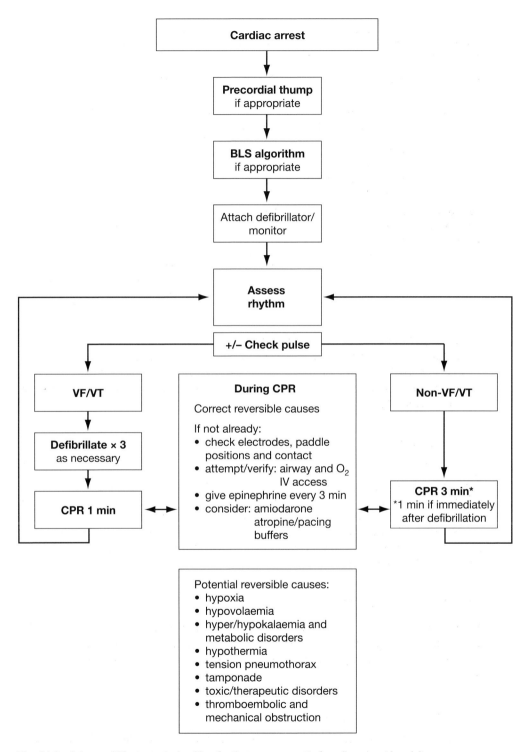

Fig. 21.3 Advanced life support algorithm for the management of cardiac arrest in adults.

pregnant woman require that an experienced/skilled intubator and equipment for failed intubation should be available.

Defibrillation

Immediate defibrillation to reverse ventricular fibrillation (VF) pulseless, ventricular tachycardia (VT) remains vital, as no other intervention will be successful in restoring a normal cardiac rhythm. The risk to the unborn baby is extremely low and is greatly out-weighed by the benefits to the mother.

Resuscitation drugs

As with the newborn baby, the principal resuscitation drug remains oxygen although other drugs are also used, such as epinephrine, to support maternal and newborn circulation during cardiopulmonary resuscitation. Drugs for maternal resuscitation are given in Table 21.4.

Emergency caesarean section

Emergency caesarean section is directly linked to both the successful resuscitation of the mother and the newborn and, therefore, it is an integral part of maternal resus-

Table 21.4   Maternal resuscitation drugs.

Drug	Dose/route	Rationale	Frequency
Epinephrine (the principal resuscitation drug and formerly known as adrenaline)	1 mg 1:10 000 intravenous (IV) or via endotracheal (ET) tube (double the dose)	To improve cerebral and coronary artery perfusion	1 mg every 3 minutes
Atropine	3 mg IV or via ET tube (double the dose)	To increase heart rate by blocking the parasympathetic nervous system	Once only
Amiodarone	300 mg IV bolus with a further 150 mg if required	To increase reversal of ventricular fibrillation (VF)/ventricular tachycardia (VT) following defibrillation	A new recommendation for resistant VF/VT
Calcium chloride	10 ml/10% solution IV only	To protect heart from hyperkalaemia or magnesium overdose	Until QRS complexes narrow
Sodium bicarbonate	1 mmol/kg (1 ml/kg of 8.4%) typically 50 ml bolus IV of 8.4%	Treatment of acidosis in intubated patients during prolonged cardiac arrest, treatment of hyperkalaemia and to treat tricyclic anti-depressant overdose	Depending on clinical situation

citation (Whitten & Montgomery, 2000). It is therefore of paramount importance that there is no delay in performing this emergency procedure. No time should be wasted in moving the mother in cardiac arrest to an operating theatre, as this will affect the performance of the BLS. Appropriate equipment should be brought to the woman.

Summary

For a midwife to be able to safely perform resuscitation of both the mother and the newborn baby a combination of training, clinical assessment skills and the ability to identify the at-risk mother/infant are a priority.

Infant resuscitation

- Anticipation of problems allows for preparation.
- Environment warm, draught free.
- Towels for effective stimulation and drying the newborn.

Airway

- Baby on firm surface, 'sniffing position'.
- Do not over suction.

Breathing

- First five breathes – (2–3 seconds) a slow, constant pressure to inflate the lungs.

Circulation

- Cardiac compressions if heart rate <100 bpm.
- Compressions rate of 3:1, preferably using the two-thumb method.
- Proceed to intubation if necessary.

Maternal resuscitation

- Rare occurrence, complicated by pregnancy.
- Emergency caesarean section aids resuscitation and may save the baby.
- Positioning – use a wedge to create a lateral tilt.

Airway

- Head tilt-jaw lift.

Breathing

- Oxygen slowly and effectively delivered.

Circulation

- Cardiac compressions at a ratio of 15:2.

Useful contact

Resuscitation Council (UK)   5th Floor, Tavistock House North, Tavistock Square, London WC1H 9HR. Telephone: 020 7388 4678. Website: www.resus.org.uk
Provides evidence-based guidelines and information for professionals.

References

American Heart Association, Resuscitation Council (UK), European Resuscitation Council *et al.* (2000) International Guidelines 2000 for cardiopulmonary resuscitation and emergency cardiovascular care – An international consensus on science. *Resuscitation* **46** (special issue) xix–xx, 293–301, 401–416.

Codero, L. & How, E. (1971) Neonatal bradycardia following nasopharyngeal suction. *Journal of Pediatrics* **78** (78), 441–3.

Ergenekon, E., Koc, E., Atalay, Y. & Soysal, S. (2000) Neonatal resuscitation course experience in Turkey. *Resuscitation* **45** (3), 225–7.

Falciglia, H. (1988) Failure to prevent meconium aspiration syndrome. *Obstetrics and Gynecology* **71**, 349–53.

Palme-Kilander, C. (1992) Methods of resuscitation in low Apgar score newborn infants – a national survey. *Acta Paediatrica* **81**, 739–44.

Royal College of Paediatrics and Child Health and Royal College of Obstetricians and Gynaecologists (1997) *Resuscitation of Babies at Birth*. BMJ Publishing, London.

Stephenson, J., Du, J. & Oliver, T. (1970) The effects of cooling on blood gas tension in newborn infants. *Journal of Pediatrics* **76**, 848–52.

Tyson, J. (2000) Immediate care of the newborn infant. In *A Guide to Effective Care in Pregnancy and Childbirth*, 3rd edn (Enkin, M., Keirse, M.J.N.C., Neilson, J. *et al.*, eds), pp. 417–28. Oxford University Press, Oxford.

Van Reempts, P. & Van Acker, K. (2001) Ethical aspects of cardiopulmonary resuscitation in premature neonates: where do we stand? *Resuscitation* **51** (3), 225–32.

Whitten, W. & Montgomery, L. (2000) Postmortem and perimortem caesarean sections: what are the indications? *Journal of the Royal Society of Medicine* **93**, 6–9.

Whyte, S., Sinha, A. & Wyllie, J. (1999) Neonatal resuscitation – a practical assessment. *Resuscitation* **40** (1), 21–5.

Zideman, D., Bingham, R., Beattie, T. *et al.* (1998) Recommendations on resuscitation of babies at birth. *Resuscitation* **37** (2), 103–10.

22 Perineal trauma and suturing

Perineal trauma

Incidence

- 70% of women giving birth vaginally sustain some degree of perineal trauma (Yiannnouzis, 2002).
- In the UK, 350 000 women undergo perineal repair annually (Kettle, 2002).
- The vast majority of maternal morbidity following perineal trauma remains unreported to health professionals (Glazener *et al.*, 1995).

Facts

- Perineal trauma is associated with postnatal morbidity (Kettle, 2002; Yiannnouzis, 2002) with tears involving the anal sphincter being underreported. The later can be associated with distressing postpartum faecal incontinence (Sultan, 2002).
- Second-degree tears vary widely from small and well aligned to complicated, extensive and misaligned (Yiannnouzis, 2002).
- There is an increasing trend for midwives to leave first- and increasingly, second-degree tears unsutured (Yiannnouzis, 2002).
- The evidence suggests that using the correct repair material and suture technique will significantly reduce postnatal pain (Kettle *et al.*, 2002).
- Unfortunately, many doctors and midwives feel they lack confidence when suturing. Staff training and supervision in suturing techniques is directly linked to increased staff confidence (Kettle, 2002).

To suture or not to suture?

There have been various small studies involving women who have sustained first- or second-degree tears which have been left unsutured. Providing the tears were not actively bleeding, they were left to heal naturally. Reports vary between positive benefits, such as reduced pain and increased comfort in non-sutured groups, as well as indifference, i.e. that there was little difference in pain levels between groups (Head, 1993; Jackson, 2000; Lundquist *et al.*, 2000). The limited evidence suggests that the act of suturing in itself may introduce infection for a minority of women. Importantly, no adverse affects in healing have been noted in unsutured tears, leading to the assumption that the body can and does heal itself effectively following childbirth.

The trend towards not suturing tears has evolved on the strength of limited evidence and Yiannnouzis (2002) suggests this has probably occurred for a variety of reasons, including increased maternal choice, increased midwifery autonomy and staffing pressures. Lundquist *et al.* (2000) suggest that non-suturing offers women choice, and avoidance of the discomfort of anaesthesia and sutures. Some clinicians speculate that in the absence of robust evidence, leaving the muscle layer unsutured could cause problems later on (McCandlish, 2001). While there is no strong evidence to support one option over another, midwives should be guided by local protocols and their own clinical judgement when advising women. Suturing should probably be recommended for: any perineal trauma that is extensive, a large second-degree tear, a third-degree tear, a fourth-degree tear, if bleeding continues, if the wound is very misaligned/complicated or the result of an unnatural, straight-edged cut from an

Table 22.1 Classification of perineal lacerations/trauma.

Degree of laceration	Description of perineal laceration
1st degree tear	Involving just the skin
2nd degree tear	Involving skin and muscle, it may be small or extensive
3rd degree tear*	Involving skin, muscle and extending into the anal sphincter. Sultan (2002) suggests this can be subdivided into: 3a: Partial tear of the anal sphincter involving less than 50% thickness 3b: Complete tear of the anal sphincter 3c: Internal sphincter also torn
4th degree tear*	Involving skin, muscle and extending into the anal sphincter and rectal mucosa

* These tears should be sutured by an experienced clinician, ideally in theatre where there is a good light source and adequate analgesia/anaesthesia for the woman. Post-repair care may involve a catheter, avoiding constipation and detailed explanations to the mother. Due to the impact such trauma can have on a woman's quality of life, the community midwife and GP should be informed and obstetric follow-up is essential (Sultan, 2002).

episiotomy. For a classification of perineal lacerations see Table 22.1. Ultimately, it should remain the woman's choice as to whether to accept or decline suturing.

Who should suture?

The RCOG (2002) suggests that practitioners who are appropriately trained are more likely to provide a consistent, high standard of perineal repair and thus will contribute to reducing the extent of morbidity and litigation associated with this procedure.

From the literature reviewed by Jackson (2000), women appear to prefer their midwife to conduct the perineal repair. This, Jackson suggests, allows for continuity and reduced waiting time. Presumably, the woman's midwife is usually female and she is familiar to them, so women may feel they can trust her over an unknown person. Lying in lithotomy can be a very vulnerable, restrictive experience, so being sutured by their own midwife is likely to help reduce their anxieties. Any complicated tear outside the midwife's remit or confidence level should be referred to an experienced clinician. Sometimes this can occur during the suturing procedure when the extent of the trauma has been clearly visualized.

Whoever completes the suturing, the midwife in attendance must ensure that the suturing clinician is sensitive, careful and responds appropriately to any pain the woman may experience.

Providing care for survivors of childhood sexual abuse

Women often do not disclose that they have been sexually abused as a child or previously sexually assaulted or raped. Symptoms exhibited by survivors of previous sexual abuse can be misinterpreted and result in women being labelled as 'difficult patients' (this was also dealt with in Chapter 16). This lack of awareness by health professionals can result in inappropriate treatment, resulting in further damage suggests Aldcroft (2001).

For such women the lithotomy position dictates that they are immobilized and at the mercy of an authoritative figure. Women may feel they are submitting to a painful, invasive and sexually threatening procedure. This can leave them feeling violated and powerless (Kitzinger, 1992). Such an experience can be negative and disempowering and can have far-reaching psychological consequences. It may affect their relationship with their baby who may inadvertently be blamed for 'putting them through this' (Aldcroft, 2001).

Suturing

Long-term perineal morbidity is associated with anatomically incorrect approximation of wounds and unrecognized trauma to the external anal sphincter which can lead to major physical, psychological and social problems (RCOG, 2003). The type of suturing material, the technique of repair, and the skill of the operator, are the three main factors that influence the outcome of perineal repair (RCOG, 2003).

Suturing materials

In studies reviewed by Kettle & Johanson (2002a) polyglycolic acid sutures (e.g. Dexon or Vicryl) were found to result in reduced short-term pain and less analgesia than other materials. However, more women required postnatal removal of their stitches by their community midwife, commonly for reasons of 'tightness' or 'irritation'.

Alternatively, rapidly absorbed polyglycolic 910 (e.g. Vicryl Rapide) degrades rapidly, reducing its tensile strength by 50% after 5 days, with no traction left after 14 days (Kettle & Johanson, 2002a). It appears to offer the advantage of reduced postnatal pain and reduces the need for suture removal in 1 in 10 women sutured (Kettle *et al.*, 2002) compared to standard polyglycolic acid suture material (e.g. Dexon or Vicryl). *Rapidly absorbed polyglycolic acid* is, therefore, the suture material of choice.

Suturing techniques and analgesia

Suturing is an aseptic technique, which should take place under adequate analgesia. The clinician must be gentle, sensitive and *never proceed if the woman is inadequately anaesthetized*. Remember local anaesthetic takes time to work properly. Women may choose to combine entonox and local or regional anaesthetic. If the woman has an epidural *in situ*, the midwife should not be reluctant to offer a 'top-up' as Saunders *et al.* (2002) found that this offers a superior degree of analgesia compared to local anaesthetic.

A study (Saunders *et al.*, 2002) which reported women's experience of pain when undergoing perineal suturing highlighted that 16.5% of women reported 'distressing', 'horrible' or 'excruciating' pain while receiving sutures. To the surprise of the reviewers women's pain scores did not diminish as the time between suturing and pain reporting increased. In particular women without regional anaesthetic were found to endure high levels of pain during this procedure (Saunders *et al.*, 2002).

The degree of tear will involve different layers (see also Table 22.1) and so will influence the type of suturing technique to be used:

- **Muscle layer**. Suturing of the muscle layer traditionally combined interrupted and/or continuous suture techniques, sometimes referred to as a two-stage technique. This is no longer recommended. Instead Kettle *et al.* (2002) and the RCOG (2003) recommend a loose, continuous non-locking technique should be used to suture vaginal tissue, as this may be beneficial in reducing short-term pain and later suture removal. See also below under 'Suturing procedure outline'.
- **Skin layer**. The use of subcuticular continuous suturing appears to be superior to interrupted sutures for the perineal skin (Kettle *et al.*, 2002; Kettle & Johanson, 2002b). See also below under 'Suturing procedure outline'.
- **Skin layer unsutured**. Studies have also evaluated leaving the skin unsutured. Again, this is preferable to interrupted sutures to the skin, resulting in a significant reduction in adverse outcomes as well as representing a cost-effective use of healthcare resources (Petrou *et al.*, 2001).

There has, as yet, been no comparison between subcuticular continuous suturing and leaving the skin unsutured.

Figure 22.1 shows a selection of suturing needle types. Needles are available in various sizes, thicknesses, shapes and types and tend to be chosen according to user preference (Ethicon, 1998). Figure 22.2 shows the basic sequence of inserting a stitch and tying a knot.

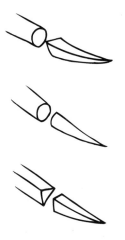

Tapercut needles offer the advantage of a cutting tip, followed by a smooth round body, therefore combining easier piercing and penetration with the minimal trauma of the rounded body.

Round-bodied needles are designed to separate the tissues and although they can be used for repairing the perineum, they can make it difficult to penetrate the skin.

Cutting needles are used for tissue that is difficult to penetrate, which is why they are sometimes chosen for the tough skin area.

Fig. 22.1   Suturing needle types.

Suturing at home

At home, midwives must be resourceful! A good fixed light source is essential. Ensure the woman can lie comfortably with her bottom on the edge of a firm bed and the midwife positioned on the floor. The woman may find it most comfortable to rest her legs on separate chairs or she can abduct them herself but this is only usually comfortable for a short time. If both the woman and the midwife attempt suturing on the floor it is very hard on the midwife's back.

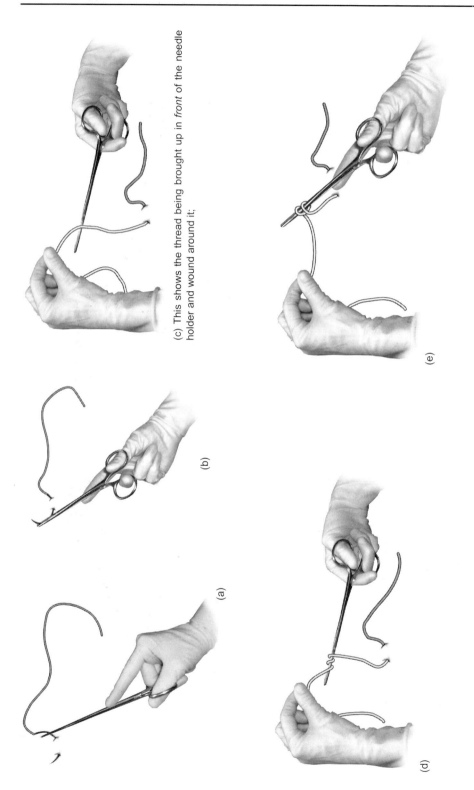

(c) This shows the thread being brought up in *front* of the needle holder and wound around it;

(b)

(a)

(e)

(d)

Fig. 22.2   Suturing and tying a knot. (a)–(m) Illustrates the step-by-step insertion of a stitch and knot tying by a right-handed individual. Left-handed individuals can use an advanced photocopier to flip the images. Knots can be hand tied if preferred.

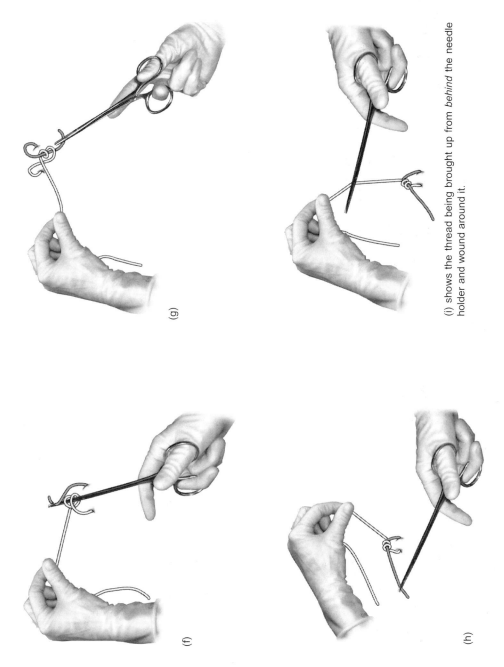

(i) shows the thread being brought up from *behind* the needle holder and wound around it.

(g)

(f)

(h)

Fig. 22.2 *Contd.*

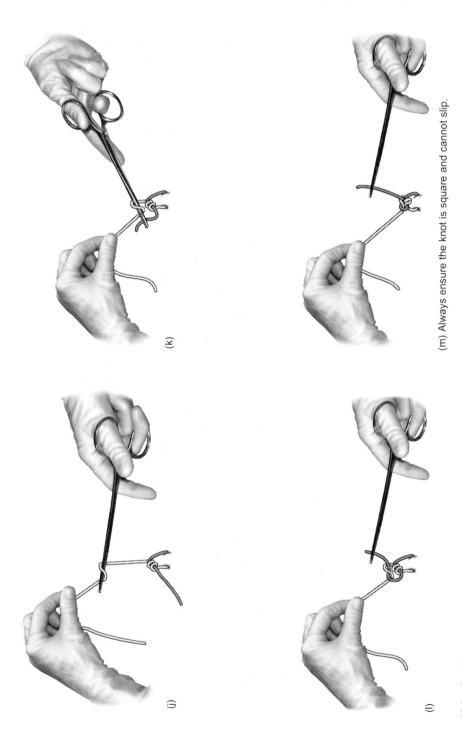

(k)

(j)

(m) Always ensure the knot is square and cannot slip.

(l)

Fig. 22.2 *Contd.*

Suturing procedure outline

Following discussion, explanations, reassurances and informed consent from the woman, the midwife can prepare everything ready for suturing, including a fixed light source, optional post-suturing analgesia (such as a diclofenac suppository) and, in hospital, the call bell within reach.

Before starting the repair address the following questions:

- Is the mother as comfortable as possible?
- Does she understand what has to be done and how long it will take?
- Can you see what has to be done?
- Can you do it?

An overview of the perineum is shown in Fig. 22.3 to help in the visualization of the morphology of the female genitalia.

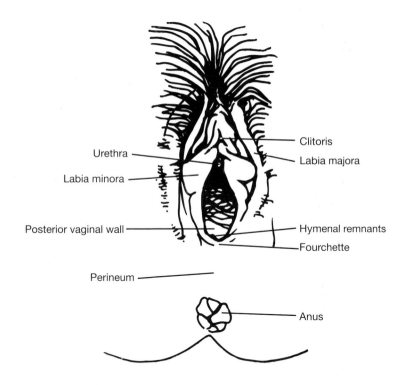

Common mistakes and long-term perineal morbidity can be associated with:

- Anatomically incorrect approximation of wounds (RCOG, 2002)
- Unrecognised trauma to the external anal sphincter (Sultan, 2002)
- Sutures placed at the skin of the fourchette
- Sutures tied too tightly (Ethicon, 1998)
- The type of suturing material (RCOG, 2002)
- The technique of repair (RCOG, 2002)
- The skill of the operator (RCOG, 2002)

Fig. 22.3 Overview of the perineum.

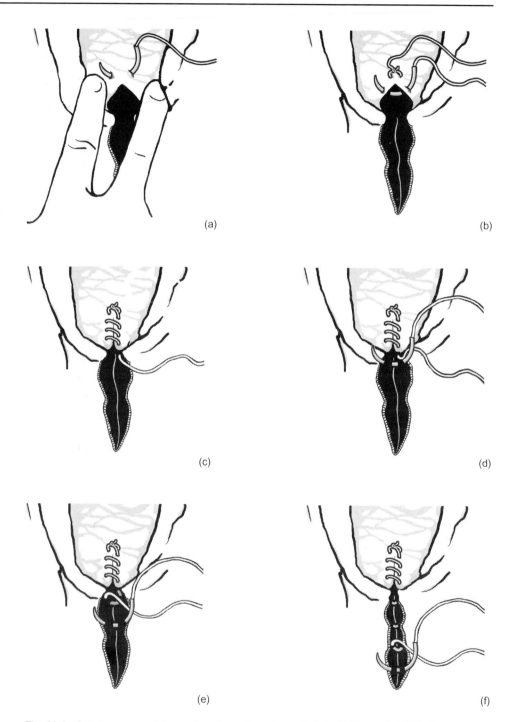

(a)

(b)

(c)

(d)

(e)

(f)

Fig. 22.4   Suturing a second-degree tear (based on a large study by Kettle *et al.*, 2002). Place the first stitch above the apex of the vaginal trauma, in order to secure any deeper bleeding points (a, b). Place loose, continuous sutures from the apex along the tear. Do not use a locking or blanket stitch, or pull sutures too tight (c). The perineum stitches are placed loosely and deeply in the subcuticular tissue (d–g)

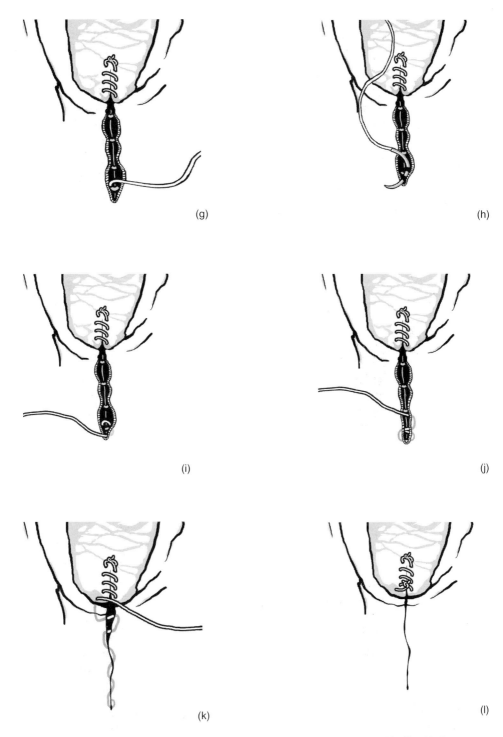

(g)

(h)

(i)

(j)

(k)

(l)

Fig. 22.4 *Contd.* ... Place subcuticular, continuous sutures just under the skin (avoid placing any sutures in the fourchette) (h–k). Finish with the thread in the vagina, where a knot is tied (l).

Placing the woman's legs in lithotomy is no longer routine practice in many hospitals. The woman may prefer to just relax her legs apart (Kettle *et al.*, 2002), resting her knees against obsolete lithotomy poles if desired. A particularly nervous woman may feel more in control with her legs resting apart and, while she may need to close them if something hurts or distresses her, the midwife's patience and sensitivity will help her through this ordeal.

- Ensure the woman is comfortable and holding/feeding her baby if possible as then she is more likely to relax and pay less attention to what is happening.
- Extend the sterile field by covering the area with sterile drapes.
- Warn the woman before touching, wiping or injecting anything. As the midwife earns the woman's confidence, the woman will begin to trust her, relax and stop anticipating pain.
- Clean only enough of the perineum to inject the local anaesthetic, otherwise this will burn and sting and is, therefore, not a good start to the procedure.
- Infiltrate local anaesthetic (the woman may wish to use entonox) and *wait for it to work*.
- Clean the area more thoroughly if required.
- Insert a tampon. This keeps the area below it blood free and visually clear. Warn the woman this is very uncomfortable, she may wish to use entonox again. Secure the tampon string to the drapes.
- Move the tear 'back together' in order to visualize significant meeting points, insure there is no anal involvement.
- Then locate the apex in the vagina, secure the first stitch just above it.
- Using a continuous suture technique, from the apex, bring the muscle layers together (see Fig. 22.4a–c).
- If a stitch(s) appears mis-placed, unfortunately it will require the needle to be cut free to allow unpicking and then a knot tied. Recommence a new set of continuous stitching from the point left off.
- For the skin either leave unsutured or use a subcuticular continuous suturing technique (Fig. 22.4d–h). Do not insert interrupted stitches to this area.
- Visually inspect the stitches before preparing the woman for the uncomfortable removal of the tampon.
- Prepare the woman before checking her rectum. Insert a lubricated finger, fleshy side up and slowly withdraw it, gently feeling for any stitches that may have gone through, for 'buttonholes' or a tear.
- If the woman wishes (and providing there are no contraindications) many clinicians give a diclofenac 100 mg suppository, rectally post suturing.
- Place a sanitary pad over the perineum and assist the woman back into a comfortable position.
- Count up and account for all needles, swabs and instruments.

Some general information can be shared with the woman over the actual suturing:

- Suggest she tries to pass urine in the bath, following suturing, as it is thought to be less painful.
- Discuss sitting, breastfeeding and comfort; pain control (such as cool packs) and if sutures become tight in several days suggest that although it may appear daunting, the removal of one can bring great relief.

- Most women do not have their bowels opened until day 3 postpartum, discuss this topic and explain that she will not 'come undone'. Advise her re hygiene and washing, wiping gently from front to back, supporting the perineum with a pad when having bowels open, etc.
- It can be appropriate to discuss the future and sex, the first intercourse after the baby and ensuring the couple both feel relaxed and aroused enough before having full intercourse.

Summary

- Suturing should probably be recommended for perineal trauma that is complicated/large/bleeding/very misaligned/third or fourth degree or from an episiotomy.
- Any tear outside the midwife's remit, or confidence level, should be referred to an experienced clinician.
- Third and fourth degree tears can go undiagnosed, with distressing side effects and morbidity for the woman.
- Ultimately, it should remain the woman's choice as to whether to accept or decline suturing.
- Non-suturing is an option for women who may wish to avoid the pain and discomfort of anaesthesia and sutures.
- Clinicians must be sensitive, careful and respond appropriately to any pain or anxieties the woman may have.
- Women tend to prefer their midwife to conduct the perineal repair.
- Lack of awareness by health professionals can result in inappropriate treatment of women who are survivors of childhood sexual abuse.

Suture materials and technique

- Suturing is an aseptic technique, which should take place under effective analgesia.
- In studies rapidly absorbed polyglycolic acid came out as the suture material of choice.
- The muscle layer should be sutured by using a continuous suture technique.
- Subcuticular continuous sutures, or leaving the skin unsutured, are both preferable to interrupted sutures for the skin.

References

Aldcroft, D. (2001) A guide to providing care for survivors of child sex abuse. *British Journal of Midwifery* **9** (2), 81–5.

ETHICON (1998) *Perineal Repair*. A Booklet for Professionals. Produced by Johnson & Johnson.

Glazener, C.M.A., Abdalla, M., Stroud, P. *et al.* (1995) Postnatal maternal morbidity: extent, causes, prevention and treatment. *British Journal of Obstetrics and Gynaecology* **102**, 286–7.

Head, M. (1993) Dropping stitches. Do unsutured tears to the perineum heal better than sutured ones? *Nursing Times* **89** (33), 64–5.

Jackson, K. (2000) The bottom line: care of the perineum must be improved. *British Journal of Midwifery* **8** (10), 609–14.

Kettle, C. (2002) Materials and methods for perineal repair. Are you sitting comfortably? Issues around perineal trauma. *RCM Midwives Journal* **5** (9) 298–301.

Kettle, C., Hills, R.K., Jones, P., Darby, L., Gray, R. & Johanson, R. (2002) Continuous versus interrupted perineal repair with standard or rapidly absorbed sutures after spontaneous vaginal birth: a randomised controlled trial. *The Lancet* **359**, 2217–22.

Kettle, C. & Johanson, R. (2002a) Absorbable synthetic versus catgut suture material for perineal repair (Cochrane Review). *The Cochrane Library* Issue 4. Update Software, Oxford.

Kettle, C. & Johanson, R. (2002b) Continuous versus interrupted sutures for perineal repair (Cochrane Review). *The Cochrane Library* Issue 4. Update Software, Oxford.

Kitzinger, J.V. (1992) Counteracting, not re-enacting, the violation of women's bodies: the challenge for perinatal caregivers. *Birth* **19** (4), 219–22.

Lundquist, M., Olisson, A., Nissen, E. & Normal, M. (2000) Is it necessary to suture all lacerations after a vaginal delivery? *Birth* **27** (2), 79–85.

McCandlish, R. (2001) Routine perineal suturing: is it time to stop? *MIDIRS Midwifery Digest* **11** (3), 296–300.

Petrou, S., Gordon, B., Mackrodt, C. *et al.* (2001) How cost-effective is it to leave the skin unsutured? *British Journal of Midwifery* **9** (4), 209–14.

RCOG (2003) *Clinical Green Top Guidelines: Methods and Materials Used in Perineal Repair* (23). Website: www.rcog.org.uk/guidelines (accessed May 2003).

Saunders, J., Campbell, R. & Peters, T.J. (2002) Effectiveness of pain relief during suturing. *BJOG: An International Journal of Obstetrics and Gynaecology* **109**, 1066–8.

Sultan, A. (2002) 'Have I missed a third degree tear?' The identification, treatment and follow-up of women who experience perineal trauma. Are you sitting comfortably? Issues around perineal trauma. *RCM Midwives Journal* **5** (9), 298.

Yiannouzis, K. (2002) Describing perineal trauma: the development of an assessment tool. Are you sitting comfortably? Issues around perineal trauma. *RCM Midwives Journal* **5** (9), 300–301.

23 Pharmacopoeia

Introduction

This pharmacopoeia encompasses some of the commonest drugs administered during the intrapartum period. This pharmacopoeia *is a guide only* and midwives should refer to local protocols and the *British National Formulary* which is updated as new evidence emerges.

- The midwife is responsible and accountable for her own actions and must be familiar with local protocols and policies, for standing orders information and in the prescribing and administration of drugs.
- Midwives practising outside their employing authority, or outside the NHS, should seek advice from their supervisor of midwives regarding any matters related to the supply, administration, storage, surrender and destruction of controlled drugs and other medicines (NMC, 2003).
- Rule 41 (NMC, 2003) states that a practising midwife shall only administer those medicines, including analgesics, in which she has been trained as to use, dosage and methods of administration.

Abbreviations in prescribing

Table 23.1   Route of administration.

Abbreviation	Route of administration
IM	Intramuscular injection
IV	Intravenous
sc	Subcutaneous
po; *per oram*	Oral
pr; *per rectum*	Rectal
pv; *per vaginum*	Vaginal

Table 23.2   Frequency of drug administration.

Abbreviation	Frequency
Stat	Immediately
bd; *bis die*	Twice a day
tds; *ter die sumendus*	Three times a day
qds; *quatre die sumendus*	Four times a day
Nocte	At night
prn; *pro re nata*	As needed
hrly	Hourly

Table 23.3 Units of measurement.

Abbreviation	Unit
μg	Microgram
ng	Nanogram
mg	Milligrams
g	Grams
kg	Kilograms
fl	Femtolitre
ml; mL	Millilitre
l; L	Litre
IU	International Units
mU	Milli units

Drug calculations

Table 23.4 Drug calculations.

$$\frac{\text{what you want}}{\text{what you have}} \times \text{what it is supplied in} =$$

Example:
100 mg of penicillin is prescribed but it comes as a preparation of 125 mg of penicillin in a 5 ml solution.

$$\frac{100\,\text{mg}}{125\,\text{mg}} \times 5\,\text{ml} = 4\,\text{ml}$$

Therefore a dose of 4 ml of the preparation will give the prescribed 100 mg of penicillin.

Drugs listing

(A) ANALGESIA AND REGIONAL LOCAL ANAESTHESIA

Drug: **Bupivacaine hydrochloride/Marcain®/ropivacaine hydrochloride**

Dosage:	Adjusted according to procedure and the patient's physical status and weight, and as prescribed by the anaesthetist
Indications:	Regional local anaesthetic for labour pain, caesarean section, post-delivery procedures (e.g. suturing, manual removal of placenta, post-operative pain relief)
Route:	Lumbar epidural/spinal route
Contraindications:	Hypovolaemia, hypotension, maternal infection, coagulation disorders or on going coagulation treatment (Banister, 1997), cardiac/respiratory impairment, epilepsy, complete heart block (Joint Formulary Committee, 2003)
Side effects:	CNS effects, respiratory depression and convulsions, hypotension, bradycardia (Joint Formulary Committee, 2003)

Drug: **Entonox®/Equanox® (nitrous oxide and oxygen)**

Dosage:	Self administered as required
Indications:	Pain in labour

Route: Inhaled via a mask or mouthpiece
Contraindications: —
Side effects: Drowsiness, nausea and vomiting, dry mouth (Banister, 1997)

Note: Rule 41 (NMC, 2003) applies: a practicing midwife shall only administer medicines including inhalational analgesics by mean of apparatus if she is satisfied that the apparatus has been properly maintained and (a) it has a CE marking or, if it does not have such a marking, (b) it is of a type for the time being approved by the NMC as suitable for use by a midwife.

Drug: Lignocaine hydrochloride or lidocaine hydrochloride

Dosage: • 5–20 ml, depending on concentration, and as per standing order
                      • 0.5%, 1%, 2%
Indications: • Local anaesthetic used prior to performing an episiotomy or for suturing
                      • This drug is also used to treat specific cardiac problems. This particular use is covered in the British National Formulary (Joint Formulary Committee, 2003)
Route: sc
Contraindications: Hypotension, hypovolaemia, bradycardia, complete heart block (Joint Formulary Committee, 2003)
Side effects: Hypotension, bradycardia, anaphylaxis (Joint Formulary Committee, 2003)
Cautions: Epilepsy, hepatic or respiratory or cardiac impairment, bradycardia (Joint Formulary Committee, 2003). **Take care to avoid intravascular injection** (Banister, 1997) Accidental intravascular injection can lead to central nervous system excitory response, including drowsiness, convulsions and respiratory arrest (Bannister, 1997; Joint Formulary Committee, 2003)

Drug: Paracetamol

Dosage: • 500 mg–1g 4 to 6 hourly
                      • Maximum 4 g daily
Indications: • Mild to moderate pain
                      • Pyrexia
Route: po, pr
Contraindications: Hepatic or renal disease, alcohol dependence
Side effects: Rarely blood disorders, rashes, overdose causes liver damage (Joint Formulary Committee, 2003)

Drug: Pethidine hydrochloride

Dosage: • 50–100 mg 1- to 3-hourly
Indications: • Short lasting analgesia for moderate pain, also has a strong sedative effect
                      • Not suitable for severe pain (Joint Formulary Committee, 2003)
Route: • Usually administered IM
                      • Also po, sc and IV injection
Contraindications: A compromised fetus, renal impairment, existing respiratory depression (Banister, 1997; Joint Formulary Committee, 2003)
Side effects: • **In the baby:** crosses the placental barrier within 2 minutes of administration. Can cause bradycardia, slow excretion by the neonatal liver, depresses sucking reflexes (Banister 1997), and causes respiratory depression, drowsiness and depressed reflexes in the newborn (Joint Formulary Committee, 2003)
                      • **In the mother:** nausea, vomiting, drowsiness, respiratory depression, bradycardia (Joint Formulary Committee, 2003)

Drug: Voltarol®/diclofenac sodium

Dosage: 75–150 mg in 24 hours, doses can be divided into 2 to 3 smaller doses to a maximum of 150 mg in 24 hours (Joint Formulary Committee, 2003)
Indications: Pain and inflammation, usually for postnatal or postoperative analgesia

Route:	po (preferably after food), or as pr or IM
Contraindications:	Asthma, pregnancy (Banister, 1997)
Side effects:	Suppositories may cause localized rectal irritation (Joint Formulary Committee, 2003), gastric irritability, ulceration, coagulation disorders leading to haemorrhage, headache, dizziness and vertigo (Banister, 1997)
Cautions:	Can interact with other drugs, including analgesics, hypertensives causing increased hypertensive effects, and in beta-blockers antagonism of hypertensive effects (Banister, 1997)

(B) ANTICONVULSANT THERAPY

Drug: Magnesium sulphate

Dosage:	• Regimes vary between hospitals: check local protocols • Loading dose of 4 g is given slowly over 5–10 minutes • 1 g hourly can be administered as a maintenance dose
Indications:	Anticonvulsant–muscle relaxant used in pre-eclampsia and eclampsia
Route:	IV injection or IV infusion
Contraindications:	—
Side effects:	Generally associated with hypermagnesaemia, nausea, vomiting, thirst, flushing of skin, hypotension, arrhythmias, coma, respiratory depression, drowsiness, confusion, loss of tendon reflexes, muscle weakness (Joint Formulary Committee, 2003)
Cautions:	Monitor for overdose. Calcium gluconate injection is used for the management of magnesium toxicity (Joint Formulary Committee, 2003)

(C) ANTIHYPERTENSIVE THERAPY

Drug: Hydralazine hydrochloride

Dosage:	• po 25–50 mg • Hydralazine is usually titrated against the woman's blood pressure in labour • 5–10 mg by slow IV injection in 10 ml fluid (Joint Formulary Committee, 2003) • Repeated every 20 minutes 5 mg IV injection, with a maximum cumulative dose of 20 mg (DoH, 2001)
Indications:	Hypertension
Route:	po, IV injection or IV infusion
Contraindications:	Idiopathic systemic lupus erythematosus (SLE), severe tachycardia, high output heart failure, myocardial insufficiency due to mechanical obstruction (Joint Formulary Committee, 2003)
Side effects:	Tachycardia, palpitations, flushing, hypotension, fluid retention, gastro-intestinal disturbances, headache, dizziness (Joint Formulary Committee, 2003)
Cautions:	Colloids are usually infused before treatment is initiated to maintain uteroplacental circulation. Anaesthetics enhance the drug's hypotensive effects (Banister, 1997)

(D) BETAMIMETIC/TOCOLYTIC THERAPY

Drug: Ritodrine hydrochloride/Yutopar®

Dosage:	• Regimes vary between hospitals: check local protocols • Commonly commenced at 50 μg/minute • Increased by 50 μg /minute every 10 minutes until contractions stop (or are less than 1:15) *or* maternal pulse reaches 140 bpm • The stabilizing dose is usually between 150–350 μg/minute • Maximum dose 350 μg /minute (Joint Formulary Committee, 2003)

Indications:	• Used to delay uncomplicated preterm delivery
	• Once the steroid course and/or transfer to a specialist unit have been completed there is no benefit from the betamimetic infusion continuing (Joint Formulary Committee, 2003)
Route:	po, IV infusion
Contraindications:	Cardiac disease, severe pre-eclampsia or eclampsia (Joint Formulary Committee, 2003). Fetal death or a fetal abnormality that is incompatible with life, or where fetal or maternal condition requires urgent delivery (Walkinshaw, 2001), active bleeding (as betamimetics relax the uterus), preterm rupture of membranes and/or infection (in which there is probably no benefit to stopping labour (Keirse, 2000))
Side effects:	Unpleasant and serious side effects include palpitations, chest pain, arrhythmias, tremor, nausea, vomiting, headache, thirst, hypokalaemia, restlessness and agitation, and, although rare, maternal death may also result (Joint Formulary Committee, 2003)
Cautions:	Betamimetics should be avoided in women with the following conditions: diabetes, as they seriously affect carbohydrate metabolism; hyperthyroidism (Joint Formulary Committee, 2003); heart disease, as they have severe cardiovascular side effects including inducing a tachycardia (Keirse, 2000; Joint Formulary Committee, 2003)
	Stop the infusion if: maternal heart rate exceeds 140 bpm, or the woman experiences any **chest pain** or **breathlessness** (Joint Formulary Committee, 2003)
	Maintain a strict fluid chart and avoid over-hydration, as fluid overload can cause pulmonary oedema (Joint Formulary Committee, 2003)
	Depending on local policy, test blood maternal blood sugar and urea and electrolytes 6–12 hourly and auscultate the woman's chest for signs of oedema 4–8 hourly

(E) CORTICOSTEROIDS

Note: while corticosteroids can be used to treat the mother for an acute medical condition in labour (e.g. an asthma attack), their use described here relates to their routine prophylactic administration to mothers at risk of preterm delivery. Every effort should be made to treat women with a course of corticosteroids prior to possible preterm delivery, whether planned or unplanned (CESDI, 2003).

Drug: Betamethasone/Dexamethasone

Dosage:	First dose 12 mg, and a second 12 mg dose 12 hours later
Indications:	Prophylactic treatment administered to the mother at risk of preterm birth to promote surfactant production in the lungs of her unborn baby (Crowley, 2002)
Route:	IM, po
Contraindications:	Systemic infection (unless responding to appropriate antimicrobial treatment). Refer also to the Joint Formulary Committee (2003)
Side effects:	Presently under investigation to ascertain if multiple doses are associated with possible endocrine defects in infants
Cautions:	Diabetes in the mother. Repeated prenatal exposure may suppress adrenal function in the baby but is rarely clinically significant (Joint Formulary Committee, 2003)

(F) OXYTOCIC AGENTS

Regime for postpartum haemorrhage (Joint Formulary Committee, 2003): in cases of excessive uterine bleeding, any placental products remaining in the uterus should be removed. In cases of bleeding caused by uterine atony, oxytocic drugs are used in turn as follows:

• Oxytocin 5–10 units by IV injection
• Ergometrine maleate 250–500 µg by IV injection. If ergometrine maleate is inappropriate (e.g. in pre-eclampsia, hypertension), oxytocin alone may be given by IM injection (unlicensed indication, Joint Formulary Committee)
• Oxytocin 5–30 units in 500 ml infusion fluid given by IV infusion at a rate that controls uterine atony.
• Carboprost (Hemabate®) has an important role in severe postpartum haemorrhage unresponsive to ergometrine maleate and oxytocin. Carboprost is not an oxytocic agent but a prostaglandin.

Drug: Ergometrine maleate

Dosage:	0.5 mg
Indications:	Postpartum haemorrhage
Route:	IM (takes $2\frac{1}{2}$ minutes to act) or IV injection (takes 45 seconds to act) (Crafter, 2002)
Contraindications:	As for Syntometrine®
Side effects:	**In the mother:** nausea, vomiting, hypertension, headaches, bradycardia, palpitations, dyspnoea, severe after-pains and rarely stroke and myocardial infarction (Joint Formulary Committee, 2003)
Caution:	**1 mg MAXIMUM of ergometrine maleate total dose**

Drug: Syntocinon® (stored in fridge)

Dosage:

For induction of labour (based on NICE guidelines, 2002):
- IV infusion 30 IU in 500 ml normal saline
- 1 ml/hr = 1 mU/min. Most women should have adequate contractions at 12 mU/min
- 20 mU/min is the MAXIMUM licensed dose
- If regular contractions not established after TOTAL of 5 IU (5 hours on suggested regime) then induction should be stopped

Postpartum (following the delivery of the baby):
- 5–10 units by slow IV injection
- Greater quantities are used in infusions

Indications:
- Induction or augmentation of labour
- Active management for delivery of the placenta. This drug is used instead of Syntometrine® or ergometrine maleate in women with hypertension
- For retained placenta (see * below under 'Side effects')
- Treatment of postpartum haemorrhage

Route:
In labour:
- IV infusion

Postpartum haemorrhage:
- IM takes $2\frac{1}{2}$ minutes to act (unlicensed route, Joint Formulary Committee, 2003)
- IV injection of slow bolus takes 45 seconds to act
- IV infusion of 5–30 units in 500 ml of intravenous fluid titrated according to the severity of postpartum haemorrhage (Joint Formulary Committee, 2003). However, Crafter (2002) notes that in practice sometimes 40 units or greater are used

Contraindications: Hypertonic uterine contractions, fetal distress, severe pre-eclampsia and cardiovascular disease (Banister, 1997)

Side effects: **Mother:** uterine hyperstimulation, hypotension, arrhythmias, nausea, vomiting, rash and anaphylaxis, placental abruption, amniotic fluid embolism, uterine spasm even at low doses

* In approved trials, Syntocinon® has been administered into the maternal side of the umbilical cord if the placenta is retained to improve the chance of its spontaneous delivery (Carroli & Bergel, 2002; see also Chapter 11 for more information)

Baby: Fetal distress, asphyxia, intrauterine death

Caution: **Interactions:** can cause severe hypotension and arrhythmias when administered during anaesthetic (DoH, 2001). It can potentiate the effects of prostaglandins (Banister, 1997)

Do not confuse intrapartum and postpartum drug regimes, as large or bolus doses would be very dangerous if accidentally administered during labour

Drug: Syntometrine® (**Syntocinon®** and ergometrine maleate) (stored in fridge)

Dosage:
- 1 ml ampoule contains 5 units/ml of Syntocinon® and 0.5 mg of ergometrine maleate
- Maximum dose 1 mg of ergometrine maleate in total in either form, i.e. Syntometrine® or ergometrine maleate

Indications: Postpartum haemorrhage

Route: IM only (Joint Formulary Committee, 2003), takes $2\frac{1}{2}$ minutes to act (Crafter, 2002)

Contraindications:	Do not give if the woman is in labour, or is hypertensive, pre-eclamptic or eclamptic, or is a severe asthmatic or has sepsis. Renal impairment, hepatic, cardiac or pulmonary disease and some medical disorders (Joint Formulary Committee, 2003)
	In cases of retained placenta, because ergometrine maleate can close the cervical os it should be avoided in postpartum haemorrhage if the placenta is still *in situ*. In this case Syntocinon® may then be preferable (Crafter, 2002)
Side effects:	Nausea, vomiting, hypertension, headaches, bradycardia, tinnitus, palpitations, chest pain, dyspnoea, severe after-pains and rarely stroke and myocardial infarction (Joint Formulary Committee, 2003)

In retained placenta:
Because these drugs can close the cervical os they should be avoided in heavy bleeding if the placenta is still *in situ*. In this case Syntocinon® would then be preferable (Crafter, 2002)

Caution:	**1 mg MAXIMUM of ergometrine maleate total dose**

(G) PROSTAGLANDINS

Drug: Hemabate®/Carboprost (stored in fridge)

Dosage:	According to Pharmacia & Upjohn (1996):
	• Initial dose 250 micrograms (1.0 ml)
	• Frequency of 1.5 hourly intervals, and doses should not be given closer than 15 minutes apart
	• **Maximum dose 2 mg (8 doses)**
Indications:	• Postpartum haemorrhage that is unresponsive to Syntocinon® or ergometrine maleate (Pharmacia & Upjohn,1996)
Route:	IM
Contraindications:	Cardio, pulmonary hepatic or renal disease, untreated pelvic inflammatory disease (Joint Formulary Committee, 2003). Should be used with caution in clients with a history of asthma, glaucoma, hypertension, hypotension, anaemia, jaundice, diabetes or epilepsy (Pharmacia & Upjohn,1996)
Side effects:	Nausea, vomiting, flushing, hyperthermia (Banister, 1997) diarrhoea, hypertension, wheezing, asthma, headaches and, very rarely, cardiovascular collapse (Joint Formulary Committee, 2003)
	This drug will probably make the woman feel very unwell. Sickness and diarrhoea are fairly common so prepare the woman in advance. Commonly transient side effects usually pass when the therapy ends (Pharmacia & Upjohn,1996)

(H) VITAMINS

Drug: Konakion® MM Paediatric/vitamin K (phytomenadione)

Dosage:	In the UK more than 97% of babies receive vitamin K after birth (Ansell *et al.*, 2001) as either a single 1 mg/0.2 ml injection or as an oral regime as follows:
	• The first oral dose following birth, the second at one week old and a final third dose is recommended for breastfed babies
	• 2–3 oral doses (Joint Formulary Committee, 2003)
Indications:	Vitamin K is thought beneficial in the manufacture of clotting factors in newborns. DoH (1998) advocates that newborns should receive an appropriate vitamin K regime but that the choice of administration (po or IM) and whether to decline it altogether should rest with the parents
Route:	• IM (single dose)
	• po (2–3 dose regime)
Contraindications:	—
Side effects:	With parenteral administration in premature infants of less than 2.5 kg there is an increased risk of kernicterus

Useful contact

The *British National Formulary* is a joint publication of the British Medical Association and the Royal Pharmaceutical Society of Great Britain aiming to give healthcare professionals up-to-date information about the use of medicines in the UK. It is published twice a year (order from Customer Services 01491 829 272). It is also available online at www.bnf.org

References

Ansell, P., Roman, E., Fear, N.T. *et al.* (2001) Vitamin K policies and midwives practice: questionnaire survey. *British Medical Journal* **322**, 150–52.

Banister, C. (1997) *The Midwife's Pharmacopoeia*. Midwife Practice Guides. Books for Midwives Press, Hale, Cheshire.

Carroli, G. & Bergel, E. (2002) Umbilical vein injection for management of retained placenta (Cochrane Review). *The Cochrane Library* Issue 4. Update Software, Oxford.

CESDI (2003) *Project 27/28: An Enquiriy into Quality and Care and its Effects on Survival of Babies Born at 27/28 Weeks*. Stationery Office, London.

Crafter, H. (2002) Intrapartum and primary postpartum haemorrhage. In *Emergencies Around Childbirth – A Handbook for Midwives* (Boyle, M., ed.), pp. 113–26. Radcliffe Medical Press, Oxford.

Crowley, P. (2002) Prophylactic corticosteroids for preterm birth (Cochrane Review). *The Cochrane Library* Issue 4. Update Software, Oxford.

DoH (1998) *Vitamin K for Babies*. PLO/CNO/998/4.

DoH (2001) *Why Mothers Die, 1997–1999. The fifth report of the Confidential Enquiries into Maternal Deaths in the United Kingdom*. Department of Health, RCOG Press, London.

Joint Formulary Committee (2003) *British National Formulary*, 45th edn. British Medical Association and Royal Pharmaceutical Society of Great Britain, London.

Keirse M.J.N.C. (2000) Preterm birth. In *A Guide to Effective Care in Pregnancy and Childbirth*, 3rd edn (Enkin, M., Keirse, M.J.N.C., Neilson, J. *et al.*, eds), pp. 214–23, 352. Oxford University Press, Oxford.

NICE (2001) Clinical Guidelines D – Induction of Labour. National Institute for Clinical Excellence, London.

NMC (2003) Midwives Rules and Code of Conduct Practice. Rule 41. Nursing and Midwifery Council (formerly UKCC), London. www.nmc-uk.org (accessed May 2003).

Pharmacia & Upjohn (2002) Hemabate sterile solution (carboprost tromethamine) drug company literature for physicians and patients. Pharmacia & Upjohn, a subsidiary of Pharmacia Corporation, Kalamazoo, MI, USA.

Walkinshaw, S.A. (2001) Preterm labour and delivery of the preterm infant. In *Turnbull's Obstetrics*, 3rd edn (Chamberlin, G. & Steer, P., eds), pp. 493–520. Churchill Livingstone, Edinburgh.

Glossary

Adrenal hyperplasia. A condition in which the sex of the baby can appear difficult to determine.

Adrenaline. A hormone secreted by the adrenal glands in response to 'stress'.

Anencephaly. A congenital abnormality where the fetus has no cranial vault and the cerebral hemispheres of the brain fail to develop. The baby may live for days, even weeks, but cannot survive extauterine life.

Anaemia. Low haemoglobin in the blood.

Anuria. No urine output from the kidneys indicating a severely compromised condition.

Apgar. A scoring system to assess neonatal well-being, respiratory effort, heart rate, muscle tone, response to stimuli and colour at birth.

Artificial rupture of the membranes (ARM). Manually breaking the waters that protect the baby *in utero*. It can be done during labour or prior to the birth as the head crowns.

Asphyxia neonatorum. Failure of the baby to breathe at birth.

Asynclitism. The condition when a baby has difficulty negotiating the pelvic inlet and the parietal bone presents first. The fetal head is tilted sideways to the left or the right.

Atony. A lack of muscle tone, in childbirth this is commonly pertaining to the uterus.

Ballottement. A term commonly used to describe the floating or moving away of the non-engaged presenting part when pushed (during a vaginal examination) or palpated (during abdominal palpation).

Bishop's score. A scoring system used to assess the cervix and identify any changes towards the onset of labour.

Bradycardia. A particularly slow heart rate.

Breech. A presentation where the baby's buttocks lie in the lower pole of the uterus, the lie is longitudinal and the baby's sacrum is the denominator.

Cannula. A flexible tube inserted into vessels, commonly into a vein, to administer fluid or drugs.

Caput. An oedematous swelling of the fetal scalp during labour, usually caused by pressure from the cervix and more common if the membranes have ruptured.

Cataracts. A cloudy opacity of the lens in the eye which adversely affects the eyesight.

Catecholamine. A term used to describe a group of hormones secreted at times of stress, including neurotransmitters such as adrenaline and dopamine.

Catheter. A flexible tube which can be inserted in various vessels or organs, such as into the bladder to drain it of urine, or into a vessel which measures the pressure in the right atrium of the heart (central venous pressure/CVP line).

Central venous pressure (CVP) line. A special catheter inserted into a blood vessel to measure the difference in pressures between the cardiac output and the venous return. This pressure is indicative of blood volume.

Cephalic. The head of the baby.

Cephalohaematoma. A swelling beneath one of the cranial bones, caused by a collection of blood. Occurs following delivery.

Cephalopelvic disproportion (CPD). Where the baby's head is in a sub-optimal position or is too large in relation to the size or shape fo the maternal pelvis, so that the baby cannot pass through it.

Changing Childbirth. A government, all-party report, advocating a change in the service provided for women during pregnancy and childbirth, aiming to increase midwifery-led care, continuity of carer, improve choice and redirect care to the community

Coagulopathy. Where clotting factors are used up/reduced and blood fails to clot.

Cone biopsy. Surgery involving the removal of a cone-shaped area of cervix, in order to remove precancerous cells.

Corticosteroids. A group of steroid hormones produced in the adrenal cortex, also created synthetically.

Crowning. The point at which the fetal head stays in position at the vulva (no longer receding between contractions) and preceding actual delivery of the head.

Cyanosis. A blueness of the extremities and face due to a low level of oxygen in the blood.

Denominator. A specific point of the presenting part that indicates its relationship within the pelvis. The occiput is the denominator in a vertex position, the sacrum is the denominator with a breech presentation and the mentum is the denominator in a face presentation.

Disseminated intravascular coagulation (DIC). Failure of the normal blood clotting mechanism.

Doula. A woman who supports another throughout labour and birth.

Electronic fetal monitoring (EFM). A device which records and makes audible the fetal heart.

Endocervix. The mucous membrane lining the cervical canal.

Endorphins. A group of hormones secreted by the brain which activate the body's opiate receptors. During labour they often have a relaxing as well as a pain-relieving effect.

Episiotomy. An invasive procedure involving a cut to the perineum of a woman prior to her baby being born.

Expectant management. Although the term 'management' implies control or intervention, expectant management is a non-intraventionalist decision where a 'wait and see' approach to care is used.

External cephalic version (ECV). The palpation of the maternal uterus to manoeuvre the baby from a malposition, such as a breech or a transverse or oblique lie, to a cephalic presentation which is more likely to result in a vaginal birth.

Fetal heart rate (FHR). The beats per minute of the fetal heart, usually averaging a range between 110 bpm and 160 bpm.

HELLP syndrome. HELLP stands for **H**aemolysis, **E**levated **L**iver enzymes, **L**ow **P**latelets. HELLP syndrome is a potentially life-threatening condition and a severe complication of pre-eclampsia.

Hydrocele. Swollen testes in the newborn caused by the accumulation of fluid. This is fairly common, benign and resolves at around 6–12 weeks of age.

Hypoglycaemia. Abnormally low blood sugar.

Hypospadias. The abnormal location of the urethral opening on the underside of the penis.

Iatrogenic. Illness, injury or morbidity caused by medical care or treatment.

Intermittent auscultation (IA). Assessing the fetal heart at regular intervals.

Intrapartum. From the onset of labour until after the delivery of the placenta.

Intrauterine death. Death of the baby while still in the womb/*in utero*.

Intravenous (IV). A route via the veins to administer intravenous fluids or drugs.

Jaundice. A yellowing of the skin caused by excessive amounts of bile pigments.

Kernicterus. In babies with severe and sudden onset jaundice there is a yellow staining of the basal ganglia of the brain which can be fatal if untreated. Often linked to Rhesus isoimmunization.

Ketones. A bi-product of fat metabolism due to low carbohydrate levels.

Ketoacidosis. An imbalance of electrolytes in the blood with high levels of ketones.

Lie. The relation of the long axis of the fetus to the long axis of the mother. When parallel to the mother's spine the lie is longitudinal, and when across is transverse or oblique.

Macrosomia. A particularly large baby for gestational age. Can be associated with maternal diabetes or obesity.

Malposition. A term used to describe the sub-optimal position of any fetal part in relation to the maternal pelvis.

Malpresentations. Any presentation of the baby other than cephalic.

Mendelson's syndrome. The fatal aspiration of the stomach contents during a general anaesthetic.

Mentum. The chin.

Morbidity. Pertaining to injury or trauma.

Mortality. Pertaining to death.

Moulding. When the bones of the fetal skull slightly overlap during the course of labour.

Multigravida. A woman who is pregnant and has had one or more previous pregnancies.

Multiparous. A woman who has previously given birth to at least one viable baby.

Neonatal intensive care unit (NICU). A unit specializing in the care of very preterm infants.

Oliguria. Very low urinary excretion.

Os. The inner opening of the cervix.

Oxytocic. A group of drugs, which cause the uterus to contract.

Oxytocin. A natural hormone produced in the body that causes the uterus to contract.

Peri-mortem caesarean section. A caesarean that is performed when the mother has collapsed such as during a cardiac arrest. This may improve the success of resuscitation attempts and may save the baby.

Placenta accreta/increta/percreta. Placenta accreta is the adhesion of the placenta to the myometrium, placenta increta is when the placenta invades the myometrium and placenta percreta is when the placenta penetrates the myometrium or deeper to the serosa of the uterus. Any of these conditions is potentially life threatening and surgical removal is essential. In invasive cases hysterectomy is often necessary to deliver the placenta and control haemorrhage.

Podalic version. Involves the internal grasping of the fetal foot, to convert a baby of transverse lie to a longitudinal lie and breech presentation.

Post-dates. See **Post-mature/post-maturity**.

Post-mature/post-maturity. A pregnancy that has extended beyond the expected date of delivery.

Post-mortem. The medical examination of a dead body with the aim of discovering the cause of death.

Post-mortem caesarean section. A caesarean following maternal death.

Postpartum haemorrhage. Significant bleeding from the uterus or genital tract in the first 24 hours following the birth may be caused by uterine atony or trauma. Secondary postpartum haemorrhage can occur later and is usually caused by retained products and/or uterine infection.

Primiparous. A woman who has born one child.

Primigravida. A woman pregnant for the first time.

Prophylactic/prophylaxis. In order to prevent/preventative treatment.

Presentation/presenting part. The part of the fetus which first enters the pelvis, most commonly cephalic but can also be breech, shoulder, brow or face presentation.

Preterm labour. Onset of labour prior to 37 completed weeks of pregnancy.

Puerperal sepsis. Infection of the genital tract following birth.

Puerperium. The period following the birth of the baby when the woman is recovering and caring for her baby.

Pyrexia/pyrexial. A raised temperature, usually above 37°C.

Restitution. The alignment of the shoulders into the anterior posterior diameter of the pelvis prior to their delivery.

Rhesus factor. The presence or absence of an antigen in the blood determines a person's blood group as being Rhesus positive or Rhesus negative.

Semi-recumbent. A posture where the person is between the lying and sitting position and which can have adverse effects during labour/birth.

Show. A cervical mucous plug that can be heavily blood stained. It may be passed via the vagina prior to the onset of labour, during labour and often at full dilatation of the cervix.

Special care baby unit (SCBU). A facility to care for preterm or unwell newborn babies.

Stillbirth. A term used to describe the birth of a baby, over 24 weeks gestation, who has died prior to delivery and whom at birth has not breathed or shown any signs of life.

Tachycardia. A particularly fast heart rate.

Temperature. The degree of heat in the body usually measured by means of a thermometer or judged by touch.

Thrombocytopenia. Platelet deficiency.

Transcutaneous electrical nerve stimulation (TENS). A small battery operated, electrical stimulation device which is secured to the woman's back in labour and may aid coping with back pain and/or painful contractors.

Trophoblastic invasion. The trophoblast is the covering of the blastocyst (fertilized ovum/zygote). It initially feeds the developing blastocyst and then invades into the decidua of the endometrium to enable chorionic and maternal circulations to develop via formation of the placenta.

Umbilical cord. The cord connecting the baby to the placenta.

Uterine atony. Uterine atony following birth can be caused by a retained placenta, excessive oxytocin use in labour and other causes. This is when the muscles of the uterus fail to contract adequately and result in a postpartum haemorrhage.

Uterine rupture. An occasional event where the walls of the uterus separate/tear apart and which can be fatal for the baby and occasionally for the mother.

Uterus. The womb.

Vacuum extractor. See **Ventouse**.

Vertex. The part of the baby's head that most commonly presents at the cervix/vulva during a cephalic labour/birth.

Ventouse. A soft, round suction cup that is secured over the baby's head and pulled to assist/augment delivery of the baby.

Vitamin K. A group of organic compounds found mainly in green vegetable matter that are necessary for the formation of prothrombin which is essential for the clotting of blood.

Appendix A
Automated blood pressure devices

Mean and standard deviation (mmHg) of differences in blood pressure measurements between standard and device (standard minus device) in pregnancy and pre-eclampsia. Acceptable standard 5(8) mmHg (Association for the Advancement of Medical Instrumentation).

Machine	Pregnancy		Pre-eclampsia	
	Systolic	Diastolic	Systolic	Diastolic
SpaceLabs 90207	3(4)	4(4)	19(8)	0.6(3)
Quiettrak	0.34(9)	1.6(8)	25(16)	18(8)
Omron Hem 705CP	0.9(10)	1.5(10)	2(10)	8(8)
Dinamap XL301	—	—	15(9)	11(7)
SpaceLabs Scout	—	—	18(10)	4(10)
Welsh Allen Lifesign	2(7)	3(6)	8(6)	6(5)

*Reproduced with kind permission from Professor Andrew Shenman.

Appendix B
Midwife ventouse practitioner log book record

Midwife Ventouse Practitioner Log Book Record

Ventouse practitioner name . . . . **Unit** . . . .
Case no . . . . Date . . . . Time of delivery . . . .
Client name . . . . Reg no . . . . Age . . . .
Address . . . .
Gestation . . . . Gravida/Para . . . .
Induction: Yes/No   Method . . . .
Augmentation: 1st stage . . . .   2nd stage . . . .

Indication for ventouse . . . .
Abdo palpation . . . .   Fifths palpable per abdo . . . .
Contractions . . . .
Vaginal examination: Dilatation . . . .   Station . . . .   Caput . . . .   Moulding . . . .

A

R ( ) L

P

Analgesia . . . .   Catheterised pre-procedure: Yes/No
Type of ventouse (e.g. silc/Kiwi . . . .   Number of pulls . . . .
Traction required: Easy / Moderate / Strong
Perineum: Intact / 1st / 2nd / 3rd / 4th degree trear / episiotomy

COMMENTS ON DELIVERY:

EBL . . . .   Baby: Male / female   Birth weight . . . .
Length of labour: 1st stage . . . . .   Meconium at delivery? Yes/No
                  2nd stage . . . .   APGARS . . . .
                  3rd stage . . . .   General condition of baby . . . .

With kind permission from Cathy Charles, West Wiltshire Primary Health Care Trust.

Appendix C
Decision to decline midwife ventouse delivery

Decision to Decline Midwife Ventouse Delivery

It is recognised that a midwife ventouse practitioner's (MVP) skill may be determined not just by successful ventouse deliveries, but also by declining to attempt ventouse extraction on unsuitable cases. MVPs should complete this form whenever asked to do a ventouse delivery, which, following assessment, they decline to perform.

A MVP may decide against ventouse delivery for any reason. It is understood that decision-making, particularly in an isolated community unit, is not always easy.

This form merely aims to monitor MVP decision-making. It should in no way inhibit midwives from calling in an MVP for an opinion.

Please note: if an MVP *actually starts* a ventouse delivery which is then abandoned, s/he should not complete this form but fill in the existing MVP log book form and complete a risk management form in the usual way.

Do not file this form in a client's maternity notes. Please send one copy to your manager and retain a copy for your ventouse practitioner logbook.

Ventouse practitioner name . . . . **Unit** . . . .
Case no . . . .   Date . . . .   Time of delivery . . . .
Client name . . . .   Reg no . . . .   Age . . . .
Address . . . .
Gestation . . . .   Gravida/Para . . . .
Induction: Yes/No   Method . . . .
Augmentation: 1st stage . . . .   2nd stage . . . .

Indication for ventouse . . . .
Abdo palpation . . . .   Fifths palpable per abdo . . . .
Contractions . . . .
Vaginal examination: Dilatation . . . .   Station . . . .   Caput . . . .   Moulding . . . .

Reason for declining ventouse:

Outcome:

Reproduced with kind permission from Cathy Charles, West Wiltshire Primary Health Care Trust.

Appendix D
Checklist following a pregnancy loss after 24 weeks

This is an example of a checklist that can be used following delivery of a stillbirth or neonatal death. Many maternity units will have devised their own form, which can be ticked, signed and dated as appropriate.

Mother's Name . . . . Partner's Name . . . .
Unit No. . . . . Telephone No. . . . .

	Please tick, sign and date where appropriate
1. Both parents informed of stillbirth death by:	Name: . . . .
2. Consultant Obstetrician and Supervisor of Midwives informed:	. . . . Consultant . . . . Supervisor
3. Parents given opportunity to see/hold the baby	
4. Momentoes offered to parents (please tick): Photographs: Other: Taken ☐ Lock of hair ☐ Accepted by parents ☐ Cot card ☐ Kept in notes ☐ Name band ☐ Foot/hand print ☐	
5. Religious advisor notified (if desired by parents). Baptism or other religious ceremony offered	
6. Consent for post-mortem requested? Consent given: Yes ☐ Declined ☐	
7. Inform mortician as soon as possible that consent for post-mortem has been obtained	
8. Date and time of post-mortem given?	
9. Post-mortem form completed by **medical staff**?	
10. GP informed: By telephone ☐ By letter ☐	
11. Notice of death form completed?	
12. Community midwife informed on day of discharge: By telephone ☐ By discharge letter ☐	

Contd.

13. Health visitor informed?	
14. Apply 'teardrop' sticker to mother's notes?	
15. Anti-D given? Yes ☐ No ☐	
16. Rubella vaccination given? Yes ☐ No ☐	
17. Bloods taken for investigation? Yes ☐ No ☐ (Note: not listed as may vary between hospitals)	
18. Mother given information regarding lactation?	

19. Contact groups discussed (if appropriate)?
    – SANDS
    – ARC
    – Miscarriage Association	

20. Parentcraft/Relaxation classes cancelled?	
20. At discharge, have TTO drugs been given? Yes ☐ No ☐ (TTO – to take out)	

22. Inform Consultant's Secretary of need for appointment as soon as possible and attach 'proforma' to notes
                    Yes ☐   No ☐
                    Date of appointment	

23. Genetic counselling appointment made (if appropriate) Yes ☐ No ☐	
24. Death or Stillbirth certificate completed, explained and given to parents. Print name of Certifying Officer on counterfoil.	
25. Information on funeral arrangements given and discussed.	

26. Parents' decision on funeral arrangements:
    Hospital:
    Burial ☐   Cremation ☐   Informal service ☐
    Private:
    Burial ☐ Cremation ☐	

27. Chapel service requested Yes ☐ No ☐	
28. Parents given information about The Book of Remembrance?	
29. Notify Bereavement Co-ordinator	
30. CESDI form completed, signed and posted.	

When completed retain this checklist in mother's notes

Note: if the pregnancy was a twin pregnancy and one twin died in utero, regardless of gestational ages, if it was delivered *after* 24/40 of pregnancy it should be registered as stillborn.

Reprinted by kind permission of Judy Byrne, Worcestershire Acute Hospital NHS Trust.

Appendix E
NICE clinical practice algorithm (EFM)

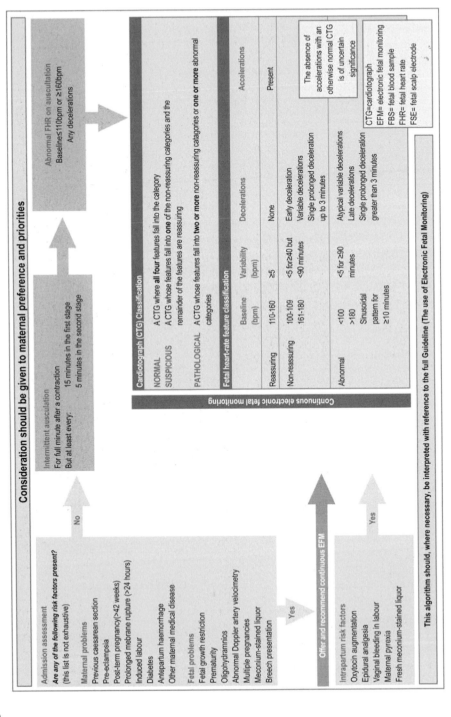

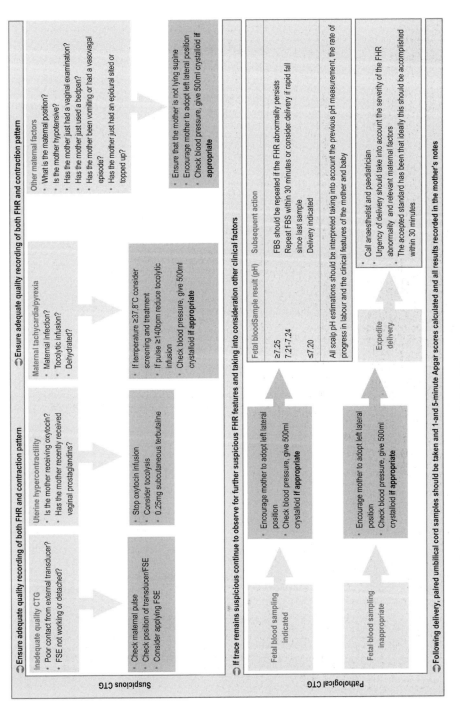

Suspicious CTG

🔊 **Ensure adequate quality recording of both FHR and contraction pattern**

Inadequate quality CTG	Uterine hypercontractility	Maternal tachycardia/pyrexia
• Poor contact from external transducer?	• Is the mother receiving oxytocin?	• Maternal infection?
• FSE not working or detached?	• Has the mother recently received vaginal prostaglandins?	• Tocolytic infusion?
		• Dehydrated?

• Check maternal pulse	• Stop oxytocin infusion	• If temperature ≥37.8°C consider screening and treatment
• Check position of transducer/FSE	• Consider tocolysis	• If pulse ≥140bpm reduce tocolytic infusion
• Consider applying FSE	• 0.25mg subcutaneous terbutaline	• Check blood pressure, give 500ml crystalloid **if appropriate**

🔊 **Ensure adequate quality recording of both FHR and contraction pattern**

Other maternal factors
• What is the maternal position?
• Is the mother hypotensive?
• Has the mother just had a vaginal examination?
• Has the mother just used a bedpan?
• Has the mother been vomiting or had a vasovagal episode?
• Has the mother just had an epidural sited or topped up?

• Ensure that the mother is not lying supine
• Encourage mother to adopt left lateral position
• Check blood pressure, give 500ml crystalloid **if appropriate**

🔊 **If trace remains suspicious continue to observe for further suspicious FHR features and taking into consideration other clinical factors**

Pathological CTG

Fetal blood sampling indicated	• Encourage mother to adopt left lateral position
	• Check blood pressure, give 500ml crystalloid **if appropriate**

Fetal blood sampling inappropriate	• Encourage mother to adopt left lateral position
	• Check blood pressure, give 500ml crystalloid **if appropriate**

Fetal bloodSample result (pH)	Subsequent action
≥7.25	FBS should be repeated if the FHR abnormality persists
7.21–7.24	Repeat FBS within 30 minutes or consider delivery if rapid fall since last sample
≤7.20	Delivery indicated

All scalp pH estimations should be interpreted taking into account the previous pH measurement, the rate of progress in labour and the clinical features of the mother and baby

Expedite delivery	• Call anaesthetist and paediatrician
	• Urgency of delivery should take into account the severity of the FHR abnormality and relevant maternal factors
	• The accepted standard has been that ideally this should be accomplished within 30 minutes

🔊 **Following delivery, paired umbilical cord samples should be taken and 1-and 5-minute Apgar scores calculated and all results recorded in the mother's notes**

Reproduced with kind permission from the National Institute of Clinical Excellence.

Appendix F
Weight conversion chart

lb oz	kg	lb oz	kg	lb oz	kg	lb oz	kg
0 1	0.028	3 9	1.616	7 1	3.203	10 9	4.791
0 2	0.057	3 10	1.644	7 2	3.232	10 10	4.819
0 3	0.085	3 11	1.673	7 3	3.260	10 11	4.848
0 4	0.113	3 12	1.701	7 4	3.289	10 12	4.876
0 5	0.142	3 13	1.729	7 5	3.317	10 13	4.904
0 6	0.170	3 14	1.758	7 6	3.345	10 14	4.932
0 7	0.198	3 15	1.786	7 7	3.374	10 15	4.961
0 8	0.227	4 0	1.814	7 8	3.402	11 0	4.990
0 9	0.255	4 1	1.843	7 9	3.430	11 1	5.018
0 10	0.283	4 2	1.871	7 10	3.459	11 2	5.046
0 11	0.312	4 3	1.899	7 11	3.487	11 3	5.075
0 12	0.340	4 4	1.928	7 12	3.515	11 4	5.103
0 13	0.369	4 5	1.956	7 13	3.544	11 5	5.131
0 14	0.397	4 6	1.984	7 14	3.572	11 6	5.160
0 15	0.425	4 7	2.013	7 15	3.600	11 7	5.188
1 0	0.454	4 8	2.041	8 0	3.629	11 8	5.216
1 1	0.482	4 9	2.070	8 1	3.657	11 9	5.245
1 2	0.510	4 10	2.098	8 2	3.685	11 10	5.273
1 3	0.539	4 11	2.126	8 3	3.714	11 11	5.301
1 4	0.567	4 12	2.155	8 4	3.742	11 12	5.330
1 5	0.595	4 13	2.183	8 5	3.770	11 13	5.358
1 6	0.624	4 14	2.211	8 6	3.799	11 14	5.386
1 7	0.652	4 15	2.240	8 7	3.827	11 15	5.415
1 8	0.680	5 0	2.268	8 8	3.856	12 0	5.443
1 9	0.709	5 1	2.296	8 9	3.884	12 1	5.471
1 10	0.737	5 2	2.325	8 10	3.912	12 2	5.500
1 11	0.765	5 3	2.353	8 11	3.941	12 3	5.528
1 12	0.794	5 4	2.381	8 12	3.969	12 4	5.557
1 13	0.822	5 5	2.410	8 13	3.997	12 5	5.585
1 14	0.850	5 6	2.438	8 14	4.026	12 6	5.613
1 15	0.879	5 7	2.466	8 15	4.054	12 7	5.642
2 0	0.907	5 8	2.495	9 0	4.082	12 8	5.670
2 1	0.936	5 9	2.523	9 1	4.111	12 9	5.698
2 2	0.964	5 10	2.551	9 2	4.139	12 10	5.727
2 3	0.992	5 11	2.580	9 3	4.167	12 11	5.755
2 4	1.021	5 12	2.608	9 4	4.196	12 12	5.783
2 5	1.049	5 13	2.637	9 5	4.224	12 13	5.812
2 6	1.077	5 14	2.665	9 6	4.252	12 14	5.840
2 7	1.106	5 15	2.693	9 7	4.281	12 15	5.868
2 8	1.134	6 0	2.722	9 8	4.309	13 0	5.897
2 9	1.162	6 1	2.750	9 9	4.337	13 1	5.925
2 10	1.191	6 2	2.778	9 10	4.366	13 2	5.953
2 11	1.219	6 3	2.807	9 11	4.394	13 3	5.982
2 12	1.247	6 4	2.835	9 12	4.423	13 4	6.010
2 13	1.276	6 5	2.863	9 13	4.451	13 5	6.038
2 14	1.304	6 6	2.892	9 14	4.479	13 6	6.067
2 15	1.332	6 7	2.920	9 15	4.508	13 7	6.095
3 0	1.361	6 8	2.948	10 0	4.536	13 8	6.123
3 1	1.389	6 9	2.977	10 1	4.564	13 9	6.152
3 2	1.417	6 10	3.005	10 2	4.592	13 10	6.180
3 3	1.446	6 11	3.033	10 3	4.621	13 11	6.209
3 4	1.474	6 12	3.062	10 4	4.649	13 12	6.237
3 5	1.503	6 13	3.090	10 5	4.678	13 13	6.265
3 6	1.531	6 14	3.118	10 6	4.706	13 14	6.294
3 7	1.559	6 15	3.147	10 7	4.734	13 15	6.322
3 8	1.588	7 0	3.175	10 8	4.763	14 0	6.350

Index